Neonatal Emergencies

Neonatal Emergencies
Early Detection and Management

Second Edition

J A Black MD, FRCP
Late Consultant Paediatrician, Children's Hospital and Jessop Hospital for Women, Sheffield

and

M F Whitfield MD, FRCP, FRCP(C)
Associate Professor, Department of Paediatrics, University of British Columbia
Neonatologist and Director, Neonatal Follow-up Programme, British Columbia's Children's Hospital, Vancouver, Canada

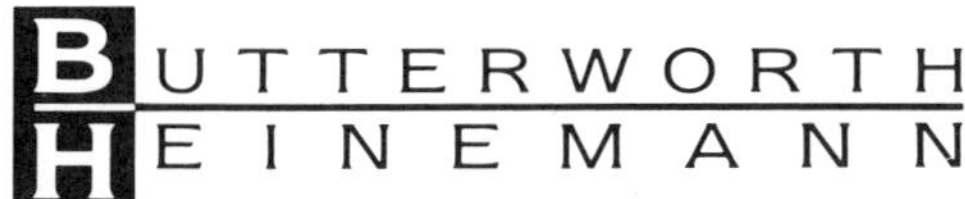

Butterworth-Heinemann Ltd
Linacre House, Jordan Hill, Oxford OX2 8DP

 | PART OF REED INTERNATIONAL BOOKS

OXFORD LONDON BOSTON
MUNICH NEW DELHI SINGAPORE SYDNEY
TOKYO TORONTO WELLINGTON

First published 1972
Reprinted 1974
Second edition 1991

British Library Cataloguing in Publication Data
Black, J.A.
Neonatal emergencies: Early detection and management. – 2nd ed.
I. Title II. Whitfield, M.
618.92

ISBN 0 7506 1313 0

Library of Congress Cataloguing in Publication Data
Black, J.A. (John Angus)
Neonatal emergencies : early detection and management / J.A. Black and M. Whitfield. — 2nd ed.
p. cm.
Rev. ed. of : Neonatal emergencies – and other problems.
Butterworths. 1972.
Includes bibliographical references and index.
ISBN 0 7506 1313 0
1. Neonatal emergencies. I. Whitfield, M. (Michael) II. Black, J. A. (John Angus) Neonatal emergencies – and other problems. III. Title.
[DNLM: 1. Emergencies—in infancy & childhood. 2. Infant, Newborn, Diseases. WS 420 B627n]
RJ253.5.B63 1991
618.92'01—dc20
DNLM/DLC
for Library of Congress 91–19266
CIP

Composition by Scribe Design, Gillingham, Kent
Printed in Great Britain at the University Press, Cambridge

Contents

Preface to the second edition

This book is intended for those who have day-to-day care of the newborn infant. We have tried to combine obstetrics and paediatrics so that the obstetrician and the neonatologist regard the neonate as an individual whose characteristics are the resultant of his or her ethnic and genetic background, and whose condition at birth is due to events during pregnancy, labour and delivery.

Since the first edition, the care of the newborn has changed out of all recognition; we have added much new material, including chapters on electrolyte disorders, hydrops fetalis, the floppy infant, practical procedures and iatrogenic disease.

We hope that the basic concept has been retained, which is that neonatal emergencies can only be successfully treated if they can be anticipated or detected at an early stage, as a result of an intelligent appreciation of all the factors that influence the health and development of the fetus and infant. For this reason we have included a number of relevant references, and some suggested background reading.

We have attempted to give prominence to the problems and anxieties of the parents, and particularly of the mother, when the fetus or infant is found to be abnormal, becomes seriously ill, or dies *in utero* or shortly after delivery.

We are grateful to our wives and families for their support and encouragement during the preparation of this book, and we would like to acknowledge the help and advice we have received from the editorial staff of Butterworth-Heinemann. We are much indebted to Dr Harold Gamsu for his help and constructive comments. We also thank Mrs Sandra Parfitt and Ms Prunella Barlow for their unfailing care and attention to detail in typing the manuscripts.

JAB
MFW

Chapter 1

The background to fetal and neonatal disease

Advances in carrier detection, prenatal diagnosis and in certain cases, prenatal treatment, have greatly improved the scope for the prevention of fetal and neonatal disease. Where a fetal abnormality has been detected but a termination is not indicated, or not acceptable, a knowledge of the diagnosis will enable postnatal treatment to be given promptly, with a reduction in severity of the disease or prevention of further deterioration. The services which should be available for prenatal and immediate postnatal diagnosis, counselling and treatment are shown in Table 1.1.

Table 1.1. Requirements for prenatal and postnatal services

Obstetrician, with knowledge of fetal and neonatal medicine
Neonatologist, with knowledge of obstetrics and fetal medicine
Obstetrician or fetal medicine specialist in diagnostic ultrasound
Clinical geneticist
Laboratories equipped to deal with specimens from prenatal investigations
Pathologist expert in fetal and neonatal pathology
Counsellors, especially for specific ethnic groups

Prepregnancy counselling and testing (also p. 28)

The best time for counselling is before conception, or in certain cases, before marriage. The discovery of a risk factor at the antenatal clinic does not allow time for proper discussion and emotional adjustment.

Table 1.2. Identifiable risk conditions before pregnancy

Increased risk of fetal abnormality
Maternal age, over 35 years
Maternal illness or treatment
Maternal drug abuse
Promiscuous sexual behaviour
Family history of known or possible genetic disease
Parental consanguinity
Ethnic group
Previous obstetric history
Increased risk of maternal morbidity or mortality
Chronic maternal illness

Modified from Connor and Whittle (1989), with permission of authors and publishers.

Risk factors can often be identified before pregnancy (Table 1.2) and each needs to be discussed with an obstetrician or a geneticist, depending upon the condition. The risks to the fetus of the appropriate prenatal investigations should also be discussed.

It may also be convenient to determine before pregnancy the woman's ABO and rhesus group, and to discover whether she is immune to rubella, toxoplasmosis and cytomegalovirus (CMV) infection or has rhesus or irregular antibodies (see Table 1.8).

Identifiable risk conditions before pregnancy

Maternal age over 35 years

In the UK, about 7% of mothers will be over the age of 35 years; the risk of a fetus with an autosomal trisomy (Trisomies 21, 18, and 13) rises from 1 in 1000 pregnancies at 20 years to 1 in 250 at 35 years, and 1 in 75 at 40 years. Advanced maternal age is also associated with an increased risk for 47XXX and 47XXY abnormalities (Ferguson–Smith and Yates, 1984). Methods of prediction are discussed on p. 16. Apart from chromosomal abnormalities, the woman over 35 years has an increased risk of hypertension, pre-eclampsia, fibroids, prolonged labour, fetal hypoxia during delivery and caesarean section.

Maternal illness and treatment

Childhood illnesses
Conditions such as rheumatic fever, which may have long-term sequelae or require continued treatment, are important. Some types of congenital heart disease may need careful management during labour, and may be associated with a risk of a cardiac lesion in the offspring (p. 20).

Conditions persisting into pregnancy
Conditions that will persist into pregnancy, such as diabetes, thyrotoxicosis and phenylketonuria, may involve modification of treatment or management in order to safeguard the fetus (p. 25). For a list of maternal illnesses present before pregnancy which may affect the fetus see Table 1.3.

Visits abroad
These should be recorded, with dates and details of countries visited, and any illnesses and treatment. Injections or blood transfusions may carry the risk of infection with hepatitis B virus (HBV), hepatitis C virus (HCV) or human immunodeficiency virus (HIV).

Drug treatment before pregnancy
Drugs given during pregnancy which may carry a risk of malformation of the fetus are discussed on p. 6. There is only one group of drugs with a sufficiently long half-life to have any effect on the fetus when given before conception. The high-potency retinoid drugs, isotretinoin (Roaccutane or (US) Accutane) and etretinate (Tigasol), if used before or during

Table 1.3. Effects on the fetus and newborn of maternal disease present before or arising during pregnancy

Maternal condition	*Fetal or neonatal effects*	*Remarks*
Cardiovascular, cardiac and renal disease		
Pre-eclampsia Hypertension	Pre-term delivery, fetal hypoxia during labour or delivery, small for gestational age (SGA) infant; progression to eclampsia with risk of fetal or maternal death	
Mitral stenosis Cyanotic congenital heart disease	SGA infant	
Valve replacement	Warfarin syndrome (p. 6)	
Chronic pyelonephritis	SGA infant	
Chronic nephritis	SGA infant	High fetal loss with hypertension and glomerular filtration rate (GFR) 60–70ml/min per 1.73 m^2: fertility reduced at GFR <40
Kidney transplant recipient	SGA infant: possible transient immunosuppression due to maternal treatment	
Haemodialysis for renal disease		Pregnancy rare
Endocrine disease		
Diabetes mellitus		See pp. 215–216
Hypothyroidism	Mother treated or untreated; no fetal effect	Untreated: reduced fertility
Goitre, endemic (iodine deficiency)	Goitre common, with or without hypothyroidism. Severe maternal deficiency causes mental defect, deafness, and spasticity	
Thyrotoxicosis	Overtreatment: fetal goitre ± hypothyroidism. Surgery, with persisting eye signs: risk of fetal thyrotoxicosis (p. 25)	
Hyperparathyroidism	Mother untreated: transient hypocalcaemia (p. 219)	
Hypoparathyroidism	Mother untreated: transient hypercalcaemia (p. 221)	
Congenital adrenal hyperplasia (21-hydroxylase deficiency) autosomal recessive (AR)	Mother treated: no fetal effect	Mother infertile if untreated. Treated: reduced fertility (polycystic ovaries)
Adrenal hypofunction (all causes)	Mother treated: no fetal effect	Mother untreated: high fetal loss
Cushing's disease	Surgery before conception: no fetal effect. Mother untreated; high fetal loss and risk of transient neonatal adrenal hypofunction	

Table 1.3.

Maternal condition	*Fetal or neonatal effects*	*Remarks*
Blood disorders		
Iron deficiency anaemia	Iron deficiency in infant. Severe cases, pre-term delivery	
Megaloblastic anaemia (nutritional or secondary to untreated coeliac disease)	Pre-term delivery: intrauterine death in severe cases	
Sickle cell anaemia (HbSS) (AR)	Mother untreated: abortion, pre-term delivery, SGA infant. Fetus does not develop condition, but risk of HbSS infant if father a carrier or HbSS	
Sickle cell trait (HbAS)	Fetus does not develop condition, but risk of HbSS infant if father is carrier or HbSS	Clinical disease very occasionally in HbSS infant (p. 81)
Sickle cell HbC disease (HbSC)	Fetal survival better than for HbSS anaemia. Fetus does not develop condition. Risk of affected infant depends upon father's carrier state	
Sickle cell-β thalassaemia	As above	
β-Thalassaemia major (homozygous) (AR)	High fetal loss if maternal anaemia uncorrected. Fetus does not develop condition. Risk of affected homozygous infant if father carrier or is homozygous	
β-Thalassaemia minor (heterozygous)	No fetal risk. Risk of homozygous infant as above	
α^{o} Thalassaemia (heterozygous) (AR)	No fetal effect if mother only is heterozygous. Both parents heterozygous: 1 in 4 risk of α^{o} thalassaemia (Hb Bart's) hydrops, with intrauterine or neonatal death (pp. 8 and 17)	
Spherocytosis	No fetal risk: 50% chance of affected infant with neonatal jaundice	25–30% mutation rate, therefore neither parent may be affected
Metabolic disorders		
Hyperammonaemia (X-linked type, ornithine transcarbamylase deficiency)	Unaffected fetus of either sex may develop brain damage from symptomless hyperammonaemia in heterozygous mother. Affected female is normal at birth; condition lethal in male	See p. 284.
Osteomalacia (severe vitamin D deficiency)	Hypocalcaemia in first week, often with X-ray evidence of rickets	Hypocalcaemia: suspect vitamin D deficiency in Asian mothers even in absence of clinical osteomalacia

Table 1.3.

Maternal condition	*Fetal or neonatal effects*	*Remarks*
Phenylketonuria (AR)	Mother untreated: risk of retarded microcephalic infant, with ocular, skeletal and cardiac defects	Dietary treatment preferably before conception likely to result in normal infant
Porphyria erythropoietica (AR)	Brown amniotic fluid described (Kaiser, 1980); also red primary dentition (Townes, 1965)	
Porphyria (acute intermittent type) autosomal dominant (AD)	Abortion and stillbirth occur, but fetal loss not high (Brodie *et al.*, 1977)	
Rickets, vitamin resistant (X-linked dominant type)	Transient hypercalcaemia if mother has been on high dosage vitamin D	Rickets rare before 1 year: both sexes affected but males more severely than females
Immunological and autoimmune diseases		
Systemic lupus erythematosus (SLE)	Abortion, intrauterine death, SGA infant. Fetal heart block (p. 21) occasionally discoid lesions, leucopenia, thrombocytopenia and haemolytic anaemia in newborn	
Idiopathic thrombocytopenic purpura (ITP) (autoimmune thrombocytopenia)	Risk of intracranial haemorrhage during delivery; see p. 26	Maternal thrombocytopenia
Isoimmune thrombocytopenia	Risk of intracranial haemorrhage before labour: see p. 26	Maternal platelet count normal
Myasthenia gravis	20% of infants are affected, see p. 281	
Unknown mechanism		
Myotonic dystrophy (AD, but see p.000)	Hypotonia, bilateral facial weakness, respiratory and feeding difficulty, talipes, (p. 23). High abortion and neonatal death rates.	Polyhydramnios common, reduced fetal movements, high incidence of pregnancy complications (p. 23)
Malignant disease		
Main fetal risk is due to maternal treatment		
Hodgkin's disease	Spread to fetus is rare	
Lymphosarcoma	As above	
Leukaemia } Multiple myeloma }	No reports of spread to fetus	
Malignant melanoma	Commonest tumour to involve fetus, but still rare; clinically hepatomegaly and anaemia	

Table 1.4. Teratogenic or potentially harmful drugs which may have to be started or continued during pregnancy

Drug	*Maternal indication*	*Fetal effects*
Warfarin, phenindione, related drugs	Thrombo-embolic episodes; cardiac valve replacement	Chondrodysplasia punctata, depressed nasal bridge, hypoplastic nails, cardiac malformation, hydrocephalus, prematurely calcified stippled epiphyses, hypotonia and developmental delay
Sodium valproate	Epilepsy	Neural tube defect, tetralogy of Fallot, oral clefting, other facial abnormalities
Lithium carbonate	Manic-depressive disease (bipolar affective psychosis)	12% risk of cardiac malformation, especially Ebstein's anomaly: goitre ± hypothyroidism, hypotonia, arrhythmias
Carbimazole or propylthiouracil or related drugs	Thyrotoxicosis	Small risk of goitre or hypothyroidism if minimal effective dose is used
Thalidomide*	Leprosy	Reduction deformities of limbs, cardiac defects, facial naevus

*Thalidomide is still used for the treatment of erythema nodosum leprosum (ENL) and can be obtained for this purpose only.

pregnancy, carry a high risk of spontaneous abortion or severe malformation (hydrocephalus, microcephaly, microtia, heart defects, facial and limb abnormalities (Lammer *et al.*, 1985). With etretinate used in the treatment of ichthyotic conditions, pregnancy should be avoided at least 1 month before, during and for at least 2 years after starting treatment; with isotretinoin, which is prescribed for acne, pregnancy should be avoided at least 1 month before, during and for at least 1 month after starting treatment (British National Formulary, 1990). Lammer *et al.* (1985) could find no evidence that isotretinoin is a teratogenic if taken before pregnancy, but it seems sensible to go by the British National Formulary suggestions. There are a few potentially harmful or teratogenic drugs (Table 1.4) which may have to be continued during pregnancy on clinical grounds, with the acceptance of the risk of fetal abnormality or side effects (p. 000).

Maternal drug abuse

Alcohol

The habitual consumption of alcohol before pregnancy is likely to continue during pregnancy. The regular weekly consumption of more than 35 units*

*1 unit of alcohol = 10 ml or 8.0 g of absolute alcohol: the following contain 1 unit of alcohol: 1 single whisky; 1 glass of sherry or fortified wine; 1 glass of table wine; ½ pint of beer or cider; ¼ pint of strong lager.

of alcohol is generally regarded as exposing the fetus to the risk of spontaneous mid-term abortion, low birth weight and the fetal alcohol syndrome (which may exhibit some of the following: low intelligence, mid-face hypoplasia, short palpebral fissure, smooth philtrum, small nails, hirsutism, microcephaly, microphthalmia, cardiac lesions).

Opiates and cocaine
The abuse of opiates or cocaine, with or without other drugs, is likely to persist during pregnancy and is associated with an increased risk to the fetus (p. 295).

Intravenous drug usage
This may result in infection with HBV or HIV, and the risk of intrauterine HIV or perinatal HBV infection of the infant (p. 297).

Promiscuous sexual behaviour

The mother may have been infected with HBV or HIV with the risk described above.

Possible genetically determined disease in the mother or her family

Genetically determined disease must be differentiated from a similar condition due to non-genetic causes (e.g. acquired deafness or blindness must be distinguished from hereditary deafness or blindness).

The mother's history or the history in her family may suggest a genetic disorder which may be inherited in an autosomal dominant or recessive or in an X-linked dominant or recessive manner. Many common conditions are, however, inherited multifactorially. In all these situations counselling will be required, and in difficult cases a clinical geneticist should be consulted.

Multifactorially inherited disorders do not follow a strictly Mendelian pattern, and empirical risks, based upon the community under consideration, must be given (Appendix 3). Neural tube defects (NTDs) and congenital heart disease (CHD) require special consideration (p. 19 and pp. 20–21).

Myotonic dystrophy, though inherited as an autosomal dominant, behaves in an anomalous manner when an affected female carries an affected fetus (pp. 23–24). Retinoblastoma and the fragile X syndrome are discussed on p. 22. Some non-recurring conditions, which might be thought to have a genetic basis are listed in Appendix 3.

Parental consanguinity

See page 25.

Ethnic groups

See pages 15–16.

Previous obstetric history

Previous termination of pregnancy
The reason for the termination should be determined, as this may have an important bearing on the mother's or both parents' attitude to future pregnancies. Cervical incompetence, due to a late termination or a technique involving excessive cervical dilatation, may predispose to preterm delivery in subsequent pregnancies.

Recurrent spontaneous abortion
A couple who have had three or more spontaneous abortions should be investigated. Possible causes are: double uterus, severe rhesus or other blood group isoimmunization, immunological rejection of the fetus, syphilis and, in a mother of South East Asian origin, homozygous α° thalassaemia (Hb-Bart's) hydrops fetalis. When these conditions have been excluded, the parents should be examined for a balanced translocation (p. 24).

Previous stillbirth or neonatal death
It is often a matter of chance whether there is a late stillbirth or an early neonatal death. Where a definite diagnosis was not made, all previous hospital records and post-mortem reports should be examined in an effort to reach a diagnosis. Possible causes of recurrent stillbirths are: severe rhesus or other blood group isoimmunization, syphilis, listeriosis, placental insufficiency and α° thalassaemia (see above). A previous neonatal death whose cause was not identified may have been due to metabolic disorder which was diagnosed as 'liver disease' or a condition which was missed by a less than thorough post-mortem examination, such as bilateral renal agenesis, adrenal hyperplasia or hypoplasia, bilateral choanal atresia, myotonic dystrophy (p. 23) and Werdnig Hoffman spinal muscular atrophy.

When, on review of the facts, a probable cause of the previous death or deaths can be established, the sequence of events leading to death should be carefully explained to both parents, and the risk of a further recurrence discussed. Where an alteration in management or treatment is likely to improve the chance of survival in a future pregnancy, these changes should be fully explained.

There are a number of situations which are most unlikely to recur: these are prolapsed cord, true knot or torsion of the cord, cord tightly round the neck, risks specific to twin or multiple pregnancy, bleeding from placenta praevia, accidental traumatic separation of the placenta, and other forms of fetal blood loss (p. 75).

Paternal risk conditions identifiable before pregnancy

Drug abuse
If there has been a history of IV usage, there is a risk that the female partner, and subsequently the infant, will be infected with HBV or HIV (p. 187).

Promiscuous sexual behaviour
Particularly with a history of bisexual intercourse, there is a risk of infecting the female partner with HBV or HIV.

Occupational exposure to radiation
The possible relationship between paternal occupational exposure to radiation before conception and the subsequent development of leukaemia or lymphoma in the child has been raised by the report in the Sellafield Reprocessing Plant in the UK (Gardner *et al.*, 1990). There is likely to be considerable anxiety in men who have been exposed to radiation in the course of their work. These justified fears should be explored, and if necessary a specialist in nuclear medicine should be consulted. The Sellafield results need to be confirmed at other sites and in other countries.

Possible genetically determined disease in the father or his family
The same considerations apply to the paternal history as to the maternal one.

Identifiable risk factors during pregnancy

The maternal risk factors are shown in Table 1.5.

Table 1.5. Indentifiable risk factors in pregnancy (in addition to those shown in Table 1.2)

Increased risk of fetal abnormality or risk to the infant
- Maternal age under 16 years
- Maternal infection
- Maternal exposure to teratogenic drugs or chemicals
- Maternal exposure to radiation
- Abnormal ultrasound appearance
- Elevated or very low maternal serum α-fetoprotein (AFP) level
- Premature rupture of the membranes
- Oligohydramnios
- Polyhydramnios

Conditions peculiar to pregnancy
- Pre-eclampsia
- Gestational diabetes
- Herpes gestationis

Increased risk of maternal morbidity or mortality
- Acute maternal illness
- Low social class

Maternal age under 16 years (see also under the Unmarried Mother, (p. 325) and Adolescent Pregnancy (p. 354)

In the UK the girl would be unmarried, because she would be below the age of consent to marriage. In addition to the risks of absent or inadequate antenatal care and of an unattended delivery causing hypoxia or hypothermia in the infant, there is an increased incidence of pre-eclampsia, intrauterine growth retardation and pre-term delivery. With some single mothers, there is the possibility that the infant may be abandoned immediately after delivery or later, and of emotional rejection, neglect or physical abuse. In very young girls the social problems, but not the obstetric ones, are reduced if she remains in the parental home and is accepted or supported (not necessarily financially) by the father of the child. There is no evidence that teenage pregnancy is associated with an increased risk of malformation.

Maternal infection (see also pp. 179–184)

Toxoplasmosis, rubella, CMV and herpes simplex do not cause recurrent abortion but may occasionally cause spontaneous abortion if a primary infection is acquired early in pregnancy. 'TORCH' (see Chapter 14 for definition) screening during pregnancy covers only some of the possible maternal infections capable of infecting and damaging the fetus.

Rubella (pp. 180 and 183)
Termination is usually advised when maternal infection has occurred at less than 16 weeks. Reinfection is uncommon and is thought to carry a risk of fetal damage of less than 5%.

Toxoplasmosis (pp. 180 and 182)
A primary infection during the first trimester carries the highest risk of stillbirth or damaged fetus and termination is usually recommended, if a primary infection can be proved.

Cytomegalovirus (CMV) (pp. 180 and 183)
Since the fetal risk is small, termination is not generally advised even with a proved primary infection. The infected newborn, whether damaged or not, is highly infective.

Syphilis (pp. 180 and 182)
Because infection may occur after routine testing in early pregnancy, it has been suggested that the test should be repeated in the third trimester when treatment of the fetus, via the mother, would still be effective (Stevens, Darbyshire and Brown, 1987).

Varicella-zoster virus (pp. 181 and 183)
About 20% of primary varicella infections in the first trimester result in limb hypoplasia, cutaneous scars, cataracts, chorioretinitis, cortical atrophy, cerebellar hypoplasia and convulsions. Maternal varicella (not zoster) infection during pregnancy may be complicated by severe, sometimes fatal, pneumonitis. Boyd and Walker (1988) advise treatment with acyclovir (15 mg/kg) for 5 days.

Chlamydia trachomatis (p. 185)
Intrauterine infection may occur with premature rupture of the membranes. In units with a high incidence of chlamydia, screening of both partners should be performed at around 36 weeks, and, if positive, treatment with erythromycin should be given to the infected partner or partners.

Parvovirus B19 (p. 183)
The fetal risk is greatest with a maternal infection in the first half of the pregnancy, when there is a 10% risk of spontaneous abortion or

intrauterine death. A rise in maternal serum α-fetoprotein (MsAFP) precedes the development of hydrops, which can be confirmed later by ultrasound. Intrauterine transfusion might be useful in the treatment of the hydropic fetus.

Listeriosis (p. 187)
This may cause intrauterine death.

Herpes simplex infection (p. 185)

Tuberculosis (p. 182)
Tuberculosis acquired transplacentally is very rare.

HIV infection (pp. 188–192)

Malaria (p. 182)

Brucellosis (p. 184)

Maternal exposure to teratogenic drugs or chemicals

The risk to the fetus, particularly in the first trimester, of drugs given to the mother are well known. A comprehensive list of drugs which may cause fetal malformation, subdivided according to fetal risk, is given by Whittle and Rubin (1989), and the whole subject has been reviewed extensively (see under Further reading).

There are, however, a few teratogenic drugs (Table 1.4) which may have to be started or continued throughout pregnancy on clinical grounds.

Maternal exposure to radiation

Therapeutic irradiation
The usual indication is pelvic malignancy; the embryo is not sensitive to irradiation below the age of 4 weeks gestation and after 17 weeks. Between 4 and 11 weeks gestation, exposure results in severe malformations, skeletal and genital abnormalities. Between 11 and 16 weeks gestation, there is growth retardation, microcephaly and mental retardation (for review see Dekaban, 1986).

Exposure to 'Atom bomb' (data from Hiroshima and Nagasaki)
There appeared to be no risk below 8 weeks gestation. From 8 to 15 weeks gestation there was a dose-related severe mental retardation (Otake and Schull, 1984) with a reduced risk from 16 to 25 weeks gestation. there was also an increased perinatal mortality rate after exposure (Mole, 1982).

Abnormal ultrasound appearance (p. 16)

Elevated or very low MsASP (p. 15)

Premature rupture of the membranes (see below)

Table 1.6. Causes of oligohydramnios

Stage of pregnancy at which detected	*Specific condition*
Present before 28 weeks	Absent, hypoplastic, or polycystic kidneys, urethral atresia or valves, bilateral hydronephrosis. Premature rupture of membranes or leak from amniocentesis
Developing after 28 weeks	Premature rupture of membranes. Placental insufficiency with growth-retarded fetus. Severe pre-eclampsia. Postmaturity.

Oligohydramnios (see Table 1.6 for causes)

If caused by a continuous leak from premature rupture of the membranes (PROM) or from an amniocentesis, the fetal prognosis is usually good. However, a prolonged leak with marked reduction in the volume of amniotic fluid may be associated with chorioamnionitis, cord compression during labour, pulmonary hypoplasia or 'dry lung' and occasionally compression deformities of the limbs. Oligohydramnios due to PROM at <25 weeks with no fluid on ultrasound is usually fatal.

Fetal determinants of oligohydramnios are severe renal disease from any cause (Table 1.6); the volume of amniotic fluid is severly reduced, and compression deformities of the limbs and Potter's syndrome are common; the prognosis for survival is poor, because of pulmonary hypoplasia and renal insufficiency. Amnion nodosum is often present.

A vaginal examination with a speculum will usually indicate leakage of fluid from PROM, and sonography will show the extent of fetal abnormality.

Polyhydramnios

Polyhydramnios may develop slowly or acutely; acute polyhydramnios in a singleton usually indicates a fetal abnormality, characteristically a hydropic fetus. Some of the causes of polyhydramnios are shown in Table 1.7. The development of polyhydramnios should prompt a systematic search for its cause, including screening for diabetes.

Conditions peculiar to pregnancy

Pre-eclampsia (synonyms, pre-eclamptic toxaemia, toxaemia, pregnancy-induced or associated hypertension, gestosis)

The risks associated with pre-eclampsia are pre-term delivery, intrauterine growth retardation, fetal hypoxia during labour or delivery, and progression to eclampsia,with fetal or occasionally maternal death.

Gestational diabetes

Gestational diabetes is defined as diabetes developing during pregnancy, whether or not the patient reverts to normal after delivery; this is associated with a raised perinatal mortality rate, but not with the same risk of malformation as with diabetes present before conception (p. 216).

Table 1.7. Causes of polyhydramnios

Category of diseases	*Specific condition*
Combined fetal and maternal disease	Diabetes mellitus (p. 215) Myotonic dystrophy (p. 23)
Obstetric conditions	Multiple pregnancy (p. 46) Cord tightly round the neck Intrauterine death
CNS abnormalities	Anencephaly Hydrocephalus (rarely) Hydrancephaly Iniencephaly Encephalocele Spina bifida (open) Microcephaly (rarely)
Gastrointestinal system	Astomia Oesophageal atresia (p. 148) Duodenal atresia Diaphragmatic hernia Exomphalus or gastroschisis Intrathoracic tumour with pressure on oesophagus
Respiratory tract	Pulmonary hypoplasia Adenomatoid hamartoma of lung Pleural effusion or chylothorax
Severe fetal anaemia	Feto-fetal transfusion (p. 82) Severe rhesus or other blood group isoimmunization (p. 117) α^{o} (Hb Bart's) hydrops (p. 82)
Cardiac causes	Fetal cardiac failure with hydrops, from any cause (pp. 20–21)
Fetal infection	Syphilis, toxoplasmosis, rubella, CMV, herpes simplex, parvovirus B19 (p. 183)
Skeletal	Arthrogryposis multiplex, osteogenesis imperfecta (severe form) (p. 362), thanatrophic dwarfism
Hydrops fetalis from any cause	Chapter 25
Miscellaneous	Congenital mesoblastic nephroma (a benign renal tumour) (Blank, Neerhout and Burry, 1978) Obstructive lesions of renal tract (rarely) Prader-Willi syndrome (rarely)

Herpes gestationis (pemphigoid gestationis)

In this benign condition, itchy papular, or bullous lesions develop in the second trimester. Rarely, the newborn infant is born with identical lesions or they may develop 1 or 2 days after birth; these resolve within a week. There appears to be a risk of intrauterine growth retardation (Holmes and Black, 1984).

Screening and prenatal diagnosis

Premarriage and preconceptual screening is usually combined with genetic counselling (Appendix 3).

Universal pregnancy screening ideally involves the testing of every pregnant woman. There are a number of well-established screening procedures whose value is accepted (Table 1.8). Obviously, the application

Table 1.8. Screening before and during pregnancy

	Urine	*Blood*	*Chorionic villus sampling*	*Amniotic fluid*	*Ultrasonography*	*Vaginal swab*
Preconception	Diabetes Nephropathy	Rh state Rubella state Haemoglobinopathy Carrier states	–	–	–	–
8–10 weeks	Bacteriuria	Syphilis Hepatitis B (HBsAg)	Karyotype Gene defects	–	At <16 weeks for gestational age	–
16–18 weeks	–	Anaemia Rh, ABO or irregular antibodies MsAFP	–	Karyotype AFP Acetylcholinesterase	Multiple pregnancy Gestational age Fetal anomaly	
28–30 weeks		Anaemia Rh, ABO or irregular antibodies Gestational diabetes	–	Haemolytic disease	Intrauterine growth retardation Placental size	
34–36 weeks	Pre-eclampsia	Anaemia Rh, ABO or irregular antibodies Pre-eclampsia (blood pressure)	–	Haemolytic disease	Intrauterine growth retardation	Herpes simplex virus, group B streptococcus. In units with high incidence of Chlamydia trachomatis, screen both partners

Table (modified) from Bull (1990) with permission of authors and publishers.

of other screening procedures depends upon the frequency of a specific condition in any particular population. Thus in Greece, Cyprus and Southern Italy every woman should be tested for β-thalassaemia, before marriage, before conception, or during pregnancy. In the UK, screening for β-thalassaemia is confined to certain ethnic groups (p. 16). Conversely, screening for NTDs using the maternal serum α-fetoprotein level (MsAFP) is universally applied in the UK as a high-incidence area, but it is not applied in low-incidence countries (p. 19).

Screening procedures

Maternal serum α-fetoprotein

This should be done between 16 and 20 weeks gestation. The level may be abnormally high (Table 1.9) or abnormally low (Table 1.10); assessment of levels should take into account the normal levels for each particular population, and the stage of gestation.

After a high MsAFP level has been found, the test should be repeated; if the MsAFP level is again raised, further investigation is indicated either by high-resolution ultrasound or by amniocentesis. If a fetal NTD can be excluded, the pregnancy should nevertheless be considered at risk for second-trimester abortion, stillbirth, pre-term delivery, low birth weight and perinatal death.

An abnormally low MsAFP is known to be associated with fetal autosomal chromosomal abnormalities (Trisomies 21, 18 and 13), but not

Table 1.9. Causes of raised MsAFP

Underestimated gestation age
Missed or threatened abortion
Multiple pregnancy
Anencephaly
Open spina bifida
Anterior abdominal wall defects (exomphalos and gastroschisis)
Chromosomal syndromes
Teratoma
Congenital nephrosis
Haemangioma of cord or placenta
Hereditary persistence of AFP
Intrauterine diagnostic procedure (feto-maternal haemorrhage or blood in the amniotic cavity)
Fetal infection (especially Parvovirus B19, p. 183)
Lower than average maternal weight

Table 1.10. Causes of low maternal serum AFP

Overestimated gestation
Non-viable fetus
Spontaneous abortion
Molar pregnancy (some)
Diabetes mellitus (some insulin-dependent cases)
Above average maternal weight
Fetal autosomal trisomy

Table (modified) from Gilmore and Aitken (1989), with permission of authors and publishers.

with sex chromosome anomalies. Prediction of an affected fetus can be improved by a combined assessment based on maternal age, MsAFP level, serum unconjugated oestriol level (reduced with a trisomy), and serum human chorionic gonadotrophin (raised), giving a prediction rate of over 60% of a Down's syndrome fetus, and reducing the rate of amniocentesis to 5% (Wald *et al.*, 1986). Table 1.10 shows other causes of a low MsAFP. In the absence of a chromosomal abnormality, ultrasound should be used to identify other fetal abnormalities.

Routine anomaly ultrasound scan

In most units in the UK a routine ultrasound scan is performed between 18 and 20 weeks. Counselling of the parents should include an explanation of the purpose of the investigation, its diagnostic potential and limitations, and a description of the procedure. At present over 200 structural abnormalities can be detected with high-resolution ultrasound, but a smaller number will be discovered on routine examination in a non-specialized unit.

Routine screening for cystic fibrosis

Routine screening for carriers is now practicable and may be advised for high-incidence populations such as the UK and most European countries in which the incidence of the mutation ΔF_{508} is high enough to make screening worth while (Editorial, Lancet, 1990); however, it has not yet been implemented (see also p. 18).

Selective screening for haemoglobinopathies

Selective screening is indicated for communities with a high incidence of specific conditions, the carrier state of which can be detected by simple tests, (e.g. β-thalassaemia, sickle cell disease). Table 1.11 shows the ethnic

Table 1.11. Ethnic groups in the UK at risk for a haemoglobin or red cell disorder

	Number in UK	*Common haemoglobinopathies*	*Affected infants/1000 pregnancies*	*Percentage of males G-6PD deficient*
Afro-Caribbeans	750 000	S>C>βth>D	3–4.5	12
West Africans	99 000	S>C>βth	0.3–19.2	20
Indians	873 000	βth>D,>E,>S	0.23–2.5	7
Pakistanis	370 000	βth>D,>E,>S	2.0	5
Bangladeshis	87 000	E>βth	0.4	3
East African Indians	221 000	βth>D,>E,>S	0.9–2.5	?7
Cypriots	180 000	βth>αth*>S	7.2	7
Middle Eastern (Iranians, Lebanese etc)	?200 000	βth>S	?	5–10
Chinese (Hong Kong, Singapore)	>250 000	αth*>βth	0.5	3
Italians	250 000	βth, αth >S	?	0.6

βth, β thalassaemia; αth, α thalassaemia.
Note: The α thalassaemia can be divided up into α^+thalassaemia and α^0 thalassaemia. α^+thalassaemia is usually harmless, and is the only form of thalassaemia found in Africa and the Indian subcontinent. Both forms of α thalassaemia occur in people from South East Asia and the Mediterranean: homozygous α^0 thalassaemia causes stillbirth or neonatal death.
Table (modified) from Modell and Modell (1990), with permission of authors and publishers.

groups in the UK at risk for various haemoglobinopathies. Screening for these disorders should be available to any individual of any age or sex and should be available through schools, and whenever a blood sample is requested for some other reason; but it is particularly important before marriage, before pregnancy, or in the antenatal clinic. Most units screen in the antenatal clinic all women who are not obviously of northern European origin; it is no longer practicable to screen for single disorders, partly because (as shown in Table 1.11) more than one disorder is found in most of the ethnic groups at risk, and partly because of the increasing number of people of mixed race.

Carrier testing for α° thalassaemia is not routinely done but parents who have had an infant with α° thalassaemia (Hb Bart's) hydrops should be tested in a specialized laboratory. Neonatal screening for sickle cell anaemia (HbSS) or the carrier state (HbAS) is the standard practice for at risk infants. Routine screening for G-6PD (glucose-6-phosphate dehydrogenase) deficiency is not indicated, but jaundiced infants in whom the cause of the jaundice is not obvious should be tested, and also their immediate family if the infant is found to have a low level of G-6PD. In communities with a high gene frequency about 10% of women are homozygous and are likely to be as severely deficient in G-6PD as the hemizygous males. The drugs which are now thought to cause haemolysis in affected individuals are listed in Table 10.2 (p. 107)

Selective screening of Ashkenazi Jews for Tay-Sach's disease (AR)

In Ashkenazi Jews (Jews of European origin) the estimated incidence of Tay-Sach's disease is 28/100000 live births, compared with 0.3 per 100000 live births in Caucasians. The carrier rate in Ashkenazis is 1 in 30 compared with 1 in 300 for other ethnic groups. Carriers can be identified by a lower than normal level of hexosaminidase in the serum or white cells. Prenatal diagnosis is also possible using material from chorionic villus

Table 1.12. Rare recessive conditions found predominantly in Ashkenazi Jews

Disorder	*Jewish parents* (%)	*Prevalence in Jews*	*General population*
Essential pentosuria	99	1 in 2500 (USA) 1 in 5000 (Israel)	Very rare
Plasma prothrombin antecedent factor (factor X1)	90	?	?
Familial dysautonomia (Riley-Day Syndrome)	99	1 in 10000 (USA) 1 in 12500 (Israel)	Very rare
Tay–Sach's disease (infantile)*	90	1 in 5000	1:400000
Niemann–Pick disease (infantile)*	50	> 1 in 100000	1:100000
Gaucher's disease (chronic adult)*	80	1 in 3500	Very rare
Abetalipoproteinaemia (Bassen–Kornzweig syndrome)	60	1 in 20000	Very rare
Dystrophia musculoram deformans	80	1 in 40000	?
Spongy degeneration of the brain	85	?	?
Bloom's syndrome	60	?	Rare

*Prenatal diagnosis possible.
Data from Goodman (1975) with permission of the author and publishers.

sampling or cultured amniotic fluid cells. Advice and testing are available at Guy's Hospital, London.

Lemna *et al.* (1990) have shown that mutation analysis on a whole population basis for cystic fibrosis would identify 57% of at risk couples in a North American population but only 9% of Ashkenazi couples.

There are a number of other rare conditions which are commoner in Ashkenazi Jews than in the general population: these are shown in Table 1.12.

Prenatal diagnosis

Investigation of the fetus must be directed to a specific condition or group of conditions, so that the appropriate investigations can be chosen (Table 1.13). Counselling (pp. 28–29) is important before any prenatal investigation. The timing, risks and time required to achieve a result are shown in Table 1.14 for amniocentesis, fetal blood sampling (cordocentesis), chorionic villus sampling (CVS) and ultrasound.

Less commonly used prenatal diagnostic methods

1. Fetoscopy is now only indicated in certain soft tissue disorders, such as the Treacher-Collins syndrome, which are difficult to detect by ultrasound. There is a 3% risk of abortion related to fetoscopy.

Table 1.13. Criteria for screening methods and the extent to which they are met for prenatal diagnosis

Screening method	*Safe*	*Simple*	*Cheap*	*Reliability*	
				False +ve	*False −ve*
For maternal infections					
Blood tests	+	+	+	Few	Few
For congenital malformations					
MsAFP* for NTD†				Many	
anencephaly	+	+	+	clinically	Nearly 0
spina bifida	+	+	+	relevant	20–30%
Detection of maternal diabetes	+	+	+	0	0
Ultrasound	+‡	0	0	Dependent on skill of operator and equipment	
For chromosomal disease					
Maternal age	+	+	+	>90%	65%
Maternal age + serum factors	+	+	+	>90%	<50%
For inherited disease					
Family history	+	0	0	Many	Many
Selection by ethnic group	+	+	+	Few	Is increasing§
Population screening for haemoglobin disorders and Tay-Sachs disease	+	+	+	Often clinically relevant	0

*Maternal serum AFP.
†Neural tube defects.
‡Safety depends on training and supervision of operator.
§The proportion of carriers of haemoglobin disorders or Tay-Sachs disease who are not identifiable as members of ethnic minorities is rising as population mixing progresses.
Table from Royal College of Physicians of London (1989*a*), with permission of authors and publishers.

Table 1.14 Present fetal sampling procedures, risks and time required to obtain a diagnosis

Obstetric aspects			*Time to diagnosis*					
Sampling procedure	*Weeks' gestation*	*Risk to pregnancy (%)*	*Karyotyping*		*Biochemistry*		*DNA*	
			Culture	*Rapid*	*Culture*	*Direct*	*Culture*	*Direct*
Amniocentesis	14–17	0.5–1	2–4wk	–	2–4wk	–	5wk	>10d*
Fetal blood sampling	>18	1–7	–	3d	–	2–7d	–	10d
Chorionic villus sampling	>9	2–4	2wk	2d	2wk	1d	–	10d
Ultrasound	~9	+†	Time to a definite ultrasound diagnosis depends on many variables. Rapid karotyping may be required.					

*New DNA methods promise to reduce the time to diagnosis to 1–2 days.
†The risk is of false positive diagnosis leading to abortion of a healthy fetus.
Table from the Royal College of Physicians of London (1986b), with permission of authors and publishers.

2. Fetal tissue sampling may be required for the diagnosis of certain skin disorders, such as tyrosinase negative albinism or epidermolysis bullosa, or in accessible fetal tumours. The risk of abortion is similar to that for fetoscopy.
3. Radiology is occasionally useful in the diagnosis of skeletal dysplasias which cannot be clearly defined by ultrasound.

A list of conditions which can be diagnosed prenatally by various methods is given in Appendices I–IV in *Prenatal Diagnosis in Obstetric Practice* (Whittle and Connor, (1989).

Situations requiring special consideration

Neural tube defects (NTD's)

Four possible situations need to be considered.

1. In areas with a high incidence (e.g. UK and Ireland) all mothers should be screened initially by MsAFP estimations, and those with repeated high levels should be investigated by amniocentesis (high amniotic fluid AFP) and ultrasound, or by ultrasound alone.
2. In low-incidence areas screening with MsAFP is not generally used, but routine ultrasound will detect cases of NTD.
3. Where there is a positive family history ultrasound is usually employed as the definitive investigation.
4. Investigation with ultrasound is also indicated in high-risk situations such as maternal treatment with sodium valproate, maternal diabetes and in monozygotic twins where there is a risk of anencephaly in one twin (Little and Bryan, 1988). There is an increased risk of anencephaly in people from the Indian subcontinent, especially Pakistanis (Balarajan, Raleigh and Botting, 1989) and Punjabis, but the incidence in Afro-Caribbeans is lower than in the general population.

Congenital heart disease (CHD)

Structural cardiac defects These account for 20% of all perinatal deaths attributable to malformations and 10% of all congenital abnormalities. The incidence of cardiac malformations is 8 per 1000 pregnancies; about half of these are minor and easily correctable.

Using the '4 chamber view' (Allan, 1989) between 18 and 20 weeks in the routine anomaly scan, the more severe malformations can be detected, but echocardiography at a specialist centre may be required to confirm the diagnosis or to detect minor abnormalities. In an at risk family, specialist echocardiography should in any case be arranged. The development of polyhydramnios due to fetal hydrops may be the first indication of a severe lesion. Apart from families in which a dominant or recessive mode of inheritance is obvious, the majority of cases of congenital heart disease (having excluded those due to infection, drugs, other environmental influences and specific syndromes (Burn, 1987, gives a very complete list of syndromes associated with congenital heart disease) are inherited in a multifactorial manner, and therefore empirical risks for the population studied must be given. The increasing number of survivors of cardiac surgery in childhood has enhanced the importance of considering recurrence risks for offspring or sibs. The overall risk of an affected parent having a child with CHD or of a normal parent having a second affected child is 1–4% but is 10% for an affected parent having a second affected child. However, overall risks are not particuarly helpful since the risk varies according to the lesion in the index case (Table 1.15).

Table 1.15. Recurrence risks (%) in siblings and offspring for different types of heart defect

Defect	*Sibs*	*Offspring*
Isomerism sequence*	5	1
Tricuspid atresia	1	5
Mitral atresia	2	5
Complete transposition	2	5
Pulmonary atresia	1	5
Aortic atresia	1	5
Anomalous pulmonary venous connection	3	5
Secundum atrial septal defect	3	4
Atrioventricular septal defects	2	5–10
Ebstein malformation	1	5
Ventricular septal defect, perimembranous	3	4
Pulmonary stenosis	2	6
Double outlet right ventricle	2	4
Tetralogy of Fallot	2	4
Aortic stenosis	3	5–10
Coarctation	2	3
Persistent patency of arterial duct	2.5	3

*Also known as situs ambiguus: in right isomerism the body has two right sides, and in left isomerism it has two left sides.
Table from Burn (1988a) with permission of author and publishers

Fetal arrhythmias A fetal arrhythmia may be detected on routine auscultation, during cardiotocography, because of the development of polyhydramnios secondary to fetal cardiac failure and hydrops; or a hydropic fetus may be detected on an ultrasound examination. In most cases the arrhythmia is only detected after 28 weeks. The normal fetal heart rate at 20 weeks is 140±20 beats per minute, and 130±20 beats per minute near term. A tachycardia of >200 per minute on two or more occasions indicates either atrial flutter or supraventricular tachycardia (SVT) or more rarely a ventricular tachycardia. Bradycardia due to heart block is indicated by a fetal heart rate of <100 beats per minute on two or more occasions.

Bradycardias are strongly associated with maternal systemic lupus erythematosus and less commonly with other collagen diseases; there is a high incidence of associated structural defects. No prenatal treatment is possible and the only postnatal treatment available would be a pacemaker.

For prenatal treatment of atrial flutter or SVT see page 26.

Karyotyping In all cases of severe or complex lesions, particularly if accompanied by malformation in other systems, karyotyping should be performed by fetal blood sampling, as an abnormal karyotype influences management and may be an indication for termination. In a recent series an abnormal karyotype was found in 21% of cases detected prenatally (Davis *et al.*, 1990).

Twins and multiple births (for reviews, see under Further reading)
The incidence of monozygotic (MZ) twins is the same for all countries for which reliable figures are available (4–5 MZ twin pregnancies for every 1000 pregnancies). There is considerable variation in the incidence of dizygotic (DZ) twinning: in Europe, Asia and most of Africa the rate is 7–11 per 1000 deliveries, but in parts of Nigeria rates of up to 45 per 1000 deliveries have been recorded (Nylander, 1970). There are no reliable figures for Afro-Caribbeans in the UK but the incidence for American blacks is greater than for American whites but not as high as in West Africa (Little and Thompson, 1988). Excluding the effects of ovulation-inducing drugs, the epidemiological data for triplets are similar to those of twinning. The intrauterine and postnatal complications of twins are discussed on pages 000–000. Malformations are more common in MZ than in DZ twins or singletons. Congenital heart disease affects 2% of all twin pregnancies (Burn, 1988) and is commoner in MZ twins, with only one affected. There is a slightly increased risk of anencephaly in one of MZ twins, but not of spina bifida. The high perinatal risk in multiple pregnancies can be reduced by selective feticide (p. 27).

Fetal uropathies
Routine ultrasound will detect most significant renal abnormalities, such as absent, hypoplastic or polycystic kidneys, and obstructive uropathies; but confirmation may be required at a specialist centre. Obstructive uropathies occur in 1 in 500 to 1 in 600 pregnancies (Thomas and Gordon, 1989). Severe renal insufficiency from any cause is usually associated with oligohydramnios, pulmonary hypoplasia, compression deformities and Potter's syndrome, and is incompatible with postnatal survival. Karyotyping should be done in all severe renal disorders, particularly in the presence of malformation elsewhere. A poor prognosis in obstructive uropathy is

indicated by a sodium concentration of >100 mmol/l in urine obtained by bladder puncture (Thomas and Gordon, 1989). Prenatal drainage operations have largely been unsuccessful and are not recommended.

Fragile X mental retardation (Martin-Bell syndrome)
After Down's syndrome the fragile X syndrome is the most common cause of severe mental retardation. It is inherited as an X-linked 'semi-dominant' recessive, in which males are more severely affected than the females.

Affected males are difficult to detect before puberty. Clinical features are large testes, a long face, prognathism and 'cluttering' speech – 'hurried repetitive sentences which come out in a rush' (Winter, 1989). Developmental quotient in boys ranges between 20 and 70%. About 30% of female carriers are mildly retarded. The fragile X chromosome is only present in 4–50% of cells in the male and less frequently in the female. In about 50% of females the abnormal chromosome cannot be detected at all. The demonstration of the abnormal chromosome requires special culture conditions for the cells. Prenatal diagnosis, in families with an appropriate pedigree, should be preceded by fetal sexing by amniocentesis; the male fetus is then tested, using lymphocytes from fetal blood sampling.

The presence of microcephaly, dysmorphic features, other than those mentioned above and abnormal neurological signs should exclude the diagnosis of fragile X syndrome.

Retinoblastoma (Kingston, 1989)
Retinoblastoma can be unilateral or bilateral; most bilateral cases and about 15% of unilateral cases are inherited as an autosomal dominant with incomplete penetrance. The retinoblastoma gene has been localized to chromosome 13q14, with the locus for red cell esterase D closely linked, as a marker. Some 80% of children with the abnormal gene develop tumours. Since tumours sometimes regress, it is important to look for retinal scars in the parents. Second malignancies at sites other than the eye occur in survivors and are more common in bilateral and familial cases (Kingston, 1989).

Prenatal diagnosis, and identification of other gene carriers, can usually be done using DNA probes. In affected families expert genetic and ophthalmological advice are required, with careful follow up by an ophthalmologist. Table 1.16 shows the risk of a tumour in a child.

Table 1.16. Percentage risk of retinoblastoma in a child according to affected relatives

	Risk (%)
Bilateral tumour	
Parent	40
Sib	8
Unilateral tumour	
Parent	6
Sib	2
Two sibs	40
Parent and another relative	40

Table from Kingston (1989), with permission of author and publishers.

Myotonic dystrophy (Harper, 1989a,b)

Myotonic dystrophy (dystrophia myotonica, myotonia atrophica) is inherited as an autosomal dominant, with a mean age of onset between 20 and 25 years. However, this pattern only applies to inheritance from an affected father. The combination of an affected mother carrying an affected fetus produces an anomalous result, the delivery of a newborn severely affected by hypotonia but without myotonia (see Table 1.17 for fetal complications. For an affected woman, whether or not the fetus is affected affected there are numerous complications during pregnancy and delivery (Table 1.18).

Table 1.17. Congenital myotonic dystrophy: major clinical features

Bilateral facial weakness*
Hyoptonia
Delayed motor development
Mental retardation
Neonatal respiratory distress
Talipes

*Must be distinguished from Möbius syndrome.
Table (modified) from Harper (1989*b*), with permission of author and publishers.

Table 1.18. Pregnancy complications of myotonic dystrophy

Increased muscle weakness (not common)
Increased spontaneous abortion rate
Reduced fetal movements
Polyhydramnios
Prolonged first stage of labour
Reduced voluntary muscular power in second stage
Retained placenta
Post-partum haemorrhage
Anaesthetic sensitivity
Increased neonatal mortality

Table from Harper (1989*a*), with permission of author and publishers.

It often happens that the delivery of an affected newborn draws attention to the diagnosis in a previously unrecognised and mildly affected woman.

Polyhydramnios developing late in pregnancy is common and usually indicates an affected fetus, though sometimes the fetus is normal and no cause can be found for the polyhydramnios. Caesarean section is often required, and may be complicated by respiratory arrest or insufficiency after the use of scoline or tubocurarine. Breech delivery is a common complication.

The affected newborn is extremely hypotonic, and may never establish spontaneous respiration. Death is common in the immediate postnatal period, but survivors show a progressive improvement in muscle tone over the next 3–4 years. Table 1.17 shows the main clinical features in the neonatal period. Talipes is a frequent finding, but more severe compression deformities, such as arthrogryposis, also occur.

In the most affected families it is now possible to make the diagnosis in the presymptomatic stage by the use of DNA probes. Prenatal diagnosis is also possible, using material from a chorionic villus biopsy. It is, however, more satisfactory, from DNA studies of all available family members, to establish before pregnancy, whether a prenatal diagnosis is going to be practicable or not. Most couples who are concerned about prenatal diagnosis have already had an affected child. Whenever possible, blood or unfixed tissue should be taken from fatal cases and stored for future reference. Termination of pregnancy is frequently requested if prenatal testing shows a high probability of an affected fetus.

Pregnancies at increased risk for a chromosomal abnormality

Though maternal age over 35 years is the most important factor governing the incidence of chromosomal abnormalities (p. 2), others must also be considered (Table 1.19). About 4% of couples with a history of recurrent spontaneous abortion (three or more) have a balanced translocation in one partner; though karyotyping the abortus is useful, the majority of those with abnormal chromosomes have a non-inherited error (Warburton *et al.*, 1987).

Table 1.19. Clues to a pregnancy at increased risk for a chromosomal disorder

Factors evident before pregnancy
Advanced maternal age (p. 2)
Parent with a balanced structural rearrangement (translocation)
Family history: mental retardation, multiple congenital malformation, recurrent miscarriages, known chromosomal abnormality
Maternal thyroid antibodies
Factors evident during pregnancy
Fetal abnormality detected by ultrasound; nuchal oedema, cystic hygroma, exomphalos, duodenal atresia, unexplained hydrops, multiple congenital abnormalities
Unexplained intrauterine growth retardation
Abnormality low maternal serum AFP (p. 15)
Incidental finding at amniocentesis for another indication
Threatened abortion

Table from Tolmie (1989), with permission of author and publishers.

Down's syndrome in a fetus or in a liveborn child is the most important association with translocation. In 95% of cases (at all ages) the abnormality is a Trisomy 21 and the parents are normal. In 4–5%, one parent has a centric fusion translocation involving chromosome 21. The most frequent rearrangement is a centric fusion of 14:21 chromosomes, less commonly 21:22 or 21:21. The risk of an unbalanced translocation (resulting in Down's syndrome clinically indistinguishable from one with Trisomy 21) is as follows: 14:21, mother 15%, father 1%: 21:22; mother 10%, father 5%: 21:21; mother or father 100%.

Since translocations may occur at any maternal age, it is important that all fetuses or infants with Down's syndrome should be investigated. In fact, the majority of cases of Down's syndrome in young mothers are due to

Trisomy 21 and the risk for a recurrence is low, but chromosome analysis of the fetus should be performed in subsequent pregnancies.

Consanguinity
Consanguinity is frequent in Pakistan, the Middle East and South India; in the Pakistani community in the UK, 55% of marriages are between first cousins, and marriages between an uncle and niece are not uncommon.

The risk in a first-cousin marriage of producing a child with a severe abnormality is about 3–5% above that (2%) in the general population. For second-cousin marriages there is an increased risk of 1%, and for uncle–niece marriages, the increased risk is 5–10%. Occasionally a recessive condition occurs which is unique to a particular couple, but a 1 in 4 recurrence risk can only be given after two affected children.

In the UK Pakistani community, the risk of β-thalassaemia is about 0.5% (1 in 200) but this will be increased if one parent or a close relative is affected. There is also an increased risk of one of the rarer metabolic disorders, lethal multiple malformations, and of multifactorially inherited conditions. Bundey (1988) in the Birmingham Birth Study found an excess of mental subnormality, deafness, visual defect and complex cardiac anomalies in the Pakistani community. The question of consanguineous marriage in Pakistanis must be handled with delicacy and understanding, and there is no place for condemnation by an 'outsider'. Genetic counselling should be done by someone from the same ethnic group.

Prenatal treatment

Prenatal treatment can be considered under the following headings.

Maternal disease

Diabetes mellitus
The incidence of malformations, macrosomia and its related obstetric complications (p. 215) and postnatal biochemical disturbances (p. 216) can be minimized by meticulous control of the diabetes, preferably starting before conception.

Phenylketonuria
Untreated maternal phenylketonuria (PKU) is associated with mental retardation, micocephaly and malformations of eye, heart and skeletal system. Careful dietary control, starting before conception, has been shown to reduce the risk of these complications. Some women with PKU, whose treatment was stopped in childhood, are unaware of the risk to the fetus of untreated PKU.

Thyrotoxicosis
In a proportion of cases the fetus develops thyrotoxicosis, though normally this is kept under partial control by the transplacental passage of antithyroid drugs such as carbimazole or propylthiouracil. However, where the mother has been rendered euthyroid surgically, and particularly if she

has persistant eye signs, the fetus may develop thyrotoxicosis, which if uncontrolled, carries a risk of fetal or neonatal death. Carbimazole or propylthiouracil should be given to the mother in a dose sufficient to maintain the fetal heart rate below 140 per minute.

Fetal disease

Risk of respiratory distress syndrome (RDS)
This can be assessed by estimation of lecithin/syphingomyelin ratio (p. 142). The fetus at risk from RDS after delivery can be treated by giving the mother dexamethasone.

Severe rhesus or other blood group isoimmunization
In the severely anaemic, and usually hydropic fetus, blood (CMV-negative) can be transfused into the umbilical vein by cordocentesis or intraperitoneally if the fetus is not hydropic. There is no need for an exchange transfusion. The state of the fetus can be assesed between 18 and 24 weeks by ultrasound which will detect hydrops, which develops when the haemoglobin falls below 40 g/l (Rodeck and Letsky, 1989). Rodeck and Letsky found that Liley's method of predicting the severity of the haemolytic process, though reliable in the third trimester, was unreliable in the second trimester and was misleading between 18 and 25 weeks. They found that fetuses suffering from anti-Kell disease had depressed erythropoiesis rather than haemolysis, and therefore no significant rise in bilirubin in the amniotic fluid.

Fetal autoimmune thrombocytopenia
In this condition the fetal thrombocytopenia is secondary to maternal antibodies which also depress the mother's platelets. The main risk to the fetus is intracranial haemorrhage during delivery. The risk to the fetus can be predicted from the mother's history; a platelet count on the fetus can be performed by fetal blood sampling at 38 weeks. If the count is less than 50×10^9/l, the infant should be delivered by caesarean section. The infant's platelet count usually returns to normal within a few days of delivery. Platelet transfusions are ineffective because of their short survival in this condition.

Fetal isoimmune thrombocytopenia (Daffos et al.*, 1984)*
Intracranial haemorrhage may occur before labour. If the platelet count on the fetus in the second or third trimester is less than 50×10^9/l, repeated transfusions with washed maternal platelets can be given. In contrast with rhesus isoimmunization, the mother's first child may be affected.

Fetal tachycardia (for prenatal diagnosis see p. 20 and postnatal treatment p. 176)
Fetal tachycardia may be detected on routine auscultation, on cardiotocography or after the development of polyhydramnios due to hydrops, indicating cardiac failure. Atrial flutter and supraventricular tachycardia can usually be controlled by giving digoxin to the mother in a dose of 0.75 mg daily, the dose being adjusted to maintain a serum concentration

of 2.6 nmol/l (Maxwell *et al.*, 1988). In the hydropic fetus a combination of digoxin and Verapamil may be required; the dose of Verapamil should start at 240 mg daily increasing as required up to 480 mg daily. Flecainide has recently been used with some success.

Fetal bradycardia (congenital heart block)
There is no prenatal treatment for this condition; for prenatal diagnosis, see p. 21.

Congenital adrenal hyperplasia (21-hydroxylase deficiency)
The object is to reduce or prevent the masculinization of the female fetus by giving dexamethasone to the mother starting at 5–9 weeks gestation (David and Forrest, (1984); this should be followed by fetal sexing to identify the female fetus, as soon as possible.

Vitamin B_{12} (cyanocobalamin)-sensitive methylmalonic acidaemia (Ampola et al, 1975).
The diagnosis of an affected fetus is made by finding an excess of methylmalonic acid in the amniotic fluid or from cultured cells obtained by amniocentesis at 19 weeks. These investigations can only be done after the birth of a previous affected child. Mental retardation can be prevented by giving large doses of vitamin B_{12} to the mother.

Methylcobalamin deficiency (Cobalamin E disease)
Rosenblatt *et al.* (1985) successfully treated an affected fetus by giving the mother hydroxocobalamin from the 25th week onwards.

Direct fetal intervention

Selective feticide

One twin with a severe malformation Selective feticide can be considered in the second trimester. This can be done by the injection of air into the umbilical vein or potassium chloride into the pericardial sac (Wapner *et al.* (1990)

Selective feticide raises difficult ethical problems, and the parents may be distressed or guilty at having given permission for the killing of a fetus. In monochorionic twins breakdown products from the dead fetus may cause cerebral infarction and microcephaly in the survivor (Burn, (1988_b).

Multiple pregnancy In multiple pregnancy, particularly with drug-induced ovulation, the perinatal outcome can be improved by selective feticide of one or more fetuses (Wapner *et al.*, 1990).

Hydrocephalus
Drainage operations for hydrocephalus have mainly been unsuccessful and are not advised at the present time.

Obstructive uropathies
Prenatal drainage operations are not recommended (Thomas and Gordon, 1989).

Cardiac defects

There has been limited and discouraging experience with direct correction of cardiac defects *in utero*.

Counselling for prenatal diagnosis and treatment and termination of pregnancy

Pre-pregnancy (pp. 1–2)

During pregnancy

Those involved with the management and treatment of the pregnant woman should be aware that, for both partners, pregnancy is a time of emotional sensitivity and instability. Whenever possible, discussions should involve both partners. Doctors and technicians performing investigations during pregnancy should receive instruction in counselling.

Investigations

Before every investigation or test the following information should be given.

1. The purpose of the investigation.
2. What it involves in the way of apparatus, injections, sedative drugs etc..
3. The risk to the fetus of the investigation (e.g. abortion).
4. What information it is hoped to obtain, and the use to which it will be put.
5. The method (telephone, letter, follow up clinic, counselling session) by which the result of the investigation will be given to the patient.
6. The normal interval between the investigation and the receipt of the result by the patient.
7. The facilities available to discuss the result.

Information about a negative result is just as important to the patient as a positive result; there is no excuse for saying, 'If you hear nothing, you can assume that everything is alright'.

Prenatal treatment

This is normally only justified if treatment is the only way of keeping the fetus alive or of avoiding serious fetal damage or subsequent handicap.In some circumstances the risk of the treatment to the fetus is considerable, in others it is negligable (see also pp. 25–27). In any case the situation should be fully explained, and treatment should only be embarked upon with the mother's (and preferably father's also) informed consent.

The responsibilities of the clinician

Before suggesting a particular prenatal investigation or treatment the clinician must inform himself on the following points.

1. That the procedure is appropriate; that it will produce the required information; and that it does not expose a possibly normal fetus to an unreasonable risk.

2. That the disorder under consideration is of sufficient severity to warrant a termination if the fetus is found to be affected.
3. That a termination of pregnancy would be acceptable to both partners.

Religious and cultural attitudes

Accurate information about the religious and ethnic group of both partners should be recorded in the notes. If the question of prenatal testing and possible termination arises, it should not be automatically assumed that membership of a particular religion or ethnic group will mean that the couple are opposed to a termination; they must be allowed to make their own decision. Though the presence of a counsellor of their own religious or ethnic group is usually helpful, this may not be the case if the couple's opinion on termination conflicts with the orthodox view.

Termination of pregnancy (for stillbirth and neonatal deaths, see pp. 349–352)

The parents should be given the opportunity of seeing the fetus, though not while it is still moving. They should be told if a post-mortem is being requested and should be told about the information that it is expected to produce.

If the parents wish to have a funeral, they should know that there is no grant if the fetus is less than 28 weeks gestation.

The parents should be offered information about relevant support groups, according to the condition affecting the fetus, or should be put in touch with Support after Termination for Abnormality (SATFA).

Normally a follow up appointment will be arranged with the obstetrician, neonatologist or clinical geneticist. The family doctor should be kept fully informed.

References

Allan, L.D. (1989) Diagnosis of fetal cardiac abnormalities. *Archives of Disease in Childhood*, **64**, 964–968

Ampola, N.G., Mahoney, M.J., Nakamura, E. and Tanaka, K. (1975) Prenatal therapy of a patient with B_{12} responsive methylmalonic acidemia. *New England Journal of Medicine*, **293**, 314–317

Balarajan, R., Raleigh, V.S. and Botting, B. (1989) Mortality from congenital malformations in England and Wales: variations by mother's country of birth. *Archives of Disease in Childhood*, **64**, 1457–1462

Blank, E., Neerhout, R.C. and Burry, K.A. (1978) Congenital mesoblastic nephroma and polyhydramnios. *Journal of American Medical Association*, **240**, 1504–1505

Boyd, K. and Walker, E. (1988). Use of acyclovir to treat chickenpox in pregnancy. *British Medical Journal*, **296**, 393–394

British National Formulary, No. 19, March (1990), pp.393–397. British Medical Association and The Pharmaceutical Press, London

Brodie, M.J., Moore, M.R., Thompson, G.G., Campbell, B.C. and Goldberg, A. (1977) Pregnancy and the acute porphyrias. *British Journal of Obstetrics and Gynaecology*, **84**, 726–731

Bull, M.J.V. (1990) Maternal and fetal screening for antenatal care. *British Medical Journal*, **300**, 1118–1120

Bundey, S. (1988) The Birmingham Birth Study. *Biology and Society*, **5**, 13–15

Burn, J. (1987) Aetiology of congenital heart disease. In *Paediatric Cardiology* (ed R.H. Anderson, F.J. Macartney, E.A. Shinebourn and M. Tynan) Churchill Livingstone, Edinburgh, Vol 1. pp.42–63

Burn, J. (1988*a*) Genetic advances in paediatric cardiology. *Current Opinion in Cardiology*, **3**, 43–49

Burn, J. (1988*b*) Monozygotic twins. In *Contemporary Obstetrics and Gynaecology* (ed G. Chamberlain), Butterworth, London, p.133

Connor, J.M. and Whittle, M.J. (1989) Genetic and pre-pregnancy counselling. In *Prenatal Diagnosis in Obstetric Practice* (eds M.J. Whittle and J.M. Connor), Blackwell Scientific, Oxford, p.2

Daffos, F., Forestier, F., Muller, J.Y., Reznikoff-Etievant, M., and Habib, B. (1984) Prenatal treatment of alloimmune thrombocytopenia. *Lancet*, **ii**, 32

David, M. and Forrest, M.G. (1984) Prenatal treatment of congenital adrenal hyperplasia resulting from 21-hydroxylase deficiency. *Journal of Pediatrics*, **105**, 799–803

Davis, K.G., Farquhar, C.M., Allan, L.D., Crawford, D.C. and Chapman, M.G. (1990) Structural cardiac abnormalities in the fetus: reliability of prenatal diagnosis and outcome. *British Journal of Obstetrics and Gynaecology*, **97**, 27–31

Dekaban, A.S. (1968) Abnormalities in children exposed to X-radiation during various stages of gestation. *Journal of Nuclear Medicine*, **9**, 471–477

Editorial (1990) Cystic fibrosis: prospects for screening therapy. *Lancet*, **335**, 79–80

Ferguson–Smith, M.A. and Yates, J.R.W. (1984) Maternal age-specific rates for chromosome aberrations and factors influencing them. Report of a Collaborative European Study on 52,965 amniocenteses. *Prenatal Diagnosis*, **4**, 5–44

Gardner, M.J., Snee, M.P., Hall, A.J., Powell, C.A. and Downes, S (1990) Results of a case-control study of leukaemia and lymphoma among young people near Sellafield nuclear plant in West Cumbria. *British Medical Journal*, **300**, 423–429

Gilmore, D.H. and Aitken, D.A. (1989) Prenatal screening. In *Prenatal Diagnosis in Obstetric Practice* (eds M.J. Whittle and J.M. Connor), Blackwell Scientific, Oxford, pp.22–32

Goodman, R.M. (1975) Genetic disorders among the Jewish people. In *Modern Trends in Human Genetics* (ed. A.E.H. Emery), Butterworths, London, Vol 2, p. 286

Harper, P.S. (1989*a*) *Myotonic Dystrophy,* 2nd edn, W.B. Saunders, p.128

Harper, P.S. (1989*b*) *Myotonic Dystrophy*, 2nd edn, W.B. Saunders, London, p. 189

Holmes, R.C. and Black, M.M. (1984) The fetal prognosis in pemphigoid gestations (herpes gestationis). *British Journal of Dermatology,* **110**, 67–72

Kaiser, I.H. (1990) Brown amniotic fluid in congenital porphyria erythropoietica. *Obstetrics and Gynecology,* **56**, 383–384

Kingston, H.M. (1989) *ABC of Clinical Genetics,* British Medical Journal, London, p.31

Lammer, E.J., Chen, D.T., Hoar, R.M., Agnish, N.D., Benke, P.J., Braun, J.J. *et al.* (1985) Retinoic acid embryopathy. *New England Journal of Medicine,* **313**, 837–841

Lemna, W.K., Feldman, G.L., Bar-Sheva, K., Fernbach, S.D. and Zevnovich, E.P. (1990) Mutation analysis for heterozygote detection and the prenatal diagnosis of cystic fibrosis. *New England Journal of Medicine,* **322**, 291–296

Little, J. and Bryan, E.M. (1988) Congenital anomalies. In *Twins and Twinning* (eds I. MacGillivray, D.M. Campbell and B. Thompson), Wiley, Chichester and New York, p.223

Little, J. and Thompson, B. (1988) Descriptive epidemiology. In *Twins and Twinning* (eds I. MacGillivray, D.M. Campbell and B. Thompson), Wiley, Chichester and New York, p.59

Maxwell, D.J., Crawford, D.C., Curry, P.V.M., Tynan, M. and Allan, L.D. (1988) Obstetric importance, diagnosis, and management of fetal tachycardias. *British Medical Journal,* **297**, 107–110

Modell, M. and Modell, B. (1990) Genetic screening for ethnic minorities. *British Medical Journal,* **300**, 1702–1704

Mole, R.H. (1982) Consequences of pre-natal radiation exposure for post-natal development. A review. *International Journal of Radiation Biology,* **42**, 1–12

Nylander, P.P.S. (1970) The frequency of twinning in a rural community in Western Nigeria. *Annals of Human Genetics,* **33**, 41–44

Otake, M. and Schull, W.J. (1984) In utero exposure to A-bomb radiation and mental retardation: a reassessment. *British Journal of Radiology,* **57**, 409–414

Rodeck, C.H. and Letsky, E. (1989) How the management of erythroblastosis fetalis has changed. *British Journal of Obstetrics and Gynaecology,* **94**, 759–763

Rosenblatt, D.S., Schmutz, S.M., Cooper, B.A., Zaleski, W.A. and Casey, R.E. (1985) Prenatal vitamin B_{12} therapy of a fetus with methylcobalamin deficiency (Cobalamin E disease). *Lancet,* **ii**, 1127–1129

Royal College of Physicians of London (1989*a*) *Prenatal Diagnosis and Genetic Screening,* Royal College of Physicians of London, London, p.13

Royal College of Physicians of London (1989*b*) *Prenatal Diagnosis and Genetic Screening,* Royal College of Physicians of London, London, p.18

Stevens, M.C.G., Darbyshire, P.J. and Brown, S.M. (1987) Early congenital syphilis and severe haematological disturbance. *Archives of Disease in Childhood,* **62**, 1073–1075

Thomas, D.F.M. and Gordon, A.C. (1989) Management of prenatally diagnosed uropathies. *Archives of Disease in Childhood, Fetal and Neonatal Edition,* **64**, 58–63

Tolmie, J.L. (1989) Chromosomal disorders. In *Prenatal Diagnosis in Obstetric Practice.* (eds M.J. Whittle and J.M. Connor), Blackwell Scientific, Oxford, p.34

Townes, P.L. (1965) Transplacentally acquired erythrodontia. *Journal of Pediatrics,* **67**, 600–602

Wald, N.J., Cuckle, H.S., Densem, J.W., Nauchahal, K., Royston, P., Chard, T. *et al.* (1988) Maternal screening for Down's Syndrome in early pregnancy. *British Medical Journal,* **297**, 883–887

Wapner, R.J., Davis, G.H., Johnson, A., Weinblatt, V.J., Fischer, L.G., Jackson, L.G. *et al.* (1990) Selective feticide in multiple pregnancies. *Lancet,* **i**, 90–93

Warburton, D., Kline, J., Stein, Z., Hutzler, M., China, A. and Hassold, T. (1987) Does the karyotype of a spontaneous abortion predict the karyotype of a subsequent abortion? Evidence from 273 women with two karyotyped spontaneous abortions. *American Journal of Human Genetics,* **41**, 465–483

Whittle, M.J. and Rubin, P.C. (1989) Exposure to teratogens. In *Prenatal Diagnosis in Obstetric Practice* (eds M.J. Whittle and J.M. Connor), Blackwell Scientific, Oxford, p.163

Winter, R.M. (1989) Fragile X mental retardation. *Archives of Disease in Childhood,* **64**, 1223–1224

Further reading

Bergsma, D. (ed.) (1979) *Birth Defects Compendium,* 2nd edn, MacMillan, London.

Brent, R.L. and Beckman, D.A. (eds) (1986) Teratology. *Clinics in Perinatology,* **13(3)**, 491–693

Bryan, E. (1983). *The Nature and Nurture of Twins.* Baillière Tindall, London

Bryan, E. (1986) The intrauterine hazards of twins. *Archives of Disease in Childhood,* **61**, 1044–1045

Elwood, J.M. and Elwood J.H. (1980) *Epidemiology of Anencephaly and Spina Bifida.* Oxford University Press, Oxford

Freij, B.J. and Sever, J.L. (eds) (1988) Infectious complications of pregnancy. *Clinics in Perinatology,* **15**(2), 163–149

Harper, P.S. (1988) *Practical Genetic Counselling,* 3rd edn, Wright, Bristol

MacArnarney, E.R. and Greydanus, D.E. (eds) (1981), Adolescent Pregnancy: a risk condition. *Seminars in Perinatology,* **5(i)**, 1–103

MacGillivray, I., Campbell, D.M. and Thompson, B. (eds) (1988) *Twinning and Twins.* Wiley, Chichester

Persaud, T.V.N., Chaudry, A.E. and Skelko, R.G. (1985) *Basic Concepts of Teratology.* Liss, New York

Phelan, J.P. and Martin, G.I. (1989) Polyhydramnios: fetal and neonatal implications. *Clinics in Perinatology,* **16**(4), 987–994

Porter, I.H.R., Hatcher, N.H. and Willey, A.M. (eds) (1986) *Perinatal Genetics: Diagnosis and Treatment,* Academic Press, New York

Schardein, J.L. (1985) *Chemically Induced Birth Defects,* Dekker, New York

Serjeant, G.R. (1988) *Sickle Cell Disease,* 2nd edn, Oxford University Press, Oxford

Weatherall, D.J. and Clegg, J.B. (1981) *The Thalassaemia Syndromes,* 3rd edn, Blackwell Scientific, Oxford

Whittle, J.M. and Connor, M.J. (eds) (1989) *Prenatal Diagnosis in Obstetric Practice,* Blackwell Scientific, Oxford

Chapter 2

Resuscitation of the newborn

Prompt adequate resuscitation of the apnoeic or hypoxic infant is the most important and most urgent of all neonatal emergencies, comparable with a cardiac arrest in an older child or adult. Appropriate immediate action may save the infant from death or neurological damage, while delayed inadequate or inappropriate action may lead to death or permanent impairment. The effectiveness of modern methods of infant resuscitation underline the necessity for adequate resuscitation facilities and availability of adequately trained personnel wherever babies are delivered. Hypoxia, although presenting in the newborn, originates *in utero* and the primary management for this problem should be prevention by previous recognition of the factors associated with hypoxia in the prenatal period, and active management of patients with fetal distress during labour. The elements of successful resuscitation are:

1. Good cooperation and communication between obstetric and paediatric staff at all levels.
2. Anticipation that an infant requiring resuscitation may be delivered.
3. Adequate resuscitation facilities in working order.
4. The presence of someone capable of intubation and other resuscitative procedures at all deliveries considered to be at risk.

Equipment for resuscitation of the newborn

1. Resuscitation trolley providing:
   (a) Facilities for open oxygen by mask and intermittent positive pressure ventilation (IPPV) by mask or endotracheal tube with an adjustable pressure-limiting blow-off valve usually set to limit pressure in the circuit to 30 cmH_2O. It should be possible to override this pressure in special situations.
   (b) Piped suction.
   (c) Stop-clock;
   (d) Padded, sloping surface on which to place the baby with head-down tilt.
   (e) Radiant overhead heater.

   Specially manufactured apparatus such as the Vickers' Resuscitaire provides these facilities.

2. Mucus extractor.
3. Suction catheters (e.g. Argyle, FG 5, 8 and 10).
4. Infant bag and mask of the reinflating type which can be connected to an oxygen line and has a reservoir bag (e.g. Laerdal Infant Resuscitator. The Jackson–Rees bagging system is recommended for use by experienced staff (see below).
5. Infant laryngoscope with term and premature blades, and spare batteries and bulbs. The straight laryngoscope blades only should be used; the Miller blade is the most suitable and is available in the appropriate sizes.
6. Infant orotracheal tubes with an open angle connector attached, such as Portex resuscitation sets 2.0, 2.5, 3.0 and 3.5 mm; Coles-type tubes with a shouldered tip are easier to insert than unshouldered straight endotracheal tubes and usually do not require an introducer as they are stiff enough by themselves. These tubes should not be used for longer-term ventilation; a straight unshouldered endotracheal tube should be used if prolonged ventilatory support is anticipated.
7. Oral airway size 0 and 00.
8. Paediatric McGill's forceps, small size.
9. Warmed towels.
10. Drugs:
    (a) Glucose, 10%, 10 ml ampoules.
    (b) Sodium bicarbonate 8.4% (1 mmol/ml), 10 ml ampoules, or 5% (0.6 mmol/ml).
    (c) Naloxone (Narcan Neonatal): 2 ml ampoules (0.02 mg/ml).
    (d) Adrenaline 1:10 000, 1 ml ampoules.
    (e) Vitamin K_1 (phytomenadione): 0.5 ml ampoules (1 mg per 0.5 ml).
11. Syringes, needles, butterfly needles, alcohol swabs, adhesive tape.
12. Equipment for umbilical catheterization.
13. Equipment for chest drain insertion.

All resuscitation equipment must be regularly checked, particularly that the oxygen cylinders are full. The above list is deliberately restricted as it is important to be able to find the equipment required quickly.

Situations requiring early intubation

Severe hypoxia or apnoea at delivery (white asphyxia)

With complete apnoea, the oxygen stores of an infant fall to zero within 3–4 minutes; the $P\text{CO}_2$ rises at 2.6 kPa (20 mmHg;torr) per minute and the hydrogen ion concentration falls by 0.1 pH unit per minute (Swyer, 1975). In many cases fetal hypoxia (fetal distress) will have been recognized before delivery by cardiotocography and/or fetal scalp pH measurements.

Recognition
The infant is pale, limp, unresponsive and apnoeic. It appears white because of severe acidaemia and circulatory collapse. The heart rate is likely to be less than 50 per minute, or inaudible, and pulses may be absent or barely palpable.

Other causes of pallor at delivery are:

1. Shock from acute fetal blood loss immediately before or during delivery. These infants may not be apnoeic but have poor pulses and feeble respiratory effort.
2. Severe chronic anaemia with heart failure (hydrops, p. 274) which may be due to rhesus isoimmunization, chronic blood loss *in utero* or other causes.

Management

Consideration of the following important questions during resuscitation helps the resuscitator to gauge how effective the infant's management has been in correcting the biochemical and physiological effects of hypoxia and in planning the present and future management.

1. For how long has this resuscitation been going on? An infant who is apnoeic at birth is very different prognostically from one who is still apnoeic at 20 minutes, despite adequate resuscitation.
2. How is the baby doing – getting better, static or getting worse? This is gauged by the items included in the Apgar score (Table 2.1). The Apgar score should be done at 1, 5, 10, 15 minutes etc. in order to obtain a continuous picture of the infant's condition.

Table 2.1 Apgar score

Sign	*Score*		
	0	1	2
Heart rate	Absent	<100	>100
Respiratory effort	Absent	Weak Gasping Irregular	Good Crying Regular
Muscle tone	Completely flaccid	Some flexion of extremities	Well flexed
Reflex irritability, e.g. response to nasal catheter	No response	Grimace	Cough Sneeze Gasp
Colour of trunk	White	Blue	Pink

3. Is the airway adequate? Does the chest expand with IPPV? Has the endotracheal tube come out?
4. Is the baby's temperature being adequately maintained?

Procedure for resuscitation of an hypoxic infant (Table 2.2)

1. At the time of delivery of the infant start the clock on the resuscitation trolley.
2. Collect the infant in a warm towel from the obstetrician and transfer to the resuscitation surface under the radiant overhead heater.
3. Apply stethoscope to the baby's chest to count the heart rate.
4. At the same time examine the larynx under direct vision, and quickly suck out any obstructing material above and below the larynx.

Table 2.2 Protocol for infant resuscitation

Time (min)	*Baby*	*Action*
0–2	Blue, becoming pink. Moderate tone Spontaneous respirations Apex more than 100/min	Start clock. Mucus extraction O_2 by face mask Dry off infant's skin and keep warm Apgar score at 1 min.
	Limp, blue, feeble respirations Apex more than 100/min	As above + observe, stimulation ± IPPV by mask Prepare to intubate
	Apex less than 100/min and slowing	Intubate trachea and initiate IPPV at 40/min pressure 25–30 cmH_2O, inflation time 1 second.
	Limp, blue or white No respiratory effort. Slow apex Heart rate less than 50/min	Infant severely hypoxic Intubate straight away ECM at 120/min
	Baby severely meconium stained and hypoxic	Thorough tracheal suctioning via ETT to clear meconium before ventilating
2–7	Intubated infant pink and active Rapid apex beat Trying to cry	Suck out pharynx Extubate Observe. Apgar score at 5 min
	Apex not picking up despite IPPV ?Tube in oesophagus	Check tube position and air entry Reintubate if necessary
	Baby does not sustain adequate respiration ?Over-ventilated ?Metabolic acidosis ?Effects of maternal sedation ?Hypoglycaemia ?Shock	 Wait longer before restarting IPPV Bicarbonate } via umbilical or Naloxone } peripheral vein Glucose } ?O rhesus negative blood or plasma
15–30	Baby does not improve with IPPV Apex still slow ?Pneumothorax ?ETT not in place or heart rate improves but baby will not breathe ?Brain damage or major anomaly ?Muscle problem	Repeat bicarbonate and glucose or blood? Diagnose and drain Check Medical decision required about advisability of continuing resuscitation

ETT, endotracheal tube; ECM, external cardiac massage; IPPV, intermittent positive pressure ventilation.

5. Pass an oral endotracheal tube.
6. Inflate the lungs with IPPV at a rate of 40 per minute, with a prolonged inspiration time of 1 second and a peak pressure of 25 cmH_2O. A long inspiration time is desirable because of the low lung compliance due to the presence of fluid within the lung.
7. If the heart rate is less than 50 per minute, start external cardiac massage.
8. If the heart beat remains absent for more than 2 minutes, inject 1–2 ml of adrenaline 1:10 000 down the endotracheal tube, or inject directly into the heart.
9. If there is a strong probability of respiratory depression by the

morphine group of drugs give naloxone (Narcan Neonatal) 2 ml into the umbilical vein (half this amount if the infant appears to weigh <2.5 kg).

10. At 5 minutes, if there is still apnoea, inject via the umbilical vein over 1–5 minutes, 5 mmol sodium bicarbonate (or 1.5 mmol/kg body weight) and 5 ml of glucose 10%. This will give a safe partial correction of a metabolic acidosis and any hypoglycaemia.
11. At 5 minutes, if the infant is showing a slow response to resuscitation, check that the endotracheal tube is correctly sited and that there is air entry on both sides of the chest. The tube may be down the right main bronchus, or have slipped into the oesophagus. In order to verify the position of the endotracheal tube, look for equal expansion during inflation and listen with a stethoscope to compare air entry at three sites – right chest, left chest and epigastrium. The breath sounds should be louder in the chest than in the epigastrium, and usually the breath sounds are of equal loudness on the two sides of the chest if the tube is correctly sited.
12. At 10 minutes, if the infant still cannot sustain spontaneous respiration, but has a good heart beat, repeat bicarbonate and glucose.
13. If the infant still shows a poor response to resuscitation with a slow heart beat and apnoea, carry out a quick physical examination of the infant, to exclude major malformations.
14. At 30 minutes:
    (a) If there is no respiration or apex beat despite effective resuscitation for 30 minutes and the pupils are fixed and dilated, IPPV and formal resuscitation should cease, as the prognosis if the infant survives is extremely poor (Steiner and Neligan, 1975; Scott, 1976; Thomson *et al.*, 1977);
    (b) If there is no respiration, but the heart beat is over 60 per minute with good colour and peripheral circulation and the pupils are of normal size, IPPV should continue while the blood gases are checked. The baby may have a severe metabolic acidosis and correction of this will permit initiation of spontaneous respiration. Consideration should also be given at this stage to the possibility of acute haemorrhage before delivery, and the infant may improve dramatically following intravenous infusion of 20 ml of group O rhesus negative packed cells (or fresh frozen plasma if blood is not immediately available) via the umbilical vein. For persistent shock that is unresponsive to blood or plasma, the use of dopamine (p. 72) should be considered;
    (c) If there is no respiration after giving intravenous bicarbonate, but the infant's condition is otherwise satisfactory, the baby should be placed on a mechanical ventilator until an adequate assessment of the situation can be made (see below).

Delayed onset of respiration

Delayed respiration may be caused by:

1. Severe hypoxic ischaemic encephalopathy with severe central depression.

2. Drug depression, usually from morphine, pethidine (meperidine), codeine (diamorphine), or occasionally due to prolonged general anaesthesia or heavy maternal sedation with barbiturates or benzodiazepines (e.g. diazepam), or magnesium sulphate if this has been used for the treatment of severe pre-eclampsia. There is no specific treatment for the infant depressed after maternal general anaesthesia other than mechanical ventilation, and it is rare for this to be a cause of apnoea.
3. Excessive manual ventilation resulting in a very low $P\text{CO}_2$ level, removing the stimulus to respiration.
4. No apparent reason.

Drug depression (morphine opiate group)

Recognition
Some degree of depression of the infant's respiration is likely if the mother has received an opiate within 4 hours of delivery, in particular within half to one hour before delivery. Such an infant may be in good condition at birth, but does not breathe immediately or takes an initial few gasps and then becomes apnoeic.

Management
If the probability of opiate drug depression is high, naloxone should be given either prophylactically or after a predetermined period of apnoea under close observation. Naloxone is a specific opiate antagonist without depressant side effects. The dose for naloxone is 0.01 mg/kg but since the weight of the infant is not known at delivery, a standard dose of 0.04 mg (2 ml) for term infants and half this dose for infants less than 2.5 kg is appropriate; this dose may be repeated if necessary after 10 minutes. Naloxone should preferably be given intravenously into the umbilical vein. The action of naloxone is short-lived (sometimes as little as 30 minutes) so the dose may have to be repeated after 30 minutes to 1 hour, and occasionally several times during the first day of life. It is therefore important to have adequate facilities for respiratory monitoring during the first 24 hours of life. Opiate depression may coexist with true hypoxia, requiring full-scale resuscitation in addition to the naloxone.

Delayed onset of respiration for no obvious reason

Whatever the Apgar score, if respiration does not start immediately after routine aspiration of the nose and mouth:

1. Oxygen should be given by mask and the heart rate counted during the first 2 minutes after delivery.
2. If there is no respiratory effort by 2 minutes, or if the heart rate drops below 100, the infant should be intubated and treated as for the severely hypoxic (Table 2.2).

Meconium aspiration

Recognition
It is not always possible to predict whether aspiration of meconium has occurred, even if the infant is covered with meconium at delivery or there is meconium-stained liquor. Infants with evidence of fetal distress before delivery, who are small for gestational age or are postmature, are particularly at risk. Meconium aspiration syndrome is a common cause of respiratory difficulties in term infants, with tachypnoea, cyanosis, indrawing and chest recession; it is frequently complicated by persistent fetal circulation (p. 172). Fetal distress in the pre-term infant, however, rarely causes the passage of meconium. A meconium-stained infant of less than 32 weeks is more likely to have suffered from intrauterine sepsis than hypoxia.

For management, see pp. 146–147.

Methods of resuscitation

Oral endotracheal intubation (for complications of endotracheal intubation, see p. 326)

1. Flex the infant's neck and extend the head ('sniffing a flower position'). Placing a rolled up napkin under the neck may assist in adopting this position in a term infant, but may make intubation more difficult in very small pre-term infants.
2. A straight-bladed infant laryngoscope (preferably the Miller type) should be used (Figure 2.1). A 'premature' blade should be used for

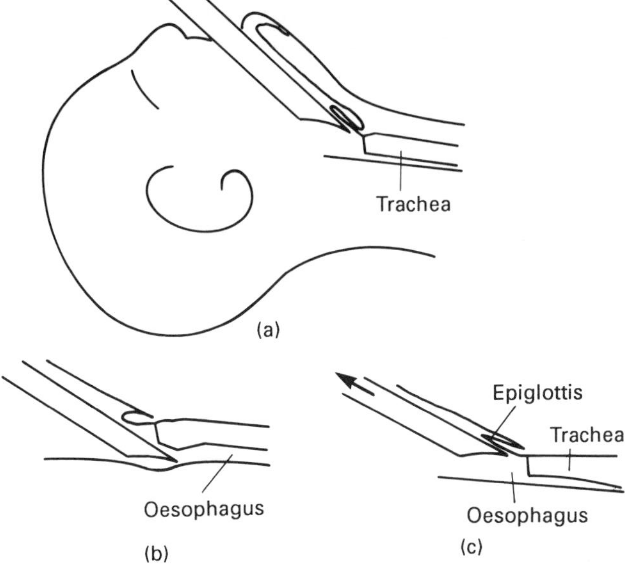

Figure 2.1 Laryngoscopy using the straight-bladed laryngoscope (for children under 6 months). Reproduced from Wilson (1987) with permission of author and publishers

infants of less than about 1.75 kg birth weight. If a 'premature' blade is used for a term baby it is impossible to see the larynx. Suction must be immediately available. The laryngoscope is inserted into the right side of the mouth and passed directly back until the uvula is seen, then moved over to the midline so that the tongue is on the left side of the laryngoscope blade. Under direct vision the blade is then advanced until the larynx comes into view. The blade tends to go into the upper oesophagus if passed too far and as the blade is gently withdrawn the epiglottis pops into view anteriorly. The tip of the blade is then used to lift up the epiglottis, permitting a straight view of the laryngeal opening. Gentle pressure on the laryngeal cartilages from the front of the neck by an assistant may help to retain the laryngeal opening more directly in view. The endotracheal tube (2.0–3.5 mm) is then passed through the laryngeal opening until the shoulder or distance mark is at the laryngeal opening and the tip of the tube 1–2 cm into the trachea. The tube is firmly secured and connected to a source of humidified oxygen with a means of providing IPPV and a safety blow-off valve at 25–30 cmH_2O. The most common reason for failure to see the laryngeal opening is over-extension of the neck. Occasionally expansion of the lungs can only be obtained by using an initial pressure as high as 60 cmH_2O, particularly in infants with severe respiratory distress syndrome (RDS), but this pressure should not be continued (pp. 140–142).

Bag and mask

Bag and mask IPPV can be used in infants who are not intubated, but in general it is less effective than IPPV by endotracheal tube. There is a tendency to inflate the stomach, particularly in infants with stiff lungs. There are two alternative types of bagging circuits:

1. A Jackson–Rees paediatric anaesthetic rebreathing bag and circuit. It takes a lot of practice and experience to use this equipment effectively, but it can be more efficient than the self-inflating type of bag described below and provides more 'feel' of lung compliance and inflation.
2. Self-inflating bag with a pressure blow-off valve, such as the Laerdal infant resuscitation bag. It is important that the mask fits adequately and that the chest moves with pressure on the bag. The resuscitation bag should have a reservoir bag attached. The neonatal size of bag is adequate only for infants up to about 3.5 kg, and the paediatric size should be used for larger infants, and older ex-premature babies. The airway is kept clear by keeping the head extended, and an oropharyngeal airway may also be useful.

Mouth-to-mouth inflation

This is indicated when no other method is available. The head is extended and the nose and mouth of the infant covered by the operator's mouth. Inflationary pressure is applied only with the cheeks, not the chest, at a rate of 40 per minute.

External cardiac massage

The infant is placed on a firm flat surface. The middle of the sternum is depressed 1–1.5 cm by the index and middle fingers at a rate of 120 per minute. Alternatively the infant's chest can be grasped by the operator's hands with the fingers at the back of the chest and the thumbs at the middle of the sternum. The sternum is then depressed by squeezing between the thumbs and fingers. It is possible in the newborn infant to obtain quite good perfusion and blood pressure readings with effective external cardiac massage.

Injection of drugs into the umbilical vein

Although it is possible in some infants to inject directly into the umbilical vein using a syringe and a No. 23 or 21 needle, this is a relatively hazardous procedure. It is difficult to keep the needle in the vein to inject the full volume of drug to be given, and inadvertent injection into an artery is likely to cause sloughing of the skin on the buttock.

The umbilical vein, therefore, should be catheterized using the following method:

1. Connect a 5 or 8 FG umbilical catheter to a three-way stopcock and 10 ml syringe filled with 0.9% NaCl. Flush through to get rid of air bubbles.
2. Using sterile precautions, the catheter is then inserted into the umbilical vein for about 5–7 cm until blood can be freely withdrawn.
3. The drug to be injected is given through the vacant stopcock inlet, and then flushed through with 0.9% NaCl.

References

Scott, H.M. (1976) Outcome of very severe birth asphyxia. *Archives of Disease in Childhood*, **50**, 712–716

Steiner, H. and Neligan, G. (1975) Perinatal cardiac arrest; quality of survivors. *Archives of Disease in Childhood*, **50**, 696–702

Swyer, P.R. (1975) *The Intensive Care of the Newly Born. Monographs in Paediatrics*, **6**, p. 36, Karger, Basel

Thompson, A.J., Searle, M. and Russell, G. (1977) Quality of survival after severe birth asphyxia. *Archives of Disease in Childhood*, **52**, 620–626

Wilson, A.M. (1987) Acute respiratory emergencies. In *Paediatric Emergencies*, 2nd edn (ed. J.A. Black), Butterworth-Heinemann, Oxford, pp. 220–224

Further reading

Dawes, G.S. (1968) *Fetal and Neonatal Physiology*, Yearbook Medical Publishers, Chicago

Hageman, J.R. (ed.) (1989) Critical issues in intrapartum and delivery room management. *Clinics in Perinatology*, **16(4)**, 785–1048

Hill, A. and Volpe, J.J. (1989) Perinatal asphyxia; clinical aspects. *Clinics in Perinatology*, **16**, 435–458

Ostheimer, G.W. (1982) Resuscitation of the newborn infant. *Clinics in Perinatology*, **9**, 177–189

Perlman, J.M. (1989) Systemic abnormalities in term infants following perinatal asphyxia: relevance to long term neurologic outcome. *Clinics in Perinatology*, **16**, 475–484

Roberton, N.R.C. (1986) Resuscitation of the newborn. In *Textbook of Neonatology* (ed. N.R.C. Roberton), Churchill Livingstone, Edinburgh, Chapter 15

Chapter 3

Injuries and complications related to birth

Because each type of delivery or obstetric complication is associated with different injuries, a knowledge of the possible injuries in each set of circumstances will assist early diagnosis and treatment. Although most birth injuries are without permanent sequelae, a full explanation of what happened and how and why it happened should be given to the parents, because what may appear relatively trivial to the obstetrician or paediatrician is of the greatest importance to the parents, both actually and emotionally, in the extremely sensitive period just after the birth of their baby.

If the damage appears disproportionate to the circumstances of the delivery, an abnormality of the infant should be suspected:

1. A bleeding tendency (usually thrombocytopenia, rarely disseminated intravascular coagulation (DIC), or a coagulation disorder should be looked for if there is diffuse bleeding into the caput or presenting part, an abnormally large cephalhaematoma or a large subaponeurotic haemorrhage. Additional evidence may be provided by petechiae, ecchymoses, bruises, oozing from the cord, injection sites or circumcision, bleeding into the respiratory or gastrointestinal tract, or evidence of internal haemorrhage (Chapter 6).
2. A fracture after a normal delivery suggests abnormal fragility of the bones, as in osteogenesis imperfecta (autosomal dominant (AD), rarely autosomal recessive (AR) (Appendix 3)), and multiple fractures confirm this possibility.
3. A subdural haematoma developing within a few days of a normal delivery may indicate an abnormally soft skull; this is found in osteogenesis imperfecta and in hypophosphatasia (AR).

Table 3.1 Birth trauma related to the size of the infant

Large infants (>4.5 kg)	*Very small infants* (<1.5 kg)
Hypoxia from long or difficult delivery Fracture of clavicle (shoulder dystocia, see text) Pneumothorax (p. 151) Rupture of liver or spleen (p. 75)	Bruising and ecchymoses from malpresentation or from handling, causing hyperbilirubinaemia (p. 103) Rupture of liver (p. 75)

ɜh the injuries commonly found with each type of delivery are ɔw, only those that require urgent attention or emergency ... are discussed. The types of birth trauma depend not only on the type of delivery, but also on the size of the infant (Table 3.1).

Delivery problems requiring urgent attention or emergency treatment

Vertex delivery

Shoulder dystocia
Shoulder dystocia, 'stuck shoulders' (Benedetti and Gabbe, 1978), occurs in large infants, commonly those of a diabetic or pre-diabetic mother, when the size of the trunk of a large fetus with a normal biparietal diameter has not been appreciated.

Shoulder dystocia may be associated with:

1. Facial plethora, as with the cord round the neck.
2. Fetal hypoxia from prolonged delivery with or without cord compression.
3. Fracture of the clavicle (p. 48).
4. Brachial plexus injury (p. 50).
5. Fracture of the shaft of the humerus (p. 49).

Precipitate delivery
Precipitate delivery, usually in an unattended or uncontrolled labour, may cause an acute supra- or sub-tentorial (posterior fossa) haematoma from tearing of the falx or tentorium (p. 94).

Fetal hypoxia
Fetal hypoxia may result from very strong sustained contractions, sometimes associated with unusual uterine sensitivity to oxytocin (Syntocinon), or too high a dose.

Face or brow delivery

The infant should be examined for any cause for the malpresentation, such as goitre or cystic hygroma, although the cord round the neck is a more common cause. Many infants, particularly after a face delivery, lie with the head extended for up to 2 weeks after delivery; this is not an indication for lumbar puncture. Conditions associated with face or brow delivery are:

1. Fetal hypoxia from prolonged labour.
2. Gross facial oedema and bruising, often with subconjunctival haemorrhages.
3. Anencephalic infant.

Breech delivery

A breech presentation may be due to a fetal abnormality, such as in anencephaly, meningomyelocele, prematurity or multiple pregnancy, or to a uterine malformation such as bicornuate or double uterus. The shape of the infant's head in some breech deliveries (or in breech presentations delivered by caesarean section) sometimes causes concern because of the elongated skull, flattened vertex and protuberant occipital bone (Sunderland, 1981). This is not moulding due to delivery and is thought to be the result of pressure of the uterine fundus. Perinatal morbidity is high in primigravidae with breech presentation and in very small pre-term infants, and it is the policy in many centres to deliver such cases by caesarean section. Complications associated with breech delivery are:

1. Fetal hypoxia from prolonged labour, often with cord compression.
2. Acute fetal hypoxia from prolapse of the cord.
3. Acute subdural haematoma (p. 96) from tear of falx or tentorium in a precipitate delivery without protection to the head.
4. Fracture of the clavicle (p. 48).
5. Brachial plexus injury (p. 50).
6. Fracture of the shaft of the humerus (p. 49).
7. Fracture through the upper humeral epiphysis (p. 49).
8. Fracture of the shaft of the femur (p. 49).
9. Fracture of the upper femoral epiphysis (p. 50).
10. Fracture of the cervical or upper thoracic spine with damage to the cord (p. 50). This is particularly common with vaginal delivery of a breech with a hyperextended head (Gresham, 1975).
11. Sternomastoid tumour, very occasionally bilateral.
12. Rupture of the liver (p. 75).
13. Shock from haemorrhage into the muscles and soft tissues of the back and buttocks (Ráliš, 1975).
14. Haemorrhagic infarction of the testes, with subsequent atrophy.
15. Increased risk of congenital dislocation of the hip in extended breech.

Forceps delivery

Forceps delivery as a 'lift-out' procedure at the end of a delivery with epidural anaesthesia, or when used to protect the head, causes little damage. Forceps delivery because of a prolonged labour or mechanically difficult delivery may be associated with the following complications:

1. Cephalhaematoma with or without a linear fracture of the skull is common. There is no point in taking an X-ray of the skull unless a depressed fracture is suspected.
2. Facial paralysis.
3. Pressure necrosis of the skin of the face, scalp or ear.
4. Subcutaneous fat necrosis of the cheek, which may be mistaken for cellulitis or an abscess.
5. Tear of the falx or tentorium as described above.

Vacuum (ventouse) extraction

Associated complications of vacuum extraction (Plauché, 1979) are:

1. Superficial damage to the scalp, which may be extensive, with sloughing of the skin.

2. Confluent subcutaneous haemorrhages into a caput, simulating a cephalhaematoma.
3. Cephalhaematoma.
4. Subaponeurotic haemorrhage (p. 79).

Caesarean section

Most of the difficulties with the newborn after an emergency section are related to the condition for which the operation was performed. Complications common to caesarean section in general are:

1. Incision into the fetus, occasionally amputation of a digit.
2. Incision into a fetal blood vessel, usually on the surface of the placenta, causing acute shock (p. 7) which may be mistaken for hypoxia.
3. Shock from blood loss due to holding the fetus above the placenta without clamping the cord (p. 74).
4. Tear of falx or tentorium as described under precipitate delivery above when there has been difficulty in delivery of the head impacted in the pelvis.
5. Fracture of the shaft of the humerus (p. 49) or femur (p. 49) when extracting the fetus from an abnormal position.

Twin pregnancy

Maternal complications in twin pregnancy (Bryan, 1983, 1986) are pre-eclampsia, polyhydramnios and pre-term delivery (see also p. 21).

Fetal complications are:

1. Intrauterine growth retardation; a twin is on average 500 g lighter than a singleton of the same gestational age.
2. Unequal growth, due to the chronic twin-to-twin transfusion syndrome, eccentric implantation of one of the cords (in monochorionic twins) or differing sites of placental implantation.
3. Increased incidence of malformations in monozygotic (MZ) twins, especially cardiac malformations.
4. Conjoined twins (MZ).
5. Intrauterine death of one (monochorionic) twin may cause DIC in the survivor, or embolic phenomena which may damage the survivor, e.g. cerebral abnormalities, aplasia cutis, intestinal atresia. The presence of a fetus papyraceus or a macerated twin should raise the suspicion of a malformation in the survivor.
6. Stillbirth of one or both twins.
7. Entanglement of the cords (monoamniotic twins), causing death of one or usually both twins.
8. Breech presentation.
9. Undiagnosed twin.
10. Fetal hypoxia in the second twin.
11. Respiratory distress syndrome, particularly in the second of pre-term twins.

The death of one twin, either *in utero* or shortly after birth, may cause unresolved mourning, guilt feelings or rejection of the surviving twin. Counselling may be required.

Antepartum haemorrhage

When this is due to placenta praevia the maternal blood may be mixed with fetal blood; the possibility of fetal haemorrhage should be considered if the infant appears shocked rather than hypoxic (p. 71). When the bleeding originates from ruptured vasa praevia, the blood will be entirely fetal and the infant may be in hypovolaemic shock (p. 71). If fetal blood loss is suspected, fetal blood can be identified whether or not mixed with maternal blood.

Accidental haemorrhage (premature separation of a normally sited placenta – abruptio placentae)

If the haemorrhage is concealed, fetal death is common. Complications of accidental haemorrhage are:

1. Fetal hypoxia.
2. Inhalation of meconium or blood from premature onset of respiration.
3. Fetomaternal haemorrhage, usually associated with traumatic separation of the placenta.
4. Vomiting of swallowed maternal blood (p. 99) usually in concealed haemorrhage when blood has entered the amniotic cavity.
5. Passage of altered or partly altered maternal blood in the stool (p. 100).
6. Rarely, DIC in the fetus (p. 91).

Complications related to the umbilical cord

1. Prolapsed cord, causing acute fetal hypoxia.
2. Haemorrhage from fetal vessels (p. 74).
3. Cord around the neck, may cause facial plethora, with or without facial petechiae and conjunctival haemorrhages. Differential obstruction to the umbilical circulation, with compression of the umbilical vein but maintenance of the umbilical arterial flow, causes hypovolaemic shock due to the fetus bleeding into the placenta (Vanhaesebrouck *et al.*, 1987); in these circumstances the infant fails to react adequately to routine resuscitation, but responds promptly to transfusion with plasma or blood. The same situation could arise with a prolapsed cord.
4. Stricture of the cord is associated with a localized absence of Wharton's jelly; torsion at the stricture may cause fetal death.
5. Rupture of the cord occurs when it is abnormally short, where it is effectively shortened by coils around the neck, or in an unattended delivery with the infant falling to the floor or into a lavatory pan. Haemorrhage is surprisingly rare, due to retraction of the torn vessels.
6. Entanglement of the cords may occur in monoamniotic twins (MZ) causing death of one or both fetuses.
7. True knot causing obstruction of blood flow (Chasnoff and Fletcher, 1977).

Local anaesthesia

In the UK, the following local anaesthetics are in general use (though other countries have different preferences): bupivacaine, for epidural (lumbar or caudal) anaesthesia and paracervical blocks, and lignocaine for spinal anaesthesia, pudendal block and infiltration of the perineum. The pharmacological effects on the fetus are similar with all three drugs. However, the various forms of local anaesthesia may harm the fetus in the following ways:

1. Fetal hypoxia caused by maternal hypotension (spinal or epidural) due either to vasodilatation or hypovolaemia from compression of the inferior vena cava if the mother is kept supine.
2. Fetal hypoxia due to maternal convulsions as a result of inadvertent intra-arterial or intravenous (particularly an epidural vein) injection of the drug. Maternal convulsions may also occur if an actual overdose of the drug is given, and this may add to fetal depression by causing a high fetal blood level.
3. Fetal depression and metabolic acidosis, with apnoea or depressed Apgar score at delivery, may result from the use of bupivacaine in paracervical block, particularly when there is a caval obstruction in the supine position, causing a higher blood level in the fetus than in the mother.
4. Direct injection of the drug into the fetal scalp or brain (paracervical, pudendal or perineal block). This results in severe convulsions which have to be controlled by intravenous diazepam (p. 205) with or without intermittent positive pressure ventilation (IPPV). If this is ineffective, an exchange transfusion may be required (p. 119).

Birth injuries requiring urgent attention or emergency treatment

All the fractures described below apart from a fractured clavicle require an orthopaedic opinion.

Fractured clavicle

Recognition
The obstetrician may hear or feel the clavicle snap. More commonly some swelling and irregularity is noticed over the clavicle, often with crepitus on pressure, and the infant does not move the affected arm. There is no Moro response on the injured side and passive movement of the arm is obviously painful. The callus which forms after 7–10 days is sometimes the first evidence of a fracture. Confirmation is by X-ray, and the infant should be carefully examined for evidence of a coexistent brachial plexus injury. Failure to move an arm may be due to the following:

1. If present from birth: fracture of clavicle, shaft or upper epiphysis of the humerus, or brachial plexus injury.
2. Developing after birth: osteitis of the humerus, septic arthritis of the

shoulder. Hemiplegia is rarely detected or detectable until some weeks or months after birth.

Management
No specific treatment is required apart from keeping the infant on its back. Healing always occurs without ultimate deformity. An orthopaedic opinion is only required if there is extreme parental concern, or the possibility of litigation.

Fracture of the shaft of the humerus

Recognition
The obstetrician is usually aware that fracture has occurred. Swelling of the middle of the upper arm is often visible or there is deformity due to medial angulation of the upper fragment. Formation of callus involving the radial nerve may cause a transient wrist drop. Confirmation is by X-ray though occasionally an X-ray immediately after birth may show no evidence of a fracture which only becomes apparent with the formation of callus.

Management
The usual treatment is to place a pad of cotton wool in the axilla and strap or bandage the arm to the chest for 3 weeks. Complete remodelling of the bone occurs in due course even when union has occurred with considerable angulation.

Fracture of the upper humeral epiphysis (epiphyseolysis)

Recognition
Swelling in the region of the shoulder joint may be visible. Confirmation by plain X-ray is difficult as the epiphysis is not ossified. An orthopaedic opinion should be requested, and an arthrogram may be necessary to show the position of the upper fragment.

Management
Realignment by the orthopaedic surgeon is important. The arm should be immobilized by a collar and cuff for 3 weeks. Long-term follow up is required as poor alignment of the epiphysis may cause deformity from asymmetrical growth.

Fracture of the shaft of the femur

Recognition
This fracture rarely goes unrecognized at delivery. Shock does not develop but the thigh is tensely swollen and tender. On X-ray the proximal fragment is usually found to be flexed.

Management
Treatment is by suspension of both legs in a gallow's splint for 3 weeks; it is important that the infant's buttocks should be kept off the mattress.

Accurate positioning of the fragments is not important as complete bone remodelling occurs and ultimately shortening is not a complication.

Fracture of the upper femoral epiphysis (epiphyseolysis)

Recognition
This is not always recognized at the time of delivery but within a few days swelling below the inguinal ligament may be obvious, with crying on passive movement of the leg. The thigh is held abducted, flexed and laterally rotated and there is usually a measurable degree of shortening. X-ray immediately after the injury is unhelpful because the epiphysis is not ossified; callus forms around the femoral neck after 7–10 days.

Management
An arthrogram is usually required to outline the position of the upper fragment. Traction may be required initially and Sharrard (1979i) recommends a hip spica after traction.

Fracture of the cervical or upper thoracic spine with spinal cord injury

Recognition
This is particularly associated with breech delivery and especially with vaginal delivery of a breech with a hyperextended head. The clinical picture (Gresham, 1975) may be:

1. Stillbirth or death at delivery.
2. Death shortly after delivery from respiratory complications.
3. Long-term survival with spasticity.
4. Survivors with minimal neurological signs, often wrongly classified as having cerebral palsy.

In those with severe injury who survive for a short time after delivery the appearance may suggest a bilateral brachial plexus injury, but on further examination it is apparent that there is a flaccid quadriplegia. Respiratory difficulty is due to paralysis of the intercostal muscles but the infant may survive for a few days if the diaphragm is functioning. Later spasticity of the legs develops, with increased reflexes and ankle clonus, if the infant lives long enough.

Brachial plexus injury

Upper plexus injury (C5 and C6) (Erb, Erb–Duchenne type)

Recognition In the more complete paralyses, the arm is adducted and medially rotated and the forearm pronated; winging of the scapula is often present and if C7 is involved the wrist and fingers are flexed. Phrenic nerve paralysis sufficient to cause respiratory distress (see below) is rare. The infant should be carefully examined to exclude other injuries associated with brachial plexus injury, such as fracture of the clavicle or humerus.

Management (Sharrard, 1979ii) X-ray should be done to exclude fracture. The upper arm should be lightly bandaged to the chest for the first week; after this the shoulder, elbow and wrist joints should be put through their full range of movements at each feed.

Recovery is usually complete within 4 weeks if damage was due to haemorrhage and oedema, but if there was rupture of nerve fibres with intact sheaths complete regeneration may take up to 2 years. Severe wasting of the paralysed muscles after 3–4 weeks indicates a poor prognosis for complete recovery. Exploration and attempted suture are difficult and unlikely to succeed. Follow up by an orthopaedic surgeon of cases with incomplete recovery by 6 weeks is important as reconstructive surgery may be required to correct deformity. The arm should *not* be abducted as the initial treatment, as was at one time advised, as this puts the plexus on the stretch and may predispose to dislocation of the shoulder joint.

Lower plexus type (C8 and T1); (Klumpke type)

Recognition There is paralysis of the intrinsic muscles of the hand (claw hand), often with Horner's syndrome (small pupil, ptosis, enophthalmos).

Management No immediate treatment is required apart from resting the arm for the first week, as described above. The outlook for complete recovery is much less good than in the upper plexus type and follow up by an orthopaedic surgeon will be required if there is paralysis persisting beyond 6 weeks.

Phrenic nerve paralysis

Recognition

This may accompany brachial plexus injury of the upper plexus type or, rarely, is due to direct pressure from a forceps blade misapplied to the neck. There is a variable degree of respiratory distress. X-ray shows an elevated diaphragm on the affected side and screening will usually be able to demonstrate paradoxical movement of the paralysed diaphragm.

Management

This is usually conservative, as complete recovery normally occurs. However, if there is severe respiratory distress, emergency plication of the diaphragm may be required.

Other types of trauma

The other types of trauma requiring emergency treatment which are considered elsewhere are:

1. Rupture of the liver (p. 75).
2. Rupture of the spleen (p. 77).
3. Subaponeurotic haemorrhage (p. 79).
4. Adrenal haemorrhage (p. 77).
5. Pneumothorax (p. 151).
6. Chylothorax (p. 158).

References

Benedetti, T.J. and Gabbe, S.G. (1978) Shoulder dystocia. *Obstetrics and Gynecology*, **52**, 526–529

Bryan, E.M. (1983) *The Nature and Nurture of Twins*, Baillière Tindall, London

Bryan, E.M. (1986) The intrauterine hazards of twins. *Archives of Disease in Childhood*, **61**, 1044–1045

Chasnoff, I.J. and Fletcher, M.A. (1977) True knot of the umbilical cord. *American Journal of Obstetrics and Gynecology*, **127**, 425–427

Gresham, E.L. (1975) Birth trauma. *Pediatric Clinics of North America*, **22**, 317–328

Plauché, W.C. (1979) Fetal cranial injuries related to delivery with the Malström vacuum extractor. *Obstetrics and Gynecology*, **53**, 750–757

Ráliš, Z.A. (1975) Birth trauma to muscles in babies born by breech delivery and its possible fatal consequences. *Archives of Disease in Childhood*, **50**, 4–13

Sharrard, W.J.W. (1979) *Paediatric Orthopaedics and Fractures*, 2nd edn, Blackwell Scientific, Oxford, Vol. 2, (i) pp. 1585–1587; (ii) pp. 1462–1466

Sunderland, R. (1981) Fetal position and skull shape. *British Journal of Obstetrics and Gynaecology*, **88**, 246–249

Vanhaesebrouck, P., Vanneste, K., de Praete, C., Van Trappen, Y. and Thiery, M. (1987) Tight nuchal cord and neonatal hypovolaemic shock. *Archives of Disease in Childhood*, **62**, 1276–1277

Further reading

Bennett, G. and Harold, A.J. (1976) Prognosis and early management of birth injuries to the brachial plexus. *British Medical Journal*, **1**, 1520–1521

Gall, S.A. (ed.) (1988) Twins. *Clinics in Perinatology*, **15**, 1–158

Sharrard, W.J.W. (1979) *Paediatric Orthopaedics and Fractures*, 2nd edn, Blackwell Scientific, Oxford, Vol. 2

Towbin, A. and Turner, G.L. (1978) Obstetric factors in fetal–neonatal visceral injury. *Obstetrics and Gynecology*, **52**, 113–124

Chapter 4

Early management of the very low birthweight infant

Low birth weight is a major risk factor for neonatal death in liveborn infants, accounting for 35% of early neonatal deaths in most perinatal population surveys (British Births, 1970). Increasing understanding of neonatal physiology and the development of techniques to support small infants have led to a dramatic improvement in mortality and morbidity rates and, with a high standard of care, the vast majority of are free of major handicaps at follow up (Vohr and Hack, 1982).

An infant may be of low birth weight because it is:

1. Born early (pre-term). Infants of 1.5 kg or less are usually 32 weeks' gestation or less.
2. Poorly grown for the number of weeks spent *in utero* (small for gestational age (SGA)) due to:
   (a) Lack of growth support due to placental insufficiency;
   (b) Lack of growth potential due to some intrinsic growth defect in the fetus, such as major multiple congenital abnormalities, chromosomal abnormality or intrauterine infection.
3. Both born early and SGA.

In order to benefit from the decrease in perinatal morbidity and mortality offered by regionalized care of small sick infants, an infant anticipated prenatally to be of very low birth weight should, if possible, be delivered in the maternity unit serving the regional neonatal intensive-care unit (NICU) so that all available high-risk obstetric and neonatal expertise and equipment are available for the management of the labour, and of the infant after delivery. Frequently, however, it is not possible to transfer the mother to the regional NICU and preparations have to be made for delivery, resuscitation and stabilization in the local maternity unit. A very small infant born in a maternity unit with less than optimal neonatal intensive-care facilities should be transferred, when stabilized, to a larger better equipped and better staffed unit.

Recognition

Size

The infant's small size is obvious at delivery, but this must be accurately documented by measurements of weight, length and head circumference soon after birth, preferably before the infant is attached to monitoring equipment, intravenous lines etc., which makes accurate weighing difficult. Every effort should be made to weigh the infant accurately, making allowance for the weight of the cord clamp, if necessary. An accurate birth weight is important particularly in infants of <1.0 kg for:

1. Prediction of mortality and morbidity;
2. Accurate dosage of drugs and intravenous fluid;
3. Measurement of true weight gain;
4. Recognition of excessive weight gain or loss due to excessive accumulation or loss of fluid.

Gestational age

This may be assessed by a combination of:

1. Obstetric dates.
2. Confirmation of obstetric dates by clinical examination and ultrasound measurements of the fetus early in pregnancy.
3. Clinical examination of the infant and the determination of gestational age by a systematic scoring system, assessing neurological and physical characteristics, such as the method of Dubowitz (Dubowitz and Goldberg 1970), or one of the later abbreviated versions (e.g. Parkin, Hey and Clowes, 1976).

Growth parameters in relation to gestational age

By plotting the measured growth parameters against the best estimate of gestational age on a suitable intrauterine growth chart (e.g. Gairdner and Pearson, 1971), the infant's appropriateness of growth may be assessed against gestational age. An SGA infant is defined as having a weight below the 10th percentile for gestational age; such an infant may be of term gestation (37–41 completed weeks), post-term (beyond 41 completed weeks' gestation) or pre-term (less than 37 completed weeks). SGA infants are less likely to get severe respiratory distress syndrome (RDS), but more likely to have acute or acute-on-chronic hypoxia at delivery, meconium aspiration syndrome and hypoglycaemia. SGA infants also exhibit neurobehavioural anomalies for several months after delivery and are at increased risk for residual neurological damage, causing behavioural and educational problems. The avoidance of hypoxia and hypoglycaemia, and the provision of prompt resuscitation at delivery, are likely to reduce the incidence of ultimate neurological sequelae. The relationship between age at onset and severity of intrauterine growth retardation and later outcome has been studied by Fancourt *et al.* (1976).

Management

The following areas are important in providing optimal emergency management for a very low birthweight infant:

1. Prevention of hypoxia and prompt resuscitation at delivery.
2. Respiratory support and blood gas monitoring.
3. Temperature homeostasis.
4. Nutrition and fluid balance.

The difficulties which the infant encounters in these areas are due to immaturity of the organ systems and homoeostatic mechanisms.

Avoidance of hypoxia and prompt resuscitation after delivery

The obstetric management of the delivery of a pre-term or SGA infant involves particular attention to the avoidance of hypoxia by selecting the optimal time and route of delivery. Before delivery of a small infant it is important to make sure that appropriate-sized endotracheal tubes and laryngoscope blades are available, with a low threshold of intervention at delivery.

Respiratory support

Any infant of 1.5 kg or less may develop respiratory symptoms and ventilatory failure in the first 24 hours of life, due to delay or incomplete adaptation of the immature lungs to life outside the uterus. The most likely causes of respiratory difficulties in the small infant are:

1. Neonatal pulmonary oedema (wet lung, transient tachypnoea of the newborn) (p. 144).
2. Respiratory distress syndrome (pp. 140–142) with or without the immature lung syndrome.
3. Pulmonary and systemic infection (usually due to group B streptococcus infection) (pp. 60 and 184).

In order to assess the adequacy of the infant's respiratory status, it is necessary to carry out repeated blood gas estimations on arterial or free flowing capillary blood if harmful degrees of hypoxia, hyperoxia, hypercapnia or acidaemia are to be avoided. An umbilical arterial catheter or an indwelling radial arterial catheter provides ready access to arterial sampling with minimal disturbance (pp. 307 and 312).

The aim is to maintain the infant's arterial Po_2 between 8.0 and 11.0 kPa (60–80 mmHg(torr)) and the pH greater than 7.3 by the use of oxygen, ventilatory assistance as continuous positive airway pressure (CPAP) or IPPV and bicarbonate. Avoidance of hypoxia, hypoglycaemia, acidaemia and hypothermia favours optimal surfactant synthesis and avoidance of the downward hypoxia–acidaemia spiral (pp. 137–138).

Temperature homoeostasis

The small immature infant loses heat very rapidly due to a large surface area/mass ratio and inadequate thermogenesis. A small infant in an incubator with a radiant heat shield requires an air temperature of 36°C to maintain a core temperature between 36.5°C and 37°C. Infants of less than 1.0 kg birth weight often require incubator temperatures of 37°C or more because of very low endogenous heat production and large transcutaneous water losses, with consequent loss of heat. Maintenance of a high humidity level inside the incubator reduces further heat loss. A skin temperature more than 0.5°C below core temperature suggests that an infant is at the lower end of the thermoneutral zone and is having to catabolize metabolic fuel to support its body temperature. A drop in core temperature below 36°C for more than a few hours results in progressive acidaemia and hypoglycaemia and poorer survival. While radiant infrared heated intensive care tables provide ready access to the infant and maintain the temperature well, they are unsuitable for the care of the very small infant for more than a few hours as they double insensible water loss (to over 100 ml/kg per 24 hours) particularly in the smallest infants with gelatinous skin (usually less than 27 weeks' gestation). At the present time, the most suitable equipment for managing a very low birthweight infant is a double-walled incubator with a proportional servocontrolled heater pack able to servocontrol the air temperature or the infant's temperature, and providing at least 70% humidity.

Nutrition and fluid balance

An adequate nutritional intake is a major priority in the management of the low birthweight infant. The absence of coordinated sucking and swallowing makes enteral feeding hazardous; gastric emptying may be delayed; and intestinal motility is reduced. Infants with respiratory problems usually have transient ileus during the first few days of life. Gastrointestinal absorption of ingested calories, particularly as fat, is unreliable during the early weeks of life. Electrolyte and blood gas disturbances, serious respiratory problems, and perhaps the presence of an umbilical arterial catheter, delay the development of peristalsis. Perinatal and neonatal events may predispose to the development of necrotizing enterocolitis (Chapter 23). For these reasons fluid and calorie requirements may have to be given entirely by the parenteral route. A low birthweight infant needs around 65 ml/kg of fluid in the first 24 hours, but this requirement may be more than doubled because of large insensible water losses due to phototherapy, tachypnoea, pyrexia, inadequately humidified respiratory gases and transcutaneous water losses. A urine osmolality of 200 mosmol/kg or less is an indication of adequate hydration. Glucose 10% via peripheral vein or umbilical arterial catheter usually provides the bulk of the infant's calorie intake over the first 48 hours, although small volumes (1–2 ml per hour, increasing) of expressed human milk or formula may be tolerated by intermittent or continuous nasogastric infusion with 3-hourly gastric aspiration to check for progressive accumulation of gastric contents and the consequent risk of feed aspiration. Infants under 1.0 kg may require glucose 5% parenterally instead of 10% because of glucose intolerance. Glucose 10% should not be given orally because it delays gastric emptying and is tolerated less well than human milk if aspirated into the lungs.

One-third to one-half of the infant's calorie requirements is provided by 65 ml/kg per 24 hours of glucose 10% and, if significant amounts of milk cannot be tolerated by the enteral route by 72 hours of age, consideration should be given to the use of total or supplemental parenteral nutrition with carbohydrate, aminoacids and fat emulsion. Inadequate nutrition in the first weeks of life delays the resumption of growth, while over-enthusiastic feeding may lead to milk aspiration, abdominal distension or apnoeic attacks, and may increase the incidence of necrotizing enterocolitis. In infants recovering from respiratory problems in the newborn period, a bolus size of more than 5 ml/kg delivered into the stomach may affect the pulmonary mechanics and the respiratory status (Yu and Rolph, 1976). Some infants tolerate the continuous infusion of milk into the stomach, duodenum or jejunum, when they will not tolerate bolus feeding into the stomach. Infants fed continuously by the jejunal route for a long time grow more slowly than those successfully fed by the gastric route (Whitfield, 1982); therefore infants fed initially by the jejunal route should be changed to conventional feeding as soon as possible.

The appearance of abdominal distension, blood in the stools, disappearance of bowel sounds and bilious gastric aspirates suggests the onset of necrotizing enterocolitis, and enteral feeds should be stopped for several days and the infant supported by parenteral nutrition (p. 335).

Timetable for management of the low birthweight infant

The following timetable gives a progressive plan of action for medical and nursing staff for managing a small infant. The aim is to maintain the infant in the best possible condition from the respiratory, blood gas, thermal, metabolic and nutritional point of view at all times.

Before birth

Preparation There should be liaison with obstetric staff; consideration should be given to the possibility of fetal therapy (e.g. dexamethasone) and the timing and route of delivery.

Medical staff Close liaison with the obstetric staff is necessary in order to be aware of prenatal problems, adequacy of intrauterine growth, the absence of fetal distress and the choice of route of delivery. Information from serial ultrasound scans may show the pattern of the infant's growth throughout the pregnancy, and amniocentesis may have been carried out to determine the lung maturity by the lecithin/sphingomyelin ratio or the presence of phosphatidylglycerol. Oligohydramnios (p. 12) suggests intrauterine growth retardation, prolonged rupture of the membranes, with or without ascending infection, renal hypoplasia or obstructive disease of the renal tract. If there was a low lecithin/sphingomyelin ratio (less than 2:1) at a maturity of less than 34 weeks, consideration should be given to giving dexamethasone or betamethasone to the mother in order to accelerate surfactant synthesis, and attempts should be made to delay delivery by the use of β-mimetics (isoxsuprine, salbutamol, ritodrine etc.). Transfer to a tertiary centre should be considered. Signs of infection in the mother, particularly if the membranes have been ruptured for more than 48 hours, are an indication for prompt delivery. The circumstances surrounding the coming delivery should be discussed with the parents, both by obstetric and paediatric staff before delivery, so that they have a clear idea of the roles of those involved.

Nursing staff Assemble and check the equipment likely to be used in the stabilization of the infant after delivery:

Equipment

1. Double-walled servocontrolled incubator or single-walled servocontrolled incubator with a Perspex semicylindrical radiant heat shield. The incubator must be prewarmed and set at maximum humidity.
2. Cardiorespiratory monitoring equipment.
3. Oxygen analyser to measure inspired oxygen concentration.
4. Check oxygen cylinders if there is no piped oxygen.
5. Tray for umbilical catheterization (p. 307).
6. Resuscitation equipment and laryngoscope (p. 33).
7. Transcutaneous Po_2 monitor or pulse oximeter.
8. Neonatal ventilator, checked and ready for use.
9. Head-box for administration of inspired oxygen.
10. Adequate lighting.
11. Baby scales.
12. Intravenous infusion pump with glucose 10% run through.

From birth to 2 hours

At birth, resuscitation is required; transfer to special care baby unit (SCBU)/NICU; this is the phase of rapid adaptation to extrauterine life.

Medical staff

1. Adequate prompt resuscitation with a low threshold for intervention (see Chapter 2): the baby may need glucose (3 ml of 10% solution), sodium bicarbonate (2 mmol) of 8.4% solution via the umbilical vein if there has been evidence of fetal acidosis.
2. Dry the infant all over with a towel early in resuscitation to prevent heat loss. Resuscitation must be done under a radiant overhead heater.
3. When the infant is breathing spontaneously it should be transferred as soon as possible to an SCBU/NICU, having first been shown to the mother. It is usually possible for a mother to hold even a small infant at this stage, provided that the infant is adequately wrapped and constantly observed by the resuscitation staff.

Nursing staff

1. The infant requires the full attention of an experienced neonatal nurse on a one-to-one basis. The baby should be weighed at the time of transfer from the resuscitation equipment to the incubator and then connected to cardiorespiratory monitoring equipment.
2. Give 30% oxygen if cyanosed in air.
3. Monitor heart rate, respiratory rate, colour, temperature and the appearance of signs of respiratory distress (nostril flaring, grunting, chest recession, tachypnoea and tachycardia). Follow transcutaneous Po_2 or saturation.
4. An intravenous infusion of glucose 10% at 65 ml/kg per 24 hours should be commenced in order to prevent hypoglycaemia.
5. Infants, when settled, must be handled as little as possible and should

be in a good light so that any change in colour or respiratory pattern can be easily seen.

6. Suck out the mouth, if mucusy.
7. Call the doctor if the infant's condition is deteriorating or if still cyanosed or arterial saturation (SaO_2) is <90% with a fractional concentration of inspired oxygen (FiO_2) of 0.3–0.35 (30–35%) before 1–1.5 hours of age. Medical staff reassess after 1–1.5 hours.
8. Is the baby getting better or worse on the basis of: colour, oxygen requirement, development of signs of respiratory distress, air entry on auscultation, stability of observations transcutaneous $P\text{O}_2$.

If there are signs of respiratory distress and requirement for a fractional inspired oxygen concentration of >0.30 (30%), the baby needs:

1. An arterial line for blood gas sampling. This may be either an umbilical arterial catheter or a radial or posterior tibial arterial line inserted with the aid of transillumination (p. 313).
2. Chest X-ray, including most of the abdomen:
   (a) To define the cause of the respiratory difficulty and/or the radiological degree of RDS.
   (b) To define the position of the tip of the arterial catheter. The tip should be just above the aortic bifurcation at around L3/4 or above the diaphragm in the thorax.
3. Blood gases from the arterial line.
4. Glucose 10% intravenously via the umbilical catheter, 65 ml/kg per 24 hours.
5. A nasogastric tube may be passed into the stomach to aspirate the stomach contents. This may be left *in situ*, provided that the nasal airway is not obstructed.

From 2 to 12 hours.

Developing respiratory failure, fluid and calorie provision If the infant has incipient respiratory difficulty, blood gases and blood glucose or Chemstrip or Dextrostix* values should be monitored 4-hourly and action taken if necessary to maintain the blood gas status by ventilatory assistance (CPAP or IPPV), and half-correction of metabolic acidosis with intravenous bicarbonate (1/6 × base deficit × body weight in kg = number of mmol of bicarbonate required for half-correction of the metabolic component of the acidosis). The blood glucose should be maintained above 2.5 mmol/l (47 mg%). An approximate account of urine output can be kept by the weight increase of preweighed disposable napkins, or urine may be collected directly with a urine bag in males. The urine output is usually low in the first 12 hours in newborn infants and particularly in infants with

*There are numerous blood glucose test strips available. In the UK: BM-TEST 1-44 (Boehringer Mannheim) (range 1–44 mmol/l; visual or meter); Dextrostix (Ames) (range 1.4–14 mmol/l; visual or meter); Exactech (Baxter) (range 2.2–25 mmol/l; meter only); Hypoguard GA (Hypoguard) (range 0–22 mmol/l; visual or meter). In North America: Chemstrip B.G (Boehringer Mannheim) (range 1–44 mmol/l; visual); Chemstrip Accu-Check (2M and 3) (range 0.5–27 mmol/l; meter).

respiratory difficulties (less than 2 ml/kg per hour). It is usually best not to feed by the gastrointestinal route an infant who has respiratory difficulties in the first 12–24 hours of life, because RDS usually worsens during this time, and pulmonary aspiration of feed must be avoided.

Because of the difficulties in excluding group B streptococcal pneumonia and septicaemia as a component of the infant's respiratory difficulty, prophylactic ampicillin 100 mg/kg per 24 hours should be given in all infants with respiratory distress, after a blood culture, gastric aspirate and differential white count have been taken, and a urine bag attached to obtain a sample for the group B streptococcal co-agglutination test. Ampicillin may be stopped if the culture reports come back negative several days later.

An infant who clearly has significant respiratory problems in the first 2–3 hours of life and is requiring an increasing inspired oxygen concentration is likely to require respiratory assistance; if these facilities are not available in the hospital where the infant is being managed, contact with the regional NICU should be made as soon as possible. If the infant does not have respiratory difficulty and does not require umbilical catheterization, feeds may be started cautiously by the nasogastric route, either as a continuous nasogastric infusion of 1–2 ml per hour with 3-hourly nasogastric aspiration to check for build-up in gastric residue, or as intermittent bolus feeds at 1- or 2-hourly intervals of a similar volume of milk. Infants of 34 weeks' gestation or more, who are appropriately grown, can usually tolerate enteral feeding well and may manage without an intravenous infusion. Infants below this gestational age are better managed with a glucose infusion to maintain the blood glucose and to reduce the temptation to increase enteral feeds too rapidly.

From 12 to 48 hours

During this period, stabilization occurs in the fluid, calorie and electrolyte balance, and there is the possibility of apnoeic attacks.

Medical staff Check on and assess:

1. Fluid intake and urine output. The fluid intake should be around 90 ml/kg per 24 hours by 48 hours of life. If the infant did not require an umbilical arterial catheter, supplemental parenteral fluids must be provided by peripheral vein infusion unless the nasogastric intake is adequate. An infant who is totally maintained on intravenous fluids should receive per 24 hours sodium chloride 2.5 mmol/kg, potassium chloride 2.5 mmol/kg and calcium gluconate 1 mmol/kg (1 g of calcium gluconate = 2.3 mmol).
2. Temperature homoeostasis.
3. Ventilatory status: oxygen requirement and adequacy of respiratory support must be assessed (Chapter 12). Infants with mild RDS are usually recovering by this stage, with a reduced oxygen requirement, lessening respiratory difficulty and a diuresis. In infants requiring IPPV, pneumothorax is more likely to occur at this stage when lung compliance is improving; sudden collapse may be due to this cause. Infants of less than 34 weeks are likely to develop apnoeic and

bradycardic episodes at this stage. These usually respond to gentle stimulation, but some infants may eventually require ventilatory assistance either as low-pressure CPAP (3 cmH_2O) or IPPV. Ventilatory assistance may be avoided in some instances by the use of intravenous aminophylline (loading dose 7 mg/kg i.v. over 20 minutes followed by a maintenance dosage of 1.4 mg/kg 8-hourly i.v. (blood level should be maintained at 8–11 μg/ml, 55–70 μmol/l).
4. Neurological state of the infant. Plan to do the first cranial ultrasound scan at 3–4 days.
5. Can the arterial catheter be removed?
6. Chest X-ray to assess progress of pulmonary disease and method of nutrition. It is usually possible to commence feeding cautiously by the nasogastric route by about 48 hours of life in infants who are recovering from respiratory distress. Small frequent feeds, or continuous feeding, are most likely to succeed.

Nursing staff The infant with developing apnoeic attacks requires careful observation and vigilance and is a source of anxiety in an understaffed nursery. Although most apnoeic attacks respond to stimulation, facilities for IPPV by mask (e.g. using a Laerdal infant resuscitator) must be available in the incubator. Frequent repeated apnoeic attacks affect cerebral perfusion and metabolism and are likely to increase the risk of neurodevelopmental handicap. Infants who have required respiratory assistance and intubation during the first 48 hours of life become an increasing problem if the endotracheal tube cannot be removed early, due to the increasing volume and tenacity of secretions; adequate humidification of respiratory gases is very important.

Survival rates in excess of 80% should be expected in the tertiary NICU for infants between 0.75 and 1.0 kg at birth, and considerably higher above this birth weight. In optimal conditions, a significant number of infants may be expected to survive below this birth weight. The management of these infants is very specialized and if avoidable mortality and morbidity are to be prevented, they must be transferred for tertiary care, preferably *in utero*. These infants present challenging problems in fluid and electrolyte balance and nutrition and are likely to develop bronchopulmonary dysplasia, and have a high risk of significant haemorrhagic or ischaemic brain injury. Details of the management of such infants are not considered in depth here.

Outcome of pre-term infants

With modern intensive-care techniques the majority of infants who survive do so without major handicaps. Handicapped infants may have cerebral palsy, mental retardation, or visual or auditory handicaps, and these are usually apparent within the first 18 months of life. Later, difficulties in coordination and educational problems may become apparent, particularly at the time of school entry, in infants who appeared to be normal at 18 months (Nickel, Bennett and Lamson, 1982).

Major handicaps (neurological abnormality or Developmental Quotient

(DQ) less than 80 at 2 years) occur in about 13% of infants less than 1.5 kg at birth. Infants of less than 1.0 kg at birth have a major handicap rate between 7 and 17% in currently published studies (Vohr and Hack, 1982). Handicap rates in the smallest infants, less than 0.8 kg birthweight, are much higher, with major handicaps in about 50% of the survivors; however, information is scarce about survivors in this weight range (Hirata *et al.*, 1983).

Infants who are both pre-term and SGA have an increased handicap rate compared with infants of the same birth weight grown appropriately (Fitzhardinge and Steven, 1972*a*,*b*). Infants with bronchopulmonary dysplasia have a high incidence of neurodevelopmental delay in the first 2 years, and grow slowly. Improvement of the pulmonary condition is usually associated with some neurodevelopmental catch-up. These infants are thought to have an increased incidence of respiratory infections and hospitalizations in the first year of life. Intraventricular haemorrhage is an important predictor of later handicap. Grade I and II haemorrhages do not appear to increase the incidence of major handicap in infants less than 1.5 kg, with about 10% having major handicaps (Papile, Munsick-Bruno and Schaefer, 1983). These haemorrhages are small and limited to the subependymal plate or extend to a limited degree into the lateral ventricles. Grade III intraventricular haemorrhage (associated with ventricular distension by blood) has been found to be associated with a 36% handicap rate, and Grade IV (with intraparenchymal extension) associated with a 76% major handicap rate. Hydrocephalus occurs with grade III or IV intraventricular haemorrhage and further increases the severity of handicap.

Cerebral ischaemia and white matter injury (periventricular leucomalacia) may occur in the absence of haemorrhage, and is identifiable on craniosonography as areas of hyperechogenicity or white matter loss. Parenchymal hyperechogenicity of the white matter persisting into the third week of life is associated with a significant incidence of cavitation by 6–8 weeks and serious neurodevelopmental sequelae; the nature of the impairment depends on the site and extent of white matter loss. Severe visual handicap due to retinopathy or prematurity is confined to a small number of infants below 1.0 kg. Strabismus and myopia occur more commonly in infants below 1.25 kg birth weight, particularly those who have developed Grade III retinopathy of prematurity. All ex-premature infants of less than 1.25 kg should be seen by an ophthalmologist in the nursery and thereafter at 6 months corrected age, to assess residual damage due to retinopathy of prematurity, refractive errors and squints. Deafness due to nerve damage is rare (2–6%) but conductive deafness is common in the first year of life (40–60%) in infants below 1.5 kg, with the higher rate in those who were ventilated. Children who appear to be free of neurodevelopmental abnormalities at 18 months should be referred for psychological assessment by a competent psychologist at 4.5 years to ensure that cognitive problems have been identified before starting school, and that schooling at an appropriate level and at an appropriate time can be arranged. Decisions about timing of school entry should be based on the expected date of delivery, rather than the birth date in children who were born prematurely.

References

British Births (1970) Volume 1. Director, Roma Chamberlain. William Heinemann Medical Books, London, 1975

Dubowitz, L.M.S., Dubowitz, V. and Goldberg, C. (1970) Clinical assessment of gestational age in the newborn infant. *Journal of Pediatrics*, **77**, 1–10

Fancourt, R., Campbell, S., Harvey, D. and Norman, A.P. (1976) Follow up study of small-for-dates babies. *British Medical Journal*, **1**, 1435–1437

Fitzhardinge, P.M. and Steven, E.M. (1972*a*) The small-for-dates infant. I. Later growth patterns. *Pediatrics*, **49**, 671–681

Fitzhardinge, P.M. and Steven, E.M. (1972*b*) The small-for-dates infant. II. Neurological and intellectual sequelae. *Pediatrics*, **50**, 50–57

Gairdner, D. and Pearson, J. (1971) *Growth and Developmental Record, Preterm to 2 Years*, Castlemead Publications, Ware, Herts

Hirata, T., Epcar, J., Walsh, A., Mednick, J., Harris, M., McGinnis, M.S., *et al.* (1983) Survival and outcome of infants 501–750 gm – a six year experience. *Journal of Pediatrics*, **102**, 741–748

Nickel, R.E., Bennett, F.C. and Lamson, F.N. (1982) School performance of children with birth weights of 1000 g or less. *American Journal of Diseases of Children*, **136**, 105–110

Papile, L-U., Munsick-Bruno, G. and Schaefer, A. (1983) Relationship of cerebral intraventricular haemorrhage and early childhood neurologic handicaps. *Journal of Pediatrics*, **103**, 273–277

Parkin, J.M., Hey, E.N. and Clowes, J. (1976) Rapid assessment of gestational age at birth. *Archives of Disease in Childhood*, **51**, 259–263

Vohr, B.R. and Hack, M. (1982) Developmental follow up of low birth weight infants. *Pediatric Clinics of North America*, **29**, 1441–1454

Whitfield, M.F. (1982) Poor weight gain of low birth weight infant fed nasojejunally. *Archives of Disease in Childhood*, **57**, 597–601

Yu, V.Y. and Rolph, P. (1976) Effect of feeding on ventilation and respiratory mechanics in newborn infants. *Archives of Disease in Childhood*, **51**, 310–313

Further reading

Scott, D.T. (1987) Premature infants in later childhood. Some recent follow-up results. *Seminars in Perinatology*, **11**, 191–199

Vohr, B.R. and Hack, M. (1982) Developmental follow-up of low birth weight infants. *Pediatric Clinics of North America*, **29**, 1441–1454

Volpe, J.J. (1989) Intraventricular haemorrhage and brain injury in the premature infant. *Clinics in Perinatology*, **16**, 361–412

Chapter 5

Transport of the sick neonate

The outcome for sick and low birthweight infants has been shown to be improved by management in a fully staffed neonatal intensive care unit (NICU) compared with management on an *ad hoc* basis in the referring hospital special care baby unit (SCBU) where it may not be possible to provide appropriate equipment and experienced round-the-clock staffing (Usher, 1977). In the last 15 years a network of regional NICUs has been set up in Europe and North America and the transport of high-risk, or potentially high-risk, patients constitutes a major area of decision making in modern perinatal paediatric practice. Neonatal intensive care management of the high-risk neonate represents only one aspect of the high-risk obstetric/neonatal combined management approach and the best results are obtained by maximum cooperation between obstetric and neonatal staff at all levels, in the referring hospital and in the regional centre.

Maternal transfer

Whenever possible, a pregnancy anticipated to give rise to an infant requiring full intensive care facilities in the newborn period should be transferred with the infant *in utero* to the high-risk obstetric unit in the NICU hospital, if this is feasible and safe for the mother. The decision to transfer the mother should be a joint one involving the paediatric and obstetric staff in the referring hospital and the staff of the regional unit. Although each patient presents a different and individual problem, and other variables such as bed availability and bad weather may affect timing of the transfer, the following should be considered indications for discussion and possible transfer of a mother from a referring hospital to the regional centre:

1. The onset of premature labour in a pregnancy of 33 weeks' gestation or less.
2. Multiple pregnancy.
3. Serious complications of pregnancy, such as significant antepartum haemorrhage or pre-eclampsia.
4. Serious coincidental maternal disease, e.g. heart disease, renal disease and diseases that may affect the fetus, such as myasthenia gravis,

idiopathic thrombocytopenic purpura or collagen diseases (pp. 5, 21 and 89).
5. Previously recognized fetomaternal problems, such as severe rhesus isoimmunization.
6. Poor intrauterine growth, as shown by clinical assessment and/or sequential ultrasound measurements of fetal growth parameters; this is usually associated with oligohydramnios in the absence of membrane rupture.
7. Fetal anomaly identified on ultrasound examination, and possibly amenable to intrauterine treatment (p. 25), or requiring urgent intensive management following delivery (e.g. diaphragmatic hernia).

Contraindications to maternal transfer

The pregnancy must be in a reasonably stable state before transfer. The mother should not be transferred if her blood pressure is out of control or if there is active bleeding. Rapidly advancing labour is a major contraindication to transfer as it may lead to delivery *en route* – a situation that must be avoided at all costs, because it is extremely hazardous for both mother and baby. The situation should be carefully assessed and the mother stabilized before transfer, after discussion with the 'high-risk' obstetrician in the regional centre. Immediately before transfer, the degree of cervical dilatation should be assessed to reduce the risk of delivery *en route*. Clear guidelines for optimal facilities for maternal transport have not yet been well established. In British Columbia maternal transfers are managed by 'paramedics', who are specially trained in perinatal care, and by an obstetrician, if necessary, and sometimes a neonatologist in addition, if delivery in the referring hospital may be required before transfer.

Neonatal transfer

Sometimes delivery in the referring hospital is inevitable because of the advanced stage of labour of the mother, continuing antepartum haemorrhage or fulminating pre-eclampsia. In this situation the most satisfactory method of delivery should be established by discussion between the obstetric staffs in the referring hospital and the regional centre; and the best possible facilities should be organized for delivery of the infant, resuscitation after delivery and subsequent stabilization before transfer.

It is the responsibility of the regional NICU to provide transport facilities for infants needing to be transferred to the regional NICU. The regional transport team acts as an extension of the NICU, providing similar facilities. The equipment used by the neonatal transport team may be in the form of a specially modified intensive care transport incubator, or a specially modified ambulance or aircraft. This transport facility must provide:

1. Facilities for adequate temperature control, such as a suitable transport incubator with warming characteristics sufficient to maintain the body temperature of an infant of less than 1.0 kg in any environmental

temperature likely to be met in the drainage area of the perinatal centre. This may be a traditional convected air incubator, preferably with a double wall, or an enclosed unit using a servo radiant heater. In a convection incubator it may be desirable to wrap the infant in warmed Gamgee and aluminium kitchen foil to prevent radiant heat loss.
2. Self-contained infant ventilator with an adequate supply of oxygen and air, and a gas mixer.
3. Continuous monitoring facilities for heart rate, core temperature and inspired oxygen concentration. Portable units are also now available for monitoring transcutaneous $P\text{O}_2$, transcutaneous $P\text{CO}_2$ and oxygen saturation.
4. Equipment for resuscitation, intravascular infusion, chest drains and chest drain valves, Chemstrip or Dextrostix (see footnote on p. 59) and ventilator connections. Intravascular infusions must be controlled by a battery-powered infusion pump (syringe or peristaltic pump).
5. Drugs; sodium bicarbonate, digoxin, dopamine, tolazoline, pancuronium, prostaglandin E, antibiotics, anticonvulsants, glucose 10% and other intravenous infusion fluids.

The neonatal transport equipment must be fully battery powered and have facilities for running off the mains electricity supply (240 or 110 V AC, or 12 V DC, as is available in most ambulances). If possible, the equipment should also be adapted to run off 24 V DC as this is the voltage frequently provided in aircraft. The equipment must be regularly checked to be in a state of readiness at all times. In different parts of the world different combinations of staff have been used to provide intensive care infant transport team facilities. Two groups of skills are required:

1. Ability to use and 'trouble-shoot' the equipment (which might be appropriately provided by a respiratory technologist, ambulance 'paramedic', doctor or nurse).
2. Ability to assess and treat the infant (which might be provided by a doctor, specially trained nurse or a specially trained ambulance 'paramedic'). The person responsible for the management of the infant must have good neonatal intensive care skills and be fully conversant with clinical assessment of the infant, and X-ray and blood gas interpretation. There must be good medical back-up by telephone, radio or video for consultation.

Indications for transfer

The following are guidelines for discussion between the physician in the referring hospital and the neonatologist in the NICU, about possible transfer.

Low birth weight (< 1.5 kg)

Although not all infants of 1.5 kg birth weight or less get into serious difficulties, a proportion develop nutritional and respiratory problems requiring intensive management which may only be available in the regional NICU. The smaller the infant the greater the chance of problems. Improvement in survival and morbidity in infants of 1.0 kg or less at birth is dependent upon regionalized management in order to minimize serious problems and complications.

Respiratory distress syndrome (RDS), meconium aspiration syndrome, pneumothorax and other forms of displaced air

If blood gas analysis is not available, infants with relatively mild respiratory problems requiring inspired oxygen concentration greater than 0.30 (30%) oxygen to abolish cyanosis or maintain arterial oxygen saturation >90% should be transferred in order to provide adequate blood gas monitoring. Infants with RDS requiring a fractional concentration of inspired ocygen in excess of 0.6 (60%) in order to maintain an arterial PO_2 of 8.0 kPa (60 mmHg:torr) should be transferred to the regional NICU because of the high incidence of ventilatory failure and requirement for ventilatory assistance, and possible pneumothorax. Infants with significant meconium aspiration requiring increased fractional inspired oxygen concentration greater than 0.3 (30%) should be transferred because they are likely to suddenly develop severe ventilatory problems in the first 48 hours due to persistent fetal circulation (see p. 172).

Life-threatening congenital abnormalities, possibly requiring urgent surgical management

These include, for example, diaphragmatic hernia, congenital heart disease, gastroschisis or exomphalos, oesophageal atresia with tracheo-oesophageal fistula, neonatal intestinal obstruction.

Diagnostic problems

These provide another indication for transfer.

Other management problems in the sick neonate

These include, for example, neonatal convulsions, intolerance of feeds, severe jaundice requiring diagnosis and/or exchange transfusion, rare metabolic disorders.

The decision about the best management should be made mutually between the referring hospital staff and the NICU staff and the condition of the infant should be stabilized soon after delivery, before the arrival of the neonatal transport team. The aim of stabilization before transfer is to improve the baby's condition to avoid problems *en route*. This involves prevention or correction of hypoxia, hypercapnia, acidaemia, hypoglycaemia and shock. The insertion of an intravenous line is usually required with intravenous glucose 10% at 60 ml/kg per 24 hours, blood gas monitoring and appropriate manipulation of inspired oxygen concentration, and ventilatory assistance, as indicated. X-rays may be required for respiratory or abdominal conditions.

The outward trip for the neonatal transport team should be a rapid one, and is a first priority in terms of utilization of ambulance staff and equipment, because the infant may continue to deteriorate after the original telephone call, despite attempts at stabilization in the referring hospital. On arrival at the referring hospital, members of the neonatal transport team assess the infant and consolidate stabilization. If ventilation is required, blood gas analysis, if this is available, should be done to assist management and before departure to confirm appropriate treatment. Endotracheal tubes must be very securely fixed for transport and it is an advantage if a chest X-ray can be carried out before departure to confirm the position of the endotracheal tube and to exclude a pneumothorax. The diagnosis of pneumothorax is particularly important if transfer in unpressurized aircraft is contemplated because a pneumothorax increases in size with decreasing external barometric pressure. Before departure from the referring hospital, the neonatal transport team collect all the relevant clinical records about the mother, the pregnancy, the delivery and the hospital course before their arrival. They should also collect the placenta, if available, and a sample of maternal blood and any relevant X-rays. The neonatal transport team must discuss the situation with the parents who must have an opportunity to see the baby before departure.

In transit the neonatal transport team monitor the baby's condition by checking heart rate, respiratory rate, colour, temperature, activity and other monitoring information, such as transcutaneous Po_2. They must also monitor the functioning of the equipment, the state of the battery pack and the adequacy of the supply of respiratory gases. If the transport involves a flight in unpressurized aircraft, the inspired oxygen concentration will have to be increased considerably in order to maintain the same arterial Po_2 in the infant. In pressurized aircraft it may be necessary to ask for a lower altitude equivalent pressurization than usual in order to improve oxygenation of the infant (Table 5.1). This is an expensive procedure because it uses more fuel. Different aircraft permit different levels of pressurization and the aircraft may have to fly at a lower altitude, and therefore through turbulence, in order to achieve the required pressurization level. On arrival in the regional NICU, the neonatal transport team hand the infant over to the intensive care staff, ensuring transfer of all relevant patient data, and contact the parents in the referring hospital to confirm safe arrival.

Liaison with the paediatrician in the referring hospital during the baby's stay in the regional NICU is important and the infant should be transferred

Table 5.1 Effect of increase in actual or pressurization altitude on inspired oxygen needs

Required inspired oxygen concentration at sea level (%)	*Equivalent oxygen concentration* (%) *to be given to patient, by pressurization altitude in feet (metres)*					
	2000(600)	4000(1200)	6000(1800)	8000(2400)	10000(3000)	12000(3600)
21	23	25	27	29	31	34
30	32.5	35	38	42	45	49
40	43	47	51	55	60	65
50	55	59	63	68	75	82
60	65	70	76	82	90	100
70	75	81	88	96	$\geq$100	$\geq$100
80	86	94	$\geq$100	$\geq$100	$\geq$100	$\geq$100
90	98	$\geq$100	$\geq$100	$\geq$100	$\geq$100	$\geq$100

A pressurization altitude of 10 000 feet (3600 m) should be assumed on pressurized commercial jets unless the pilot states otherwise.
Data calculated from Liebman *et al.* (1976).

back to the referring hospital as soon as intensive-care management is no longer needed.

Special situations

Diaphragmatic hernia

Infants with diaphragmatic hernia (see also p. 156) frequently present with severe respiratory insufficiency in the first hours after delivery. The situation is aggravated by gaseous distension of the bowel in the left hemithorax by swallowed air. The infant's vigorous respiratory efforts confound attempts at effective ventilation, and high negative intrapleural pressure excursions encourage passage of more bowel from the abdomen through the hernia into the left hemithorax. It is important, if possible, not to give IPPV by mask, as this inflates the gastrointestinal tract and aggravates the situation. As soon as the condition is recognized, a large-bore Replogle tube should be passed into the stomach and attached to continuous suction. Before transfer the baby should be intubated and IPPV initiated; the baby should be paralysed with pancuronium 0.1–0.3 mg/kg per dose for transport to prevent struggling.

Gastroschisis/exomphalos

In infants with major gastroschisis or exomphalos, the diagnosis is obvious at delivery. The exposed bowel provides an immense surface area for heat and fluid loss. This can be prevented by covering the bowel with sterile Gamgee or swabs soaked in warm saline and covering the swabs with plastic cooking foil, such as Saran Wrap. In addition, a nasogastric tube should be passed and attached to continuous suction as inflation of the exteriorized bowel by swallowed air makes its replacement in the abdomen at operation much more difficult.

Tracheo-oesophageal fistula with oesophageal atresia (see also pp. 148–150)

In the most common form of tracheo-oesophageal fistula, the diagnosis may be suspected prenatally because of polyhydramnios, and confirmed at delivery by the inability to pass a nasogastric tube beyond 10 cm in a term infant. In general, this lesion is correctable, with a low mortality rate, but the major risks are from inhalation of saliva from the upper gastrointestinal tract, and reflux of gastric contents into the respiratory tract via the lower end of the oesophagus through the fistula. Adequate suction of the pharynx is important to prevent aspiration from above, and the baby should be kept in a head-up position, lying semiprone on the right side, to reduce the risk of aspiration of stomach contents into the lungs.

References

Liebman, J., Lucas, R., Moss, A., Cotton, E., Rosenthal, A. and Ruttenberg, H. (1976) Airline travel for children with chronic pulmonary disease. *Pediatrics*, **57**, 408–410

Usher, B. (1977) Changing mortality rates with perinatal intensive care and regionalisation. *Seminars in Perinatology*, **1**, 309–319

Further reading

Blake, A.M., McIntosh, N., Reynolds, E.O.R. and St. Andrew, D. (1975) Transport of newborn infants for intensive care. *British Medical Journal*, **4**, 13–17

Chance, G.W., O'Brien, M.J. and Swyer, P.R. (1973) Transportation of sick neonates, 1972: an unsatisfactory aspect of medical care. *Canadian Medical Association Journal*, **109**, 847–851

Chance, G., Matthew, J.D., Gash, J., Williams, G. and Cunningham, K. (1978) Neonatal transport: a controlled study of skilled assistance. *Journal of Pediatrics*, **93**, 662–666

Greene, W.T. (1980) Organization of neonatal transport services in support of a regional referral centre. *Clinics in Perinatology*, **7**, 187–195

MacDonald, M.G. and Miller, M.K. (eds) (1989) *Emergency Transport of the Perinatal Patient*, Little Brown, Boston

Chapter 6

Shock and acute blood loss

Shock

Sudden deterioration or 'collapse' is the presentation of most severe and life-threatening conditions in the newborn period. The more common causes are given in Tables 6.1–6.5. Sudden deterioration from any of these causes is accompanied by circulatory insufficiency or 'collapse' and may progress to respiratory insufficiency or respiratory arrest. The term 'shock' is used for this type of circulatory insufficiency. These cardiorespiratory abnormalities are frequently secondary to underlying problems, but may become so rapidly progressive that the first priority in treatment has to be cardiorespiratory resuscitation, with the search for and treatment of the primary cause relegated to second, but still very important order of priority.

Table 6.1 Causes of shock which may occur without obvious signs or symptoms

Acute internal blood loss (p. 750)	Necrotizing enterocolitis (Chapter 27)
Septicaemia (p. 192)	Intracranial haemorrhage (p. 94)
Pneumothorax (p. 000)	Severe hypoglycaemia (p. 210)
Cardiac failure, some types (p. 170)	Severe hypoxia (p. 134)

A critically important component in the causation of circulatory insufficiency is loss of fluid from the circulating space. This is sometimes obvious where there is external loss of blood (e.g. haemorrhage from the cord) or fluid (e.g. gastroenteritis). In most instances, however, the fluid lost from the circulation is due to the passage of extracellular fluid from the vascular space into the interstitial space due to a sudden increase in capillary permeability (so-called 'third spacing'). This results in a situation where there is no obvious external loss of blood or fluid but the infant becomes severely hypovolaemic and develops circulatory failure.

Recognition

The infant develops:

1. Greyish pallor with peripheral cyanosis, progressing to blotchy cyanosis.

2. Tachycardia with a thin thready pulse and sluggish capillary refilling, progressing to bradycardia.
3. Hypothermia.
4. Hypotension and oliguria.
5. Lethargy.
6. Deteriorating respiratory status progressing to apnoea.

Management

The infant may be extremely ill from a cause which may not be immediately apparent. Consider rapidly correctable causes of likely immediate death such as major haemorrhage, pneumothorax or pneumopericardium, or endotracheal tube blockage or dislodgement in a ventilated baby. If there is no immediately obvious cause, treatment of the shock is the first priority.

1. Consider ventilation of the infant if the breathing is laboured or irregular. The baby will probably have significant metabolic acidosis (i.e. a base deficit of 15 mmol (p. 137)) and will need bicarbonate and/or THAM (tris-hydroxyaminomethane) before the blood gas results are available. The baby should be ventilated before being given bicarbonate otherwise the bicarbonate may cause a sudden steep rise in $P\text{CO}_2$, precipitating CO_2 narcosis and sudden apnoea. The baby should also be ventilated if THAM is to be given as it causes apnoea in infants.
2. Venous access is the second most important priority. The baby will require a considerable volume expansion to re-establish effective circulation. Effective tissue perfusion is critically important as this will stop the spiral of progressive acidaemia and circulatory fluid loss. Management may be assisted by a central venous pressure line. Fresh frozen plasma (FFP) is the most useful circulatory volume replacement fluid, though blood may be preferable, if immediately available, in the most severely ill babies or those who have had a significant haemorrhage. FFP should be given quickly (10 ml/kg over 5 minutes followed by another 10 ml/kg over the next 10 minutes.)
3. The next priority is to search for a cause, concentrating on the treatable causes first (see Tables 6.1–6.5). Exclusion of a pneumothorax, taking a blood culture, and starting antibiotics are important first steps.
4. An arterial line should be inserted if possible as this will simplify management.
5. If the baby is not showing signs of improvement in circulatory status following volume expansion, ventilation and bicarbonate, dopamine should be started at a dose of 10 mcg/kg/min (see also p. 170 for further discussion of the use of dopamine) to increase myocardial contraction, and a further 20 ml/kg of FFP should be given.
6. Blood investigations to assess adequacy of treatment and to investigate the cause should include arterial blood gases, glucose, electrolytes, full blood count including white cell and platelet counts, and coagulation studies. The use of FFP tends to pre-correct any coagulation abnormalities but in severe bacterial shock exchange transfusion may be needed to correct disseminated intravascular coagulation (see Chapter 8).

7. Urine output must be monitored carefully and the urine should be tested for blood, as its presence is an important indication of acute renal injury. A renal output of >2 ml/kg per hour confirms adequate renal perfusion after volume replacement.

Acute blood loss

This can conveniently be divided into blood loss occurring before or during delivery and blood loss occurring after delivery. Where bleeding has occurred before or during delivery the infant is likely to be pale and shocked at birth, and the differential diagnosis of pallor at delivery is important (Table 6.2).

Table 6.2 Pallor at delivery

Feature	*Severe hypoxia*	*Acute blood loss*	*Severe chronic anaemia*
Fetal heart rate	Tachycardia → bradycardia (type II dips)	Tachycardia if bleeding has occurred before or during labour	Tachycardia
Apnoea at birth	+	No primary apnoea	Only in severe hydrops
Pallor	+	+	++
Cyanosis	++	+ mainly peripheral	No
Cord	Collapsed	Collapsed	Distended
Cord pulsation	Feeble or absent	Feeble or absent	Normal
Heart rate	Slow (<60 per min)	Rapid → slow	Rapid
Brachial pulse	Weak or impalpable	Weak or impalpable	Normal or feeble
Hypotonia	++	+	Only in severe hydrops
Abdomen	Normal	Normal	Distended from hepatosplenomegaly ± ascites
Skin haemorrhages	No	No	In severe rhesus isoimmunization

In severe intrapartum hypoxia (White asphyxia) there is, unless there is hypoxic brain damage, a rapid response to appropriate resuscitation (p. 34), but plasma (see above) may be required in addition to resuscitation. In severe chronic anaemia resuscitation is not usually required except in severely hydropic infants in whom there is pulmonary oedema, with or without pleural effusions and ascites, which require removal (p. 277). In shock due to haemorrhage, treatment for hypoxia causes only slight or transient improvement.

Acute blood loss before or during delivery

Recognition

If the diagnosis of acute blood loss is obvious, treatment can be started immediately; often the diagnosis of haemorrhagic shock is suspected on

Table 6.3 Acute blood loss before or during delivery

Time	*Cause*	*Diagnostic investigation*	*Cause discoverable at delivery*
During pregnancy	Acute twin-to-twin bleed	Appearance of twins, examination of placentae; Hb on twins	Yes (also p. 81 for chronic twin-to-twin haemorrhage
	Injury at amniocentesis, intrauterine transfusion, or fetoscopy	Blood-stained amniotic fluid Puncture mark on infant. Torn fetal vessel or placenta	Yes
During pregnancy or labour	Acute fetomaternal bleed	Kleihauer test on mother's blood	No (also p. 81 for chronic fetomaternal haemorrhage)
	Fetal bleeding with placenta praevia	Fetal blood mixed with maternal antepartum haemorrhage detectable with special tests Examination of placenta	No
	Fetal bleeding in accidental haemorrhage; may be combined with fetomaternal bleed	As above	No
During labour or delivery	Injury to fetal vessel at caesarean section; rupture of vasa praevia, vessels in velamentous insertion of cord (Kouyonmdjian, 1980) or supplying accessory lobe of placenta	Examination of fetal vessels and placenta	Yes
	Bleeding from scalp, puncture from electrode or fetal blood sampling	Examination of infant	Yes
	Differential compression of prolapsed cord or knot in cord with venous but not arterial obstruction (p. 47)	Hb on infant	No
During delivery	Rupture of cord	Examination of cord	Yes
	Draining blood into placenta at caesarean section (p. 46)	Ask about operative procedure	No
	Internal haemorrhage (brain or abdominal viscus)	Depends upon physical signs: intracranial haemorrhage (p. 194), rupture of liver or spleen (p. 75)	No

clinical grounds or because of a poor response to routine treatment for hypoxia, and an inspection of the placenta, fetal vessels or the infant will give the answer. Where the cause of the blood loss is not obvious, acute fetomaternal haemorrhage or internal haemorrhage should be considered. The commoner causes of bleeding are given in Table 6.3.

Management

As soon as it is recognized that the infant is in a state of shock, the cause should be sought (Table 6.3); any continuing source of blood loss should be identified and the bleeding should be stopped by whatever method is appropriate to the cause.

The subsequent management is as described on p. 76.

Acute blood loss after delivery

The more common causes of acute haemorrhage occurring after delivery and during the neonatal period are given in Table 6.4 and the more important causes are considered individually.

Table 6.4 Acute blood loss after delivery

0–24 hours	*24–36 hours*	*36–72 hours*	*2–7 days*	*Any time*
Fetal scalp puncture from electrode or blood sampling	Rupture of liver* (0–5 days)	Adrenal haemorrhage (0–4 days)	Haemorrhagic disease (up to 6 weeks in rare cases)	Renal vein thrombosis
Cord haemorrhage (loose ligature)	Subaponeurotic haemorrhage*	Acute subdural haemorrhage	Intraventricular haemorrhage	Bleeding into giant haem-angioma, with thrombocyto-penia
Cephal-haematoma*	Bleeding into muscle and soft tissues in breech delivery	Bleeding into mesentery of intestine		
Rupture of spleen* (usually in rhesus iso-immunization)	Pulmonary haemorrhage (haemorrhagic pulmonary oedema, p. 155)			

Times refer to interval after birth: figures in parentheses give extreme limits.
*If bleeding is excessive and continues in spite of transfusion and appropriate local treatment, and especially if there is evidence of skin haemorrhages, petechiae, bleeding or bruising elsewhere, investigation for thrombocytopenia or coagulation disorder is essential (pp. 86–92).

Important causes of acute blood loss after delivery

Rupture of the liver

Recognition Sudden rupture with immediate bleeding into the peritoneal cavity is rare and is more likely to occur in very small infants. More commonly, in large infants, a subcapsular haematoma forms which ruptures suddenly into the peritoneal cavity about 24–36 hours after delivery. Symptoms are those of intraperitoneal haemorrhage:

1. Sudden shock.
2. Vomiting and abdominal distension.
3. Rarely, a bluish tinge develops in the region of the umbilicus or in one or both scrotal sacs if the processus vaginalis is patent.
4. Rapidly falling haemoglobin and haematocrit; these may already be low before rupture into the peritoneum because the blood in the subcapsular haematoma is outside the vascular compartment.
5. In an erect plain X-ray the intestines may be seen floating above a horizontal fluid level of blood in the pelvis. This is not a constant sign.
6. Confirmation of the diagnosis is by aspiration of blood from the left iliac fossa using a large-bore needle.

Management (in sequence)

1. If shock is severe and the infant appears moribund, use the most immediately available of the commonly used electrolyte solutions or plasma expanders and give at the rate of 20 ml/kg, over half an hour while blood is being obtained. As soon as blood is available (see below) and can be given at the right temperature complete the transfusion with blood up to a total of 40 ml/kg of blood in 1 hour, neglecting the volume of electrolyte solution if this was less than 10 ml/kg but counting plasma expanders in the 40 ml/kg.
2. Investigate for thrombocytopenia or coagulation defect if appropriate (pp. 86–92).
3. It may be necessary to transfuse up to a total of 60 ml/kg before shock is relieved, and transfusion should then be continued slowly during laparotomy (see below).
4. Give 2 mg of vitamin K_1 (phytomenadione) intravenously if possible, otherwise intramuscularly.
5. Correct thrombocytopenia or coagulation defect.
6. Laparotomy, with suture of liver.

Use of blood and cross-matching in emergencies

1. In an acute emergency where immediate use of blood is life-saving, it is justifiable to use group O rhesus negative blood without previous cross-matching, although a formal cross-match taking 2 hours should be set up when the transfusion is started; this should include cross-matching against the mother's serum.
2. In less urgent situations group O rhesus negative blood can be used after an emergency cross-match which takes half an hour; a formal cross-match should also be set up as described above.
3. If there is time, blood of the infant's own group can be given, again with formal cross-matching.
4. Blood should *not* be given cold as this may cause arrhythmias or cardiac arrest. Blood should not be heated by immersing the bottle in hot water, nor by hanging hot water bottles round it. A warming coil can be used, as for exchange transfusion (p. 122).

Rupture of the spleen

Recognition This is less common than rupture of the liver, and occurs without any latent period. Shock therefore develops within a few hours of delivery. Occasionally a normal spleen is ruptured, but more commonly rupture occurs in an enlarged spleen in rhesus isoimmunization in which thrombocytopenia and coagulation disorders are likely in severely affected infants. Symptoms and signs are those of intraperitoneal haemorrhage and are identical with those seen in rupture of the liver.

Management Treat shock and correct blood disorders as described above for the liver. Splenectomy is invariably required. Maintenance treatment with oral penicillin will be needed until the age of 5 years, and parents and family doctor should be informed of the reason for this and the risk of septicaemia in the young child with no spleen.

Adrenal haemorrhage

Small haemorrhages into one or both adrenals are common and of no significance. Predisposing causes of a large adrenal haemorrhage are:

1. Traumatic delivery with abdominal compression.
2. Severe hypoxia.
3. Septicaemia.
4. Coagulation disorder (including the effects of anticoagulant drugs) or thrombocytopenia.

Symptoms of acute adrenal failure only occur when both glands are almost completely destroyed and are likely to be combined with those of acute blood loss, or septicaemia, or both. The right adrenal is more commonly affected. However, when the left adrenal is affected a clot extending back into the renal vein may cause renal vein thrombosis (see below) and conversely left renal vein thrombosis may extend back to involve the adrenal gland, so that on the left side there is a greater likelihood of both kidney and adrenal being involved in similar processes. On the right-hand side, kidney and adrenal veins open separately into the inferior vena cava.

Bleeding is usually confined within the capsule of the gland, with some retroperitoneal haemorrhage and rarely a small amount of intraperitoneal blood.

Recognition

1. Acute stage: initial symptoms are those of acute haemorrhage and shock. At this stage or a few hours later a large mass may be felt in the loin on one or both sides. This mass has to be distinguished from a kidney enlarged by a renal vein thrombosis (Table 6.5) or less commonly from a haemorrhage into a neuroblastoma (Murthy, Irving and Lister, 1978); ultrasound is helpful in diagnosis.
2. Later symptoms may be those of septicaemia and jaundice, which is due to the infection or to reabsorption of blood from the gland.
3. Occasionally a large mass in the loin may be found without any obvious preceding symptoms.

Table 6.5 Adrenal haemorrhage and renal vein thrombosis: differential diagnosis

	Adrenal haemorrhage	*Renal vein thrombosis*
Predisposing maternal conditions	Anticoagulant treatment, except heparin	Maternal diabetes
Age of onset	36–72 hours, up to 4 days	Any time
Septicaemia	Common	Rare
Shock	Usually	Sometimes
Anaemia	Always	Sometimes
Haematuria	None or a few red blood cells	Usually obvious
Proteinuria	None or trace	Marked
IVU*	Kidney on affected side displaced downwards with flattening of the upper calyces	Affected kidney does not excrete
Ultrasound	May distinguish between adrenal and renal mass	See under adrenal haemorrhage

*IVU, intravenous urogram.

Management (in sequence)

1. Treat as for acute haemorrhage in rupture of the liver (p. 76).
2. Give hydrocortisone 100 mg i.v. initially, followed by 25 mg 6-hourly i.m. until condition has improved, then reduce dose gradually to 25 mg twice daily, then 5 mg daily in three divided doses (2.5, 1.25, 1.25 mg).
3. Give vitamin K_1 (phytomenadione) 2 mg i.m. and repeat in 12 hours.
4. Give antibiotics if septicaemia is suspected.
5. Follow blood transfusion by intravenous glucose 5% in 0.9% sodium chloride at maintenance rate (p. 329) if electrolyte changes suggest acute adrenal failure.
6. Give sodium-retaining hormone as described for sodium-losing crises (p. 000) if indicated (see above).
7. As soon as the infant's condition permits, do an intravenous urogram (IVU) (see Table 6.5) or ultrasound examination.
8. Exploration is not helpful unless there is genuine suspicion of a neuroblastoma (confirmed by a positive vanillylmandelic acid (VMA) test), and adrenalectomy is never indicated in uncomplicated haemorrhage because it removes residual functioning tissue which is usually present.
9. Follow-up:
   (a) If the diagnosis of adrenal haemorrhage is correct the enlarged adrenal will shrink rapidly within a few days, and within 2–3 weeks a plain film of the abdomen will show a ring of calcification which shrinks slowly over the next few months to form a more dense area of calcification with the shape of the original gland (Black and Williams, 1973). This shrinkage excludes a tumour;
   (b) Within a few weeks of recovery a formal test of adrenal function should be carried out as acute adrenal failure may occur in periods of stress or infection;
   (c) Follow-up should continue for some years as hypertension may develop if one of the kidneys (usually the left) was involved in a venous thrombosis (see below).

Renal vein thrombosis
Predisposing factors appear to be maternal diabetes, dehydration or plethora (excessively high haemoglobin level) from any cause. Usually only one kidney is affected.

Recognition A thrombosis of the renal vein is equivalent to a large bleed into the kidney; shock is often an initial symptom, with haematuria, and the development of a large mass in the loin. If both kidneys are involved, there will be anuria or prolonged oliguria with a rising blood urea.

Management

1. Treat shock, and dehydration if present.
2. Do an IVU or ultrasound as soon as the infant is fit enough.
3. Try to establish whether renal output has been maintained. An initial suprapubic puncture may be necessary to obtain a specimen of urine but some of the urine in the bladder may have been formed before the acute episode, so the information obtained is of limited value.
4. If no urine has been passed within 4 hours of recovering from shock, a second suprapubic puncture should be performed. If the bladder is empty and there is clinical or radiological evidence that both kidneys are involved, treat as an organically determined anuria.
5. Exploration of a single affected kidney is not indicated but in bilateral cases venography may indicate whether there is a clot in the inferior vena cava, which can be removed surgically.
6. Follow-up: prolonged follow-up with serial IVUs or ultrasound should be performed and regular measurement of the blood pressure, because hypertension is a rare complication (Perry and Taylor, 1940).

Gastrointestinal haemorrhage

1. For haematemesis from all causes (p. 99).
2. For haemorrhagic disease (p. 87).
3. Bleeding into the mesentery produces a large laterally mobile mass which, on X-ray, displaces the intestines laterally. Shock can be severe and urgent transfusion is required.

Subaponeurotic haemorrhage
Though this is usually the result of vacuum extraction (p. 45), it may occur after an apparently normal delivery, and where this is the case a coagulation disorder or thrombocytopenia should be suspected.

Recognition The subaponeurotic layer forms a potential space over the whole skull, with bloodstaining visible in the upper eyelids. However, when there is a large bleed the shape of the head is deformed (turban-shaped) and there is pitting oedema of the scalp. Extension of the swelling laterally above the zygoma may be mistaken for a parotid swelling. Early recognition is important, because shock develops rapidly. This condition is more common in infants of African or Afro-Caribbean origin.

Management There is no surgical treatment. Shock should be treated as previously described (p. 72) and vitamin K_1 (phytomenadione) should be given intravenously if possible. When the condition develops after a normal delivery, a platelet count and screening test for a coagulation disorder should be done (p. 86).

Other causes

1. Acute subdural haematoma (p. 96).
2. Intraventricular haemorrhage (p. 98).
3. Pulmonary haemorrhage near term (p. 155).
4. Bleeding into giant haemangioma (p. 92).
5. Soft-tissue haemorrhage in breech delivery (p. 45).

References

Black, J. and Williams, D.I. (1973) Natural history of adrenal haemorrhage in the newborn. *Archives of Disease in Childhood*, **48**, 183–190

Kouyoumdjian, A. (1980) Velamentous insertion of the cord. *Obstetrics and Gynecology*, **56**, 737–742

Murthy, T.V.M., Irving, I.M. and Lister, J. (1978) Massive adrenal haemorrhage in neonatal neuroblastoma. *Journal of Pediatric Surgery*, **13**, 31–34

Perry, C.B. and Taylor, A.L. (1940) Hypertension following thrombosis of renal veins. *Journal of Pathology and Bacteriology*, **51**, 369–374

Further reading

Lister, J. and Irving, I.M. (eds) (1990) *Neonatal Surgery*, 3rd edn, Butterworths, London

Chapter 7

Severe anaemia

Severe chronic anaemia in the neonatal period may be due to the following prenatal and postnatal causes.

Prenatal causes

1. Haemolysis due to severe rhesus isoimmunization, or rarely other forms of blood group incompatibility. In homozygous α°-thalassaemia (Hb Bart's) hydrops fetalis there is a haemolytic element (see also p. 82 and (3) below).
2. Continued blood loss due to chronic fetomaternal haemorrhage, or twin-to-twin haemorrhage in identical twins.
3. Failure to make adequate amounts of haemoglobin, as in homozygous α°-thalassaemia. Congenital red cell hypoplastic anaemia (Blackfan-Diamond type) rarely, if ever, presents as anaemia at delivery and is only apparent by the age of a few weeks or months.
4. Congenital intrauterine infection (pp. 179–184).
5. Rare congenital malignant conditions such as leukaemia, neuroblastoma or with the very rare spread of secondary spread from a maternal malignancy (p. 5).
6. Iatrogenic causes such as haemorrhage following amniocentesis, intrauterine fetal blood sampling or fetoscopy.

Postnatal causes

1. Continued haemolysis in unrecognized rhesus or other isoimmunization, severe ABO incompatibility, or rarely in homozygous sickle-cell anaemia (Hegyi *et al.* (1977).
2. Congenital red cell hypoplastic anaemia (see under (3) of prenatal causes).
3. Unrecognized haemolysis in spherocytic jaundice, glucose-6-phosphate dehydrogenase (G-6PD) deficiency or other rare forms of haemolytic red cell disorders (e.g. pyruvate kinase deficiency).
4. Early anaemia of prematurity, in which the anaemia develops slowly, usually becoming obvious by the age of 5–6 weeks, or earlier if there

have been numerous blood samples, or there is haemolysis due to vitamin E deficiency which may develop in very-low-birth-weight infants with inadequate vitamin supplementation on continued total parenteral nutrition (TPN), or with malabsorption.

Recognition

At delivery

1. Anaemia from severe rhesus isoimmunization is distinguished (apart from serological and other evidence; 116–119) from other forms of anaemia at delivery by the rapid development of jaundice which is usually obvious within an hour of delivery.
2. α°-Thalassaemia may not be easy to recognize as these hydropic infants usually die shortly after delivery; in such cases, an adequate autopsy is necessary to establish the diagnosis. However, the blood film may show red cell inclusions and electrophoresis shows haemoglobin Bart's. There may be a history of similarly affected infants. Invariably both parents are Chinese or of a related race; their blood should be examined for evidence of the heterozygous state, but the diagnosis is not easy, and may require a specialized laboratory.
3. In chronic fetomaternal haemorrhage the infant may resemble one with severe rhesus disease, even to the extent of having hepatosplenomegaly and being hydropic. However, jaundice does not develop; a blood film shows evidence of iron deficiency. When this diagnosis is suspected, the mother's blood should be examined as soon as possible for the presence of fetal red cells (Kleihauer test) and for α-fetoprotein.
4. In chronic twin-to-twin transfusion the anaemic twin has a similar appearance to that in chronic fetomaternal haemorrhage (see (2) above). The recipient twin has a plethoric appearance. Examination of the placenta generally shows that it is clearly divided into a pale area supplying the anaemic twin and a dark red area supplying the plethoric twin; subsequent examination shows the presence of the vascular connection. In twin-to-twin haemorrhage the difference between the haemoglobin levels of the two infants is at least 30 g/l but often greater.
5. Infants with congenital infections rarely show severe anaemia, but jaundice, petechiae and hepatosplenomegaly are common (pp. 179–180) and in rubella and cytomegalovirus (CMV) disease, raised purpuric skin lesions are common.
6. In congenital leukaemia, and in neuroblastoma firm raised pinkish-purple skin lesions may occur which are similar to those in congenital listeriosis, rubella and CMV. In neuroblastoma there is a large abdominal mass, and, in leukaemia, hepatosplenomegaly is usual. Blood films and a bone-marrow examination should confirm the diagnosis.
7. In iatrogenic haemorrhages the previous history is usually adequate evidence, but a careful examination of the placenta, fetal vessels and the infant should be made to detect puncture marks.

Postnatal anaemia

Increasing pallor, poor feeding and poor weight gain are the usual signs of a severe anaemia developing in the postnatal period. The cause is usually obvious in the very low birthweight infant, but where there is a history of prolonged or severe jaundice the infant should be investigated for evidence of haemolysis (serum bilirubin, reticulocyte count) and specifically for spherocytic jaundice or G-6PD deficiency, although investigation of the parents or sibs may be more helpful.

Management

1. Blood should be taken before transfusion for haemoglobin level, ABO and rhesus grouping, reticulocyte count, bilirubin, Coombs' test and serum for antibody testing for blood group incompatibility and intrauterine infections. Red cells should also be kept for testing for G-6PD deficiency, pyruvate kinase deficiency and similar disorders.
2. Rhesus disease and ABO incompatibility (pp. 116–130 for management).
3. Fetomaternal haemorrhage and twin-to-twin haemorrhage: any infant with a haemoglobin of less than 70 g/l requires an urgent transfusion with packed red cells. Those with hydrops in addition should be treated in the same way as the infant with hydrops due to severe rhesus disease (see p. 117).

Any infant with a haemoglobin of less than 80 g/l should be transfused even if asymptomatic, using the calculations given below; packed cells should be used for preference. If the haemoglobin is more than 80 g/l and there is satisfactory weight gain and a reticulocyte response of more than 5%, there is no urgency about transfusion. If the infant is not progressing well, the haemoglobin should be kept above 100 g/l; this applies particularly to very low birthweight infants.

Sick low birthweight infants should be transfused whenever their haematocrit falls below 0.35.

Calculation of the volume of blood required to be transfused

Using packed red cells* with a haematocrit of around 0.66, the volume of blood required is as follows:

The required rise in haemoglobin × 2 × weight in kg; i.e. 2 ml/kg of packed cells will raise the haemoglobin level by 10 g/l.
Example: A 3.0 kg infant: required rise in haemoglobin is from 70 g/l to 140 g/l. Volume required is 3 × 2 × 7 ml = 42 ml.

In a severely anaemic infant, blood should not be given more quickly than 10 ml/kg per hour. In the presence of cardiac failure, frusemide should be

*If only whole blood is available, 6 ml/kg will be required to raise the haemoglobin level by 10 g/l, but the rate of 10 ml/kg per hour should not be exceeded, and if necessary the transfusion should be given in two stages.

given intravenously or intramuscularly before the start of transfusion (p. 277).

Route to be used for transfusions

In severely ill infants where speed is essential and handling must be reduced to a minimum, the umbilical vein should be used, providing an opportunity for measuring the central venous pressure. Otherwise a peripheral vein should be used.

Management of the plethoric twin in twin-to-twin haemorrhage

Normally no treatment is required, though there is an immediate risk of cardiac failure from an excessively large blood volume, or of hyperbilirubinaemia. If the haematocrit is more than 0.65 there is an increased risk of cerebral or renal vein thrombosis or necrotizing enterocolitis, and an exchange transfusion using 15 ml of plasma/kg should lower the haematocrit to 0.65. Frusemide should not be given in these infants as it will further raise the haematocrit.

References

Hegyi, T., Delphin, E.S., Bank, A., Polin, R.A. and Blanc, W.A. (1977) Sickle cell anaemia in the newborn. *Pediatrics*, **60**, 213–216

Further reading

Letsky, E. (1986) Anaemia in the newborn. In *Textbook of Neonatology* (ed. N.R.C. Roberton), Churchill Livingstone, Edinburgh, Chapter 19 (Part II), pp. 449–464

Oski, F.A. and Naiman, J.L. (1982) *Haematologic Problems in the Newborn*, 3rd edn, Saunders, London

Chapter 8

Bleeding and clotting disorders

The newborn may bleed from a coagulation disorder or thrombocytopenia, or from a combination of both. Although a clinical distinction between these possibilities is not always possible the following points are useful:

1. Generalized petechiae are a certain indication of thrombocytopenia; in disseminated intravascular coagulation (DIC) in which both thrombocytopenia and coagulation disorders occur, there are skin haemorrhages and oozing from puncture sites, as well as petechiae.
2. Large soft tissue or subcutaneous haemorrhages without petechiae usually indicate a coagulation disorder.
3. Purple papules with hepatosplenomegaly, without severe anaemia, occur with rubella or cytomegalovirus (CMV) disease, with anaemia in severe rhesus isoimmunization, or leukaemia, and with hepatomegaly in congenital neuroblastoma.

Family history

In any infant, particularly males, suspected of having a coagulation disorder, the family history is important in respect of affected male relatives on the mother's side; both haemophilia A and haemophilia B or Christmas disease are inherited as X-linked recessives. Von Willebrand's disease, which rarely causes symptoms in the neonatal period, is inherited as a dominant, but in 30% of cases there is no family history.

Maternal factors

Drug treatment

Drug treatment of the mother may be important in the following cases:

1. Coagulation disorders in the infant may be due to anticonvulsant treatment of the mother with phenobarbitone or anticoagulants such as the coumarin group (warfarin, or phenindione), but not heparin.
2. Thrombocytopenia in mother and infant may be due to maternal treatment with the thiazide drugs, quinine or methyldopa. This is really a form of immune thrombocytopenia (see below).

Immune thrombocytopenia

This may be due to:

1. Transplacental passage of platelet antibodies from a mother with idiopathic thrombocytopenic purpura (ITP), and in drug-induced thrombocytopenia.
2. The formation of maternal antibodies specifically against the platelets of the infant, analogous to the mechanism in rhesus isoimmunization.

Management of the bleeding infant: general principles (in sequence)

1. Exclude swallowed maternal blood in cases of haematemesis or passage of blood in the stool (Appendix 2).
2. If there is shock, or serious continued bleeding, transfuse at once with stored blood (15–20 ml/kg) with the knowledge that this will replace none of the defective factors. If there is no shock but the haemoglobin is <100 g/l, give packed cells (for calculation see p. 83).

Or

3. In severe anaemia (haemoglobin <70 g/l) with hydrops and cardiac failure, do a partial exchange transfusion, as in severe rhesus disease (p. 131).
4. Investigate the cause of the bleeding (Table 8.1).

Table 8.1 Screening tests of haemostasis in the newborn

Disorder	*Platelets*	*PT*	*PTTK*	*TT*
Immune thrombocytopenia*	Abn	N	N	N
Disseminated intravascular coagulation	Abn	Abn	Abn	Abn
Vitamin K deficiency	N	Abn	Abn	N
Afibrinogenaemia	N	Abn	Abn	Abn
Factor XIII deficiency†	N	N	N	N
Haemophilia and Christmas disease	N	N	Abn	N
Liver disease	N	Abn	Abn	Abn

Abbreviations: Abn = abnormal; N = normal; PT = prothrombin time; PTTK = partial thromboplastin time with kaolin; TT = thrombin time.
*See Table 8.2.
†Requires special tests.
This table is reproduced from Chessells (1987) with permission of the author.

5. Replace the defective factors discovered by the screening test: fresh frozen plasma (FFP, see p. 88) in a dose of 10–15 ml/kg, is the more useful for this purpose because it will cover most of the likely deficiencies, but will not stop severe haemorrhage in haemophilia (see p. 88).

Or

6. Treat with vitamin K_1 if the disorder is vitamin K responsive.
7. Treat the primary condition.

Recognition and management of some specific disorders

Haemorrhagic disease of the newborn (vitamin K deficiency)

Recognition
Haemorrhage from this cause does not occur in the first 24 hours after delivery but usually between the second and seventh days of life, although occasionally as late as 6 weeks (Cooper and Lynch, 1979). Vitamin K deficiency is normally confined to breast-fed infants, but may occur in those fed on cow's milk if absorption of vitamin K from the intestine is defective or bacterial synthesis is inhibited by antibiotics. Bleeding may be from a single or multiple sites, with or without skin or subcutaneous haemorrhages. The most common single site is the gastrointestinal tract, where shock may develop before a blood-containing stool has been passed; in such cases the abdomen is slightly distended with loops of bowel, either visible or palpable. The diagnosis can usually be confirmed by finding red or dark blood on the finger after rectal examination. Haemorrhagic disease may be complicated by internal haemorrhage, of which intracranial haemorrhage, including extradural haemorrhage (Cooper and Lynch, 1979), is the most serious. For confirmation of the diagnosis, see the screening tests in Table 8.1.

Management (in sequence)

1. Replace acute blood loss, using packed cells in anaemia (haemoglobin <100 g/l) or whole blood if there is shock.
2. Give 1 mg vitamin K_1 (phytomenadione) intravenously. This takes about 4 hours to act and, if it is necessary to stop the bleeding more quickly, 10–15 ml of fresh frozen plasma/kg should be given.

Hepatic disease with failure of synthesis of clotting factors

Recognition
The primary condition must be identified: possible causes include congenital infections, galactosaemia, fructose intolerance, hepatitis, tyrosinaemia, biliary atresia and α_1-antitrypsin deficiency.

Management (in sequence)

1. Replace acute blood loss (as above); remember in calculating the volume of blood to be given that, in addition to blood, specific factor concentrates or FFP may have to be given to stop the bleeding, and overloading of the circulation must be avoided.
2. Give FFP: 10–15 ml/kg.
3. Treat the primary condition where possible. In galactosaemia or fructose intolerance with a severely ill child with liver failure, an exchange transfusion will remove the circulating galactose or fructose very rapidly, although with little immediate effect on the hepatic failure (also p. 290).
4. Give 2 mg of vitamin K_1 intravenously if there is still a tendency to bleed. The response in liver disease is unpredictable but vitamin K_1 is worth giving.

Coagulation disorders caused by maternal drug treatment

Recognition

Bleeding usually occurs within the first 24 hours after delivery. Drugs likely to cause a coagulation defect are phenobarbitone (as an anticonvulsant) and the anticoagulant drugs, warfarin, phenindione and the coumarin group.

Management (in sequence)

1. Replace acute blood loss (as above).
2. FFP should be given, as described above.
3. There may be some response to vitamin K_1 (especially when due to phenobarbitone) which should be given in two doses of 2 mg i.m. or i.v., 12 hours apart.

Congenital deficiency of clotting factors (Factor VIII in haemophilia A; Factor IX in haemophilia B (Christmas disease) and afibrinogenaemia)

Recognition

Factor VIII and IX deficiencies are confined to male infants: afibrinogenaemia (very rare) is probably inherited as a recessive, with a variant with inactive fibrinogen which is a dominant. All three conditions may present with acute haemorrhage from the cord, after circumcision, or with haemorrhage at any other site.

Management (in sequence)

1. If transfusion is required, take blood for investigation (Table 8.1) at the time of setting up the intravenous line and before giving anything to correct the coagulation disorder.
2. If the haemoglobin is <100 g/l and there is no shock, give packed cells (for calculation see p. 83). If shock is present, give whole blood in a volume just sufficient to restore adequate tissue perfusion (usually 10–15 ml/kg), making allowance for the possibility that FFP* may have to be given later in a volume of 10–15 ml/kg; the volumes required with Factor VIII or IX concentrates are much smaller (see below).
3. If a coagulation disorder is suspected on clinical grounds and confirmed by screening tests (Table 8.1), in males an urgent request should be made for estimation of blood levels of Factor VIII or IX as required; in females less common disorders may be present.
4. Any infant requiring replacement treatment with specific coagulation factors should be transferred, when clinically fit, to a unit with easy access to specific factor concentrates and where the effects of replacement treatment on the levels of Factor VIII or IX can be frequently measured.
   (a) Factor VIII deficiency (haemophilia A) (XR). It is unlikely that FFP will stop spontaneous or severe bleeding and Factor VIII

*FFP contains all the coagulation factors (but see above for fibrinogen) and should not be confused with freeze-dried plasma which contains no Factor VIII. Purified plasma protein fraction (PPF) consists mainly of albumin and will not correct *any* coagulation disorder.

cryoprecipitate or concentrate will be required to raise the level of Factor VIII above 20% normal to stop bleeding. One unit of Factor VIII per kg will raise the blood level by 2%, and the minimum amount required will be 10 units per kg. One bag (usually 10–20 ml) of cryoprecipitate usually contains 60 units of Factor VIII (approximately 4 units/ml) and the volume required will be about 2.5 ml/kg. Factor VIII concentrate contains 10–20 units/ml and the volume required would then be 1 ml/kg. However, the levels in both these preparations are extremely variable and the effect of treatment must be monitored by frequent estimations of Factor VIII in the recipient's plasma. Also the half-life of Factor VIII in the body is 12 hours and treatment may have to be repeated at 12-hourly intervals, again with frequent Factor VIII estimations;

(b) Factor IX deficiency (Christmas disease) (XR) can usually be corrected by FFP in a dose of 10–15 ml/kg but, if bleeding is severe and overloading of the circulation is likely, a concentrate of Factor IX should be used: bleeding can usually be stopped by 10–15 units of Factor IX concentrate/kg in a volume of 1 ml/kg;

(c) Von Willebrand's disease (AD): bleeding can usually be controlled by FFP or Factor VIII preparation as for haemophilia.

5. If a complex or rare disorder is suspected, because of the results of screening tests, the absence of Factor VIII or IX deficiency in a male, failure of response to treatment, or a coagulation disorder in a female, the infant should be transferred to a specialist centre as soon as possible. As an emergency measure, FFP can be given empirically because it is likely to correct temporarily most of the rarer coagulation disorders except afibrinogenaemia in which actual fibrinogen (100 mg/kg) is required. Before giving FFP the specialist centre should be consulted about the type of blood specimens they would like taken.

Thrombocytopenia

Thrombocytopenia alone secondary to congenital infections, or to severe rhesus isoimmunization, is easily recognized and rarely requires treatment; however, DIC may occur, especially in generalized herpes infections. (see Table 8.2 for a classification.)

Immune thrombocytopenia with maternal disease

Recognition Neonatal thrombocytopenia can be expected when the mother is known to have ITP or systemic lupus erythematosus (SLE) or has been receiving treatment with drugs of the thiazide group, methyldopa or quinine. The infant is rarely affected in drug-induced thrombocytopenia and the severity of neonatal thrombocytopenia with maternal ITP is related to the mother's platelet count except where she has had a splenectomy or has been on high-dosage steroids. If symptoms are going to develop they usually do so within the first 48 hours with the appearance of extensive purpuric haemorrhages and petechiae with or without bleeding elsewhere.

Table 8.2 Thrombocytopenia in the newborn

Mechanism	*Examples*
Platelet production decreased or abnormal	Thrombocytopenia with absent radii, Wiskott–Aldrich syndrome, infections
Immune thrombocytopenia	
Passive	Maternal ITP Maternal systemic lupus erythematosus (SLE) Maternal drug ingestion
Active	Isoimmune neonatal thrombocytopenia
Intravascular coagulation	
Generalized (DIC)	Asphyxiated, hypothermic, acidotic infants Rhesus isoimmunization (Chapter 11) Respiratory distress syndrome (Chapter 12) Necrotizing enterocolitis (Chapter 23) Congenital infections, syphilis, rubella, CMV, toxoplasmosis, herpes hominis (Chapter 14)
Localized	Cavernous haemangioma Renal vein thrombosis (p. 79) Catheter thrombus

This table is reproduced from Chessells (1987) with permission of the author.

Management The diagnosis should be confirmed by a platelet count on the mother and infant. There is no evidence that steroids have any useful place in the management of the infant. In the absence of bleeding, no treatment is required but the possibility of internal haemorrhage must always be kept in mind. Platelet transfusions (see below) are practically useless because of their immediate destruction, but may be considered in an extreme emergency as a life-saving measure.

Exchange transfusion (p. 119) using fresh heparinized blood is the most effective way of removing the circulating antibody and partially replacing platelets.

For prenatal treatment, see p. 26.

Isoimmune thrombocytopenia

Recognition If a previous infant has been affected, the diagnosis is simple. In contrast with rhesus isoimmunization the first infant may be affected. In the absence of any history of thrombocytopenia, the diagnosis should be suspected when there is thrombocytopenia in the infant but the mother has a normal platelet count. The clinical picture is as described above under Immune thrombocytopenia. Confirmation of the diagnosis will require the help of a laboratory specializing in platelet disorders.

Management This is as for the management of immune thrombocytopenia with maternal disease (see above), except that washed maternal platelets may be used as replacement therapy. Recently, isoimmune thrombocytopenia has been successfully treated with intravenous immunoglobulins 400 mg/kg per day for 5 days (Derycke *et al.*, 1985).

For prenatal treatment, see p. 26.

Disseminated intravascular coagulation (DIC)

Disseminated intravascular coagulation may occur as a complicating factor in infants severely ill with septicaemia, acute neurological injury, such as hypoxic ischaemic encephalopathy, persistent fetal circulation, necrotizing enterocolitis, severe heart failure and sclerema. Pathological activation of the coagulation cascade results in consumption of platelets and coagulation factors. Secondary fibrinolysis produces accumulation of fibrin degradation products (FDPs) which are themselves anticoagulant. There is frequently an associated haemolytic anaemia which may produce a dangerously rapid rise in bilirubin level requiring exchange transfusion for jaundice.

Recognition
The infant is severely ill from one of the predisposing causes mentioned above, and develops bleeding from puncture sites, mucous membranes and skin haemorrhages.

Laboratory findings

1. Platelet count: low ($<100 \times 19^9$/l) or falling.
2. Fibrinogen level: low (<1.5 g/l) or falling.
3. Fibrin degradation products raised (>10 mg/l).
   All three of these findings usually occur together but false elevations of FDPs may occur with poor renal function or extensive bruising at delivery.
4. Prolongation of thrombin and prothrombin times. Partial thromboplastin time (PTT) is not usually helpful.

There may be jaundice and haemoglobinuria.

Management (in sequence)
1. Every attempt must be made to establish the primary cause and treat this vigorously. This usually involves an infection screen and antibiotic treatment in addition to other measures. Inability to identify the primary cause, however, must not delay further treatment.
2. Metabolic abnormalities (glucose, sodium, calcium, fluid and electrolyte balance) and particularly acidaemia and hypotension should be sought and rapidly corrected.
3. Accurate measurement of urine output is important in fluid and electrolyte management as most infants developing DIC also have incipient renal failure, which may be renal from microthrombosis or prerenal from hypotension.
4. Correct thrombocytopenia by platelet transfusion. The platelets from one unit of blood are usually concentrated in 40–50 ml, and may on special request be further concentrated to 20–25 ml (superconcentrate). The usual dose is 10 ml/kg of the normal platelet concentrate given intravenously over half an hour. The platelet count should be checked 1 hour after completion of the infusion, and a low post-transfusion level (less than 50×10^9/l) suggests very rapid consumption and that further transfusions should be of greater volume or should be of platelet superconcentrate.
5. Give FFP (10 ml/kg) to replace coagulation factors.

6. The platelet count and fibrinogen levels should be monitored 4- to 6-hourly and further transfusions given to correct thrombocytopenia and to achieve a fibrinogen level consistently above 1.0 g/l. Repeated transfusions may be needed over several days until the primary cause comes under control.
7. Repeated single volume exchange transfusions should be considered when:
   (a) It is not possible to correct the coagulation status by the above measures.
   (b) The infant develops renal failure and cannot tolerate the intravascular volume load administered by repeated platelet and FFP transfusions. An alternative in these situations may be plasma ultrafiltration;
   (c) Exchange transfusion may be indicated as treatment for the other concurrent problems (e.g. septicaemia with severe neutropenia, anaemia and jaundice from intravascular haemolysis). The exchange transfusions should be adjusted to the infant's needs using packed cells reconstituted with FFP with 'chasers' of platelet concentrate and white cell concentrate, as indicated.
8. Routine heparinization of infants with DIC in an attempt to stop continued consumption of coagulation factors has not been shown to be of benefit in the newborn period and further complicates management, and may increase the risk of intracranial haemorrhage. Heparinization may, however, be considered on the advice of a haematologist if major thrombosis has occurred, with threatened infarction of an internal organ. The dose is around 25 units/kg per hour as a continuous infusion or around 100 units/kg intermittently every 4–6 hours intravenously with 12 to 24-hourly checks of the thrombin time and appropriate dose adjustments (Chessells, 1987).

Localized intravascular coagulation

For renal vein thrombosis see p. 79; replacement of platelets is not usually required. The treatment of sequestration of platelets in a large cavernous haemangioma depends on the severity of the bleeding. As an emergency measure platelet replacement can be used. Local excision of the haemangioma under platelet cover may be practicable. Alternatively embolization of the arterial supply is safer, if done in a unit with experience in the technique. In less urgent situations there is some evidence (Fost and Esterly, 1968) that prednisone or other corticosteroids may be effective.

References

Chessells, J.M. (1987) The bleeding neonate. In *Pediatric Emergencies*, 2nd edn (ed. J.A. Black), Butterworths, London, pp. 676–678

Cooper, N.A. and Lynch, M.A. (1979) Delayed haemorrhagic disease of the newborn with extradural haematoma. *British Medical Journal*, **i**, 164–165

Derycke, M., Dreyfus, M., Ropert, J.C. and Tchernia, G. (1985) Intravenous immunoglobulin for neonatal isoimmune thrombocytopenia. *Archives of Disease in Childhood*, **60**, 667–669

Fost, N.C. and Esterly, N.B. (1968) Successful treatment of juvenile haemangiomas with prednisone. *Journal of Pediatrics*, **72**, 351–357

Further reading

Turner, T.L. (1986) Coagulation disorders of the newborn. In *Textbook of Neonatology* (ed. N.R.C. Roberton), Churchill Livingstone, Edinburgh, Chapter 19 (Part I), pp. 439–446

Willoughby, M.L.N. (1977) *Paediatric Haematology*, Churchill Livingstone, Edinburgh

Chapter 9

Bleeding from one site

Although bleeding may be apparently from one site, this does not exclude a bleeding or coagulation disorder.

For description of Apt's test to differentiate between fetal and maternal blood, see Appendix 2.

Intracranial haemorrhage (Table 9.1)

Evidence of an intracranial haemorrhage is rarely so specific that the diagnosis is immediately obvious, and it is easy to mistake the symptoms and signs for a deterioration in the primary condition, e.g. apnoeic attacks in respiratory distress syndrome (RDS), or fits after a difficult or hypoxic delivery.

In some cases the presence of a bleeding or coagulation disorder may cause severe haemorrhage after a small dural tear or other injury which would otherwise have been symptomless and unimportant.

Conditions which may cause or be associated with an intracranial haemorrhage

Mechanical causes (trauma)

In such cases there is tearing of the falx with bleeding from its venous sinus or from the major veins draining into it, or a tear of the tentorium with bleeding from the lateral sinus. Blood from a torn falx accumulates over the surface of one or both parietal lobes while bleeding from the lateral sinus may result in a haematoma in the middle fossa or below the tentorium in the posterior fossa. In all these situations the rapid accumulation of blood results in acute subdural haematoma.

1. Rapid deformation of the skull without time for stretching (moulding) to occur.
   (a) Any precipitate or uncontrolled delivery;
   (b) Rapid delivery of the head in a breech presentation, particularly in the absence of protective forceps.
2. Prolonged and difficult delivery with severe moulding, sufficient to cause rupture of one of the dural sinuses.

Table 9.1 Symptoms and signs of intracranial haemorrhage

Symptoms and signs		Other causes	Type of intracranial haemorrhage
Non-specific	Apnoeic attacks Cyanotic attacks Persistent cyanosis	Congenital heart disease Acute respiratory disease Hypoglycaemia	Intraventricular haemorrhage (IVH) or acute subdural haematoma
	Lethargy Hypotonia Poor feeding	Septicaemia Severe infection	
	Focal or generalized fits	Meningitis Hypoglycaemia Hypocalcaemia Hypomagnesaemia	
	Tonic fits	Meningitis	
Raised intracranial pressure	Tense or bulging fontanelle Enlarging head	Late meningitis Hydrocephalus	Acute subdural haematoma particularly in posterior fossa; acute cerebellar haemorrhage
Meningeal irritation	Head retraction or neck stiffness	Late meningitis Acute increase in intracranial pressure (see above)	Subarachnoid haemorrhage, rapidly developing hydrocephalus from any cause
Acute blood loss	Shock, hypotension, falling haematocrit and Hb level	Any acute haemorrhage external or enclosed	Large IVH or rapidly accumulating subdural haematoma
Localizing neurological signs	Fixed dilated pupil	None	Tentorial herniation of temporal lobe into the middle fossa on side of dilated pupil
	Nystagmus	None	IVH; acute subdural haematoma in posterior fossa; acute cerebellar haemorrhage

(a) Any prolonged delivery, particularly after a difficult application of forceps;

(b) A prolonged delivery due to uncorrected occipitoposterior position, or with a face or brow presentation.

3. An abnormally soft skull:

(a) In small pre-term infants, particularly after a breech delivery without protective forceps;

(b) A normal delivery of an infant with the severe form of osteogenesis imperfecta, or with hypophosphatasia (AR);
(c) Unrecognized hydrocephalus, after a difficult vaginal delivery.

4. Deformation of the occipital bone, causing diffuse cerebellar haemorrhage (see under Acute cerebellar haemorrhage, p. 97).

Bleeding or coagulation disorders
As described above, what would have been a symptomless minor bleed may become a major one in the presence of:

1. One of the congenital (genetically determined) coagulation disorders (p. 88).
2. Thrombocytopenia from any cause (p. 90) or very rarely one of the congenital disorders of platelet function.
3. Disseminated intravascular coagulation (p. 91).

In the presence of any of these conditions an intracranial haemorrhage may be the first indication of a bleeding or coagulation disorder, although there is usually other clinical evidence such as bruising, petechiae or oozing from puncture sites.

Respiratory disorders with hypoxia and hypercapnia
In the small pre-term infant with respiratory difficulties, usually RDS, there is clear evidence that episodes of apnoea, respiratory obstruction or other hypoxic episodes predispose to the development of an intraventricular haemorrhage.

Types of intracranial haemorrhage

Acute subdural haematoma (Abroms, McLennan and Mandell, 1977)

Recognition See above for predisposing causes. Symptoms usually develop from one up to several days after an initial improvement from the infant's poor condition at birth; less commonly symptoms develop within a few hours of delivery.

Supratentorial haematoma over the parietal lobes
The usual presenting symptoms are apnoeic attacks, apathy, poor feeding and hypotonia, often with fits which may be focal, generalized or tonic. The fontanelle becomes tense or bulging. Shock with hypotension, and a falling haematocrit and haemoglobin level are usual.

Supratentorial haematoma in the middle fossa
The haematoma may cause herniation of the tip of the temporal lobe through the tentorium, with pressure on the nucleus of the third nerve; bilateral haematomas are less likely than with those over the surface of the parietal lobe. Initial symptoms are as described above, but with the development of herniation through the tentorium, the pupil on the same side as the lesion becomes fixed and dilated. Shock is common.

Subtentorial haematoma (posterior fossa) (Pitlyk, Miller and Stayura, 1967)
Initial symptoms are similar to those described for the parietal lobe haematoma, but an acute obstructive hydrocephalus rapidly develops, followed by medullary compression which may be fatal unless the pressure is promptly relieved. The fontanelle becomes tense and serial measurement of the head circumference shows that the head is enlarging rapidly. Computerized tomography (CT) or ultrasound scan will demonstrate symmetrical enlargement of the lateral ventricles but scans are of limited value in showing the haematoma in the posterior fossa. If a scan is not available, 5–10 ml of air injected into one lateral ventricle will demonstrate the degree of hydrocephalus.

Management

Parietal lobe haematoma
Shock should be treated by blood transfusion. The site of the haematoma should be confirmed by a CT scan. Unless the situation is very critical, a neurosurgeon is the best person to evacuate the blood. If neurosurgical help cannot be obtained, a short-bevelled needle should be inserted at the lateral angle of the anterior fontanelle on both sides, and blood should be allowed to drip out without aspiration. A lumbar puncture should not be done.

Middle fossa haematoma, with fixed dilated pupil (Abroms, McLennan and Mandell, 1977)
Urgent intervention is required as progression to fatal brain-stem compression is often very rapid. No time should be wasted with scans, but a tap should be carried out through the lateral angle of the fontanelle on the side of the lesion in the hope of reaching the haematoma. If this is unsuccessful, a burr hole should be made over the middle lobe. The contralateral side should not be touched until the pupil has returned to its normal size and reactivity. A lumbar puncture should not be done.

Subtentorial haematoma (posterior fossa)
Since the initial diagnosis may be that of supratentorial haematoma this should be excluded by bilateral taps or burr holes as described above. Failure to demonstrate a haematoma above the tentorium should initiate investigation for dilated lateral ventricles (see above) and, if confirmed, burr holes should be made in the occipital bone on either side of the midline. **A lumbar puncture should not be done.**

Acute cerebellar haemorrhage (Pape, Armstrong and Fitzhardinge, 1976)

Recognition

1. Haemorrhage into the cerebellum may occur in the term infant after prolonged and difficult breech delivery. Symptoms are similar to those in a posterior fossa haematoma.
2. Acute cerebellar haemorrhage may occur in the pre-term infant under treatment with continuous positive airway pressure (CPAP) for RDS

with a mask secured by a harness, causing a deformation of the occipital bone. Symptoms are non-specific.

Management In the term infant the management should be as for the posterior fossa haematoma: in the pre-term infant there is probably no specific treatment.

Chronic subdural haematoma

Chronic subdural haematoma is not considered here because it is rarely obvious during the neonatal period and does not normally constitute an emergency.

Intraventricular haemorrhage (Volpe, 1979)

Recognition This condition is virtually confined to low-birth-weight infants with RDS or other respiratory disorders and appears to be related to a preceding episode of hypoxia and hypercapnia. The haemorrhage may occasionally develop before delivery but usually occurs between 1 and 5 days after birth. Two types of haemorrhage have been described.

Catastrophic haemorrhage

Catastrophic haemorrhage, in which there is a sudden deterioration over minutes or hours, in which shock develops with a falling haematocrit and haemoglobin level. The infant may become unconscious. Other signs are apnoeic attacks or respiratory irregularity, decerebrate spasms, tonic seizures and a flaccid quadriplegia. The pupils may become fixed and the fontanelle is usually full or tense. Metabolic disorders such as metabolic acidosis, hyponatraemia and hyperglycaemia may occur. Even when treated promptly (see below), death is usual. The most satisfactory and least traumatic way of demonstrating an intraventricular haemorrhage is by CT or ultrasound scan. A lumbar puncture should only be performed if other evidence suggests the possibility of meningitis.

Intermittent type

In this type the symptoms and signs are much less severe and progress in an irregular manner with gaps of a few hours or days between new symptoms. Initially the level of consciousness may be altered, with hypotonia and deviation of the eyes. This may be followed by an apparent improvement which is succeeded by a similar episode or episodes. However the infant usually recovers but may develop obstructive hydrocephalus or evidence of neurological damage, or both. Confirmation of the diagnosis is by CT or ultrasound scan which can be used to follow the progression of the haemorrhage.

Management Treatment of both types of intraventricular haemorrhage consists of:

1. Treatment of shock or anaemia by blood transfusion.
2. Attempts at improving ventilation and maintaining an adequate $P\text{O}_2$ and $P\text{CO}_2$.
3. Correction of metabolic acidosis or hyponatraemia.

When there is evidence of the development of hydrocephalus, repeated lumbar punctures may be used to control the ventricular dilatation until it becomes clear whether the block will resolve or the insertion of a valve will be required. Serial scans are the best way of following the progress of the hydrocephalus.

Subarachnoid haemorrhage

Recognition Small bleeds occur in pre-term and term infants, often without any obvious trauma. A clinical distinction between a subarachnoid haemorrhage and meningitis may be impossible, and a lumbar puncture must be performed as well as the rest of the infection screen procedures (p. 193). In some infants both conditions appear to develop at the same time and it is important that a blood-stained cerebrospinal fluid (CSF) should be examined by white cell count, Gram film and culture. A large subarachnoid haemorrhage may present similar symptoms and signs to an acute subdural haematoma (see above) but a subdural tap will produce a few drops of blood-stained fluid or nothing at all.

Management Once meningitis has been excluded, little active treatment is required. There seems no place for surgical intervention with burr holes or craniotomy unless it is obvious that raised intracranial pressure is due to the accumulation of a very large amount of blood. After recovery from the acute stage, obstructive hydrocephalus commonly occurs (see under Intraventricular haemorrhage above).

Haematemesis

1. Within the first 24 hours after birth:
   (a) Vomiting of maternal blood swallowed before delivery occurs in accidental haemorrhage, generally concealed. The diagnosis is usually obvious from the obstetric history, but maternal blood can be identified by Apt's test (Appendix 2) provided that all the blood has not been altered (coffee grounds vomit) by contact with gastric hydrochloric acid. Blood may continue to be passed in the stool for 3 or 4 days after birth (see below);
   (b) Less common causes are oesophageal atresia, duodenal atresia or stenosis.
2. From the second to the seventh day and occasionally much later haemorrhagic disease should be considered (p. 87).
3. During the first week and later the breast-fed infant may vomit blood swallowed during feeds, due usually to a cracked nipple and less commonly to mastitis, papilloma, or an early carcinoma of the breast. As with accidental haemorrhage the vomited blood, if sufficient in amount, can be identified as being of maternal origin, but examination of the mother's breasts and her expressed milk is essential.
4. Haematemesis from hiatus hernia may occur at any time although usually not before the first week. Fresh or altered blood may be brought up. Diagnosis is confirmed by barium swallow.

5. An acute peptic ulcer may develop in a hypoxic or infected infant, or as a result of an indwelling gastric or transpyloric tube, and occasionally as a complication of tolazoline treatment for pulmonary hypertension (persistent fetal circulation; p. 172), or from indomethacin given in an attempt to close the ductus arteriosus in the pre-term infant.
6. Haemoptysis from a massive pulmonary haemorrhage (acute haemorrhagic oedema) (p. 155) may be mistaken for vomited blood, but is usually bright red and frothy.

Blood in the stool

Any of the conditions described above may cause obvious blood in the stool. The stool may consist of a mixture of blood and faecal contents or apparently wholly of blood. Blood passes so rapidly through the infant's intestinal tract that the stool is either red or beetroot colour. In the presence of unaltered blood it is possible to distinguish fetal from maternal blood by Apt's test (Appendix 2). The more important conditions causing blood in the stool, apart from those discussed under haematemesis, are:

1. Haemorrhagic disease without haematemesis (p. 87).
2. Blood mixed with the stool, or fresh blood and mucus, or a loose stool with blood may all be early signs of necrotizing enterocolitis (p. 256) in the small pre-term infant. This is rare before the second day or after the first month.
3. Meckel's diverticulum, volvulus, duplication of the intestine, intussusception, which are all uncommon.
4. Acute bacterial infections of the gastrointestinal tract, usually salmonella or shigella infections; and occasionally due to an enteropathogenic organism, e.g. *Escherichia coli.*
5. Streaks of fresh blood round a formed stool may occur without any obvious cause but are sometimes due to anal fissure or trauma from a rectal thermometer.

Haematuria

In the first 24–48 hours a salmon pink stain on the napkin usually indicates urate crystals. The distinction can easily be made by testing the deposit on the napkin for blood or examining it under the microscope.

Vaginal bleeding (withdrawal bleeding) towards the end of the first week can be mistaken for haematuria when it stains the napkin. The diagnosis is easily made by examination of the vagina.

Genuine haematuria may be due to:

1. Any bleeding (thrombocytopenia) or coagulation disorder (pp. 85–92).
2. Renal vein thrombosis (p. 79).
3. Arterial infarction of the kidney, related to umbilical artery catheterization (p. 310).
4. Trauma from suprapubic puncture.
5. Acute bacterial infection of the renal tract, usually with a malformation such as hydronephrosis.

6. Rare causes are: Wilms' tumour, usually with blood detectable only on microscopy, tyrosinaemia (AR), polycystic disease (infantile form, AR), obstruction of the bladder neck or hydronephrosis, medullary sponge kidney (Emanuel and Aronson, 1974).

Haemoptysis

This may be due to:

1. Massive pulmonary haemorrhage (acute haemorrhagic pulmonary oedema) (p. 155).
2. Staphylococcal pneumonia (rarely).
3. Intrathoracic gastrogenous cyst (Chang *et al.*, 1976).
4. Traumatic intubation of the trachea.

References

Abroms, I.F., McLennan, J.E. and Mandell, F. (1977) Acute subdural haematoma following breech delivery. *American Journal of Diseases of Children*, **131**, 192–194

Chang, S.H., Morrison, L., Shaffner, L. and Crowe, J.E. (1976) Intrathoracic gastrogenous cysts and haemoptysis. *Journal of Pediatrics*, **88**, 594–596

Emanuel, B. and Aronson, N. (1974) Neonatal haematuria. *American Journal of Diseases of Children*, **128**, 204–206

Pape, K.E., Armstrong, D.L. and Fitzhardinge, P.M. (1976) Central nervous system pathology associated with mask ventilation in the very low birth weight infant: a new etiology for intracerebellar haemorrhages. *Pediatrics*, **58**, 473–483

Pitlyk, P.J., Miller, R.H. and Stayura, L.A. (1967) Subdural haematoma of the posterior fossa: report of a case. *Pediatrics*, **40**, 436–439

Volpe, J.J. (1979) Intracranial haemorrhage in the newborn: current understanding and dilemmas. *Neurology (Minneapolis)*, **29**, 632–635

Further reading

Glader, B.E. (1984) Bleeding disorders in the newborn infant. In *Schaffer's Diseases of the Newborn*, 5th edn (eds M.E. Avery and H.W. Taeusch), Saunders, Philadelphia, Chapter 64

Hill, A. and Volpe, J.J. (1986) Intracranial haemorrhage. In *Textbook of Neonatology* (ed. N.R.C. Roberton), Churchill Livingstone, Edinburgh, Chapter 21, (Part V), pp. 559–570

Turner, T.L. (1986) Coagulation disorders in the newborn. In *Textbook of Neonatology* (ed. N.R.C. Roberton), Churchill Livingstone, Edinburgh, Chapter 19 (Part I), pp. 439–448

Chapter 10

Jaundice

Jaundice as an emergency

Three possible emergencies may arise in relation to jaundice:

1. The danger of kernicterus at a critical level of unconjugated bilirubin, irrespective of the cause.
2. Jaundice as a manifestation of an acute septicaemic illness.
3. Jaundice as a manifestation of certain metabolic disorders.

The ways in which these situations may arise are:

1. In the management of acute haemolytic jaundice, commonly rhesus isoimmunization or ABO incompatibility, spherocytic jaundice (AD), glucose-6-phosphate dehydrogenase (G-6PD) (XR) deficiency and other less common forms of red cell abnormality. Many conditions that can cause jaundice in the newborn can be predicted by prenatal testing or anticipated because of a previously affected child.
2. Where jaundice develops unexpectedly within the first 24 hours of life.
3. Rapidly increasing jaundice starting from the second day onwards without previous indication of cause.

Some of the conditions likely to be encountered as a cause of neonatal jaundice are given in Figure 10.1 although not all of these constitute emergencies.

Factors that may contribute to hyperbilirubinaemia and the risk of kernicterus

Particularly in the pre-term infant, severe hyperbilirubinaemia may result from the summation of a number of factors, although each one alone might not cause anything more than a moderate degree of jaundice. It is for this reason, and also because the threshold level of serum bilirubin at which kernicterus can develop is lower in proportion to the degree of prematurity, that the pre-term infant is at much greater risk for kernicterus (see p. 110 for clinical features) than in the term infant.

The most common factors that contribute to jaundice are:

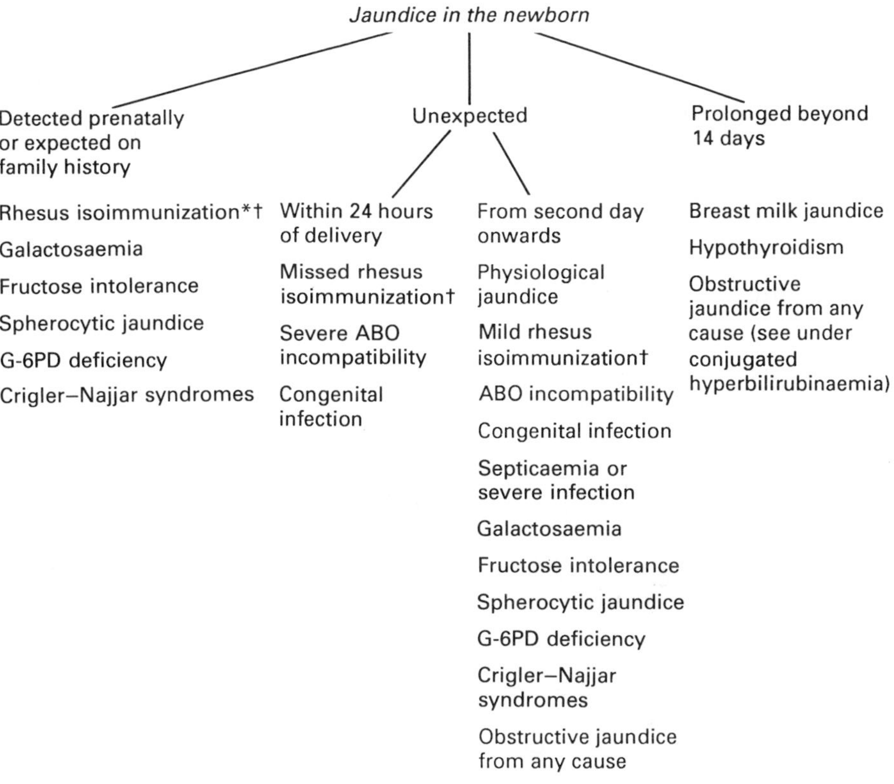

Figure 10.1 Jaundice in the newborn. Conditions that may require emergency treatment are in italic. *Can be detected prenatally. †Also other forms of blood group isoimmunization

1. Pre-term infant.
2. Reabsorption of blood from an enclosed haemorrhage or soft-tissue bruising, and possibly of swallowed blood.
3. Infection.
4. Respiratory distress syndrome and respiratory acidosis.
5. Infant of the diabetic mother.
6. Dehydration and metabolic acidosis.
7. Abnormally high haemoglobin level, as in the plethoric twin in twin-to-twin transfusion or after delayed clamping of the cord.
8. Breast milk in certain cases.
9. Hypothyroidism.
10. Haemolysis from any cause; rhesus and other blood group isoimmunization, ABO incompatibility, spherocytic jaundice, G-6PD deficiency and very rarely sickle-cell disease in the newborn (p. 82).
11. Hypoglycaemia from any cause.

Factors that lower the threshold for the development of kernicterus are:

1. Pre-term infant.
2. Hypoxia and acidosis.

3. Drugs that compete for binding sites for bilirubin: sulphonamides, salicylates, frusemide, ethacrynic acid, parenteral preparations of diazepam containing sodium benzoate* and intralipid.
4. Hypothermia.
5. Infection.
6. Hypoalbuminaemia.

Difficulties in the clinical detection or estimation of jaundice

It is difficult to estimate the degree of jaundice:

1. In artificial light.
2. In pre-term infants with a red skin.
3. In dark-skinned infants.
4. During phototherapy.
5. After phototherapy because the bilirubin in the skin exposed to the light is bleached more than the bilirubin in the circulating plasma.

Jaundice of rapid onset developing unexpectedly within the first 24 hours of life

The most likely causes are:

1. Missed rhesus isoimmunization which may be due to:
   (a) Inadequate antenatal testing;
   (b) Rhesus antibodies developing late in pregnancy; however, this rarely results in severely affected infants;
   (c) Failure to test for antibodies after amniocentesis, fetoscopy, chorionic villus sampling, or spontaneous or therapeutic abortion in a previous pregnancy;
   (d) Failure to screen for unusual antibodies, such as c(ba), Duffy, Kell etc.
   (e) The development of antibodies in a rhesus-positive woman; this may occur after a transfusion, often because of a postpartum haemorrhage, most commonly resulting in antibodies against E, ē or c̄.
2. Unusually severe ABO incompatibility.
3. Chronic intrauterine infection (pp. 179–184).
4. Galactosaemia (p. 288), rarely as early as 24 hours after birth.

Recognition

If there is skin pallor due to anaemia, the development of jaundice is easily detected. Hepatosplenomegaly is common in rhesus isoimmunization but not in ABO incompatibility.

Management (in sequence)

1. Blood is taken from the infant, preferably using the umbilical vein as this makes the specimen more comparable with a cord blood specimen

*Diazemuls (KabiVitrum) 2 ml ampoules 5 mg/ml does not act in this way (see also p. 205).

upon which the predictions of the severity of rhesus disease are based (capillary blood samples usually have a haemoglobin level of about 30 g/l higher than cord or venous blood and therefore may fail to predict some infants who will require exchange transfusion). The blood is tested for haemoglobin, rhesus and ABO group, Coombs' test, serum bilirubin. Where ABO incompatibility appears likely, appropriate testing is performed on the infant's red cells and serum (p. 118). Some blood should be retained for further testing.

2. Blood is taken from the mother for rhesus and ABO grouping and rhesus antibody testing, and is screened for other antibodies and for anti-A or -B haemolysins. Sufficient blood should be retained for cross-matching or other investigations.
3. If an exchange transfusion is not immediately required, serum bilirubin levels should be measured at 4-hourly intervals initially; a rate of rise of 8.5 mmol/l per hour (0.5 mg% per hour) indicates that an exchange transfusion may be required (pp. 119–120).
4. An upper limit that must not be exceeded without doing an exchange transfusion should be fixed, the limit being dependent upon the maturity of the infant and other factors (p. 119).
5. If an exchange transfusion is necessary and the diagnosis is still not known, the first 10–20 ml of the infant's blood removed should be kept for subsequent investigation.

Table 10.1 Indications for phototherapy

Gestation (weeks)	*Serum bilirubin level [μmol/l (mg %)] at which phototherapy should be started*
≤30	150 (8.8)
31–33	170 (10.0)
34–36	260 (15.2)
>37	320 (18.8)

These are guidelines only and should be considered with other factors, e.g. rate of rise, birth weight, presence of bruising, general condition.

6. Phototherapy (Table 10.1) should be started unless an immediate exchange transfusion is required (Table 11.1, p. 117 gives standard indications). In any case phototherapy can be started while blood is being cross-matched.
7. If there is no evidence of blood group isoimmunization or ABO incompatibility, further investigation will be required, particularly for galactosaemia and for chronic intrauterine infection (see below).

Rapidly increasing jaundice starting from the second day onwards without previous indication of cause

The possible causes include those already considered above with additional ones described below. Physiological jaundice in the term infant may develop on the second or third day of life but does not increase rapidly.

1. Physiological jaundice in the pre-term infant with additional factors (p. 103).
2. Septicaemia } In these conditions the infant is ill,
3. Metabolic disorders } with the onset of jaundice.
4. Chronic intrauterine infection (pp. 179–184).
5. Haemolytic anaemias.
6. Disorders of bilirubin glucuronidation (Crigler–Najjar syndrome type I) (AR).

Physiological jaundice in the pre-term infant

Recognition
The presence of one or more of the additional factors listed on p. 000 may convert a mild physiological hyperbilirubinaemia into severe jaundice, requiring an exchange transfusion, or lower the threshold at which this is required. The additional factors are usually obvious but it may be necessary to exclude mild ABO incompatibility in particular; a normal reticulocyte count will exclude this and also other types of haemolytic jaundice, apart from a few cases of G-6PD deficiency.

Septicaemia

Recognition
The onset of the illness is usually sudden, with decreased activity, pallor, poor feeding and apnoeic attacks in the small pre-term infant. Hypothermia is commoner than a rise in temperature. The liver is often moderately enlarged and the jaundice is due mainly to a rise in unconjugated bilirubin; however, time should not be wasted in doing liver function tests, but, immediately a septicaemia is suspected, a complete infection screen (p. 193) should be carried out, including a white cell count.

Metabolic disorders

The two most common conditions to be considered are galactosaemia and fructose intolerance. It should be noted that galactosaemia and possibly fructose intolerance may be accompanied by a septicaemia.

Recognition of galactosaemia and fructose intolerance
For symptoms, diagnosis and management, see pp. 288–291.

Chronic intrauterine infection (pp. 179–184)

Recognition
The infant is rarely very ill but there is a moderate anaemia and usually marked hepatosplenomegaly. Petechiae are common and there are raised purpuric skin lesions in rubella and cytomegalovirus disease. Both fractions of bilirubin are increased. For further details of diagnosis, see p. 180).

Haemolytic jaundice

The haemolytic disorders which develop in the first few days after delivery include rhesus and other blood group isoimmunization and ABO incompatibility, which have already been considered and are also dealt with on pp. 102–104.

Other causes of haemolytic anaemia to be considered are:

1. Spherocytosis (AD).
2. G-6PD deficiency (XR).
3. Pyruvate kinase deficiency (AR) and other less common red cell abnormalities.

Spherocytosis
Although this diagnosis is not easy to confirm in the newborn, parents and sibs should be investigated as they may be affected but unrecognized, and confirmation may be easier by this indirect method. However, in 25% of cases no affected family members can be detected, presumably because the disorder is due to a mutation in the affected infant.

G-6PD deficiency (see also p. 17)

Recognition The Mediterranean and Far Eastern types behave in a similar manner in their response to drugs, infections, acidosis etc. (Table 10.2). Spontaneous haemolysis in the newborn infant occurs in the

Table 10.2 Drugs and other situations that can cause haemolysis in G-6PD-deficient individuals*

Antimalarials Primaquine Pamaquine ?Chloroquine	Sulphones Dapsone Antibiotics Nitrofurantoin Nalidixic acid ?Chloramphenicol
Sulphonamides (most) Includes trimethoprim–sulphamethoxazole mixtures such as Septrin and Bactrim)	Vitamin K analogues except Vit.K_1 (phytomenadione)
	Also, warn about any contact with broad beans (*Vicia faba*): acute infections, especially hepatitis A and pneumonia, may cause haemolysis

*Also HbH disease (unstable haemoglobin).

Mediterranean and Far Eastern types, possibly due to the hypoxia of a normal delivery, but the shortened half-life of the affected red cells contributes to the hyperbilirubinaemia. In the African type, jaundice may occur in the neonatal period due to chemicals in cord applications, possibly menthol (Olowe and Ransome-Kuti, 1980); and occasionally it occurs spontaneously in the term infant.

In the neonatal period in affected infants the maximum bilirubin usually occurs between the second and fifth day of life, while the haemoglobin level may be normal, or as low as 70–80 g/l. A reticulocytosis is usual but not always present. On the blood film, fragmented red cells can be seen, and Heinz bodies may be present in the recovery phase. The definitive diagnostic test is a reduced level of G-6PD in the red cells, but misleadingly high levels may be found in the reticulocytes and regenerated cells in the recovery phase, or obscured if a transfusion has been required. Investigation of other family members may help in the diagnosis.

Pyruvate kinase deficiency
Pyruvate kinase deficiency and other red cell abnormalities are mainly inherited as autosomal recessives, and the diagnosis may require the help of a specialist haematologist.

Disorders of bilirubin glucuronidation: Crigler–Najjar syndromes types I (AR) and II (AR or AD; mode of inheritance uncertain) (Mowat, 1985(i)).

Recognition
These very rare conditions are due to a deficiency of hepatic uridine diphosphoglucuronate transferase (UDP transferase), and present with unconjugated hyperbilirubinaemia without evidence of haemolysis. In type I, jaundice usually develops within 48 hours of birth, while type II has a more gradual onset, during the first week, or later. In the absence of a family history, the diagnosis should be suspected when jaundice continues for longer than 4 weeks, during which the other more common diagnoses should have been excluded. Confirmation of the diagnosis is by assay of UDP transferase on liver biopsy (Mowat, 1985(i)).

Management (in sequence) of rapidly increasing jaundice from the second day onwards, without previous indication as to cause

1. Using the standard criteria (Table 11.1, p. 117), an exchange transfusion may be required; the first 10–20 ml of blood removed from the infant should be retained for further investigation if the diagnosis is not clear.
2. Phototherapy should be started, using the usual criteria (p. 110) if an exchange transfusion is not immediately required. Phototherapy should also be started after an exchange transfusion.
3. If septicaemia is suspected, an infection screen should be done and treatment started with appropriate antibiotics (p. 193). In a severely ill septicaemic infant, an exchange transfusion using fresh blood is often helpful, even if the level of bilirubin does not indicate an exchange transfusion.
4. If a metabolic disorder is suspected, feeds which contain neither lactose, sucrose nor fructose should be given; or temporarily 0.18% sodium chloride in glucose 4% can be given orally. Intravenous fructose should not be given (p. 291). If the infant is severely ill from suspected or proved galactosaemia or fructose intolerance an exchange transfusion should be carried out immediately (see also p. 287). A haemorrhagic tendency should be corrected by intravenous vitamin K_1, with the addition of fresh frozen plasma if required.
5. (a) For rhesus isoimmunization or ABO incompatibility see Chapter 11;

(b) G-6PD deficiency: An exchange transfusion may be required. The parents and other sibs should be investigated and a list of drugs likely to cause haemolysis (Table 10.2) should be given to them and to their family doctor (see also p. 107);
(c) Pyruvate kinase deficiency and other haemolytic anaemias may also require an exchange transfusion in the neonatal period;
(d) Crigler–Najjar types I and II: type I may require an exchange transfusion or may be controlled by phototherapy alone for up to 15 hours per day to maintain the serum bilirubin below 340 μmol/l (20 mg%). Phenobarbitone has no effect on type I, but in type II it will lower the bilirubin level if given in a dose of 5 mg/kg per day (Mowat, 1985(i)).

Prolonged non-obstructive jaundice

This is arbitrarily defined as jaundice lasting longer than 14 days after birth. In many cases the diagnosis has already been made, and the usual clinical problem is that of an infant who appears well and in whom what was thought to be physiological jaundice continues into the third week. The absence of severe anaemia and presence of an enlarged liver or spleen would indicate a chronic infection or a missed haemolytic condition. The two conditions which have to be considered are breast milk jaundice and hypothyroidism.

Breast milk jaundice

Recognition
Obviously confined to infants receiving breast milk, it does not occur when pooled breast milk is used. The condition appears to be due to an undefined substance in the milk of certain mothers and tends to occur in some or all of the infants of such a mother. The level of unconjugated bilirubin seldom rises above a peak of 255 μmol/l (15 mg%) during the second week but jaundice may persist for as long as 5 or 6 weeks and then slowly fades even when breast feeding is continued. Confirmation of the diagnosis can be provided by the rapid fading of the jaundice within 2–3 days of stopping breast feeding and its return if it is restarted; however, this is not a necessary or desirable form of management.

Management
In the term infant no treatment, apart from reassurance of the mother, is required. In the pre-term infant the bilirubin level may go high enough to constitute a risk of kernicterus, and in such circumstances cow's milk or breast milk from another mother or pooled breast milk should be used. In all cases, where screening for hypothyroidism has not been carried out, this diagnosis should be excluded (see below).

Hypothyroidism

Recognition
Neonatal screening for hypothyroidism is now widely practised, and undiagnosed cases should be extremely rare. Apart from infants in whom

hypothyroidism is present at birth, due to overtreatment of the mother with antithyroid drugs or chronic self-treatment with iodides, prolonged jaundice is often the first evidence of hypothyroidism. The bilirubin is usually unconjugated and in the absence of contributory factors the levels reached do not constitute any risk of kernicterus, but occasionally the conjugated fraction is also raised (p. 111). Minor indications of hypothyroidism, once suspicion has been aroused, are sluggish behaviour, slow feeding, constipation and a wrinkled forehead. In the term infant an X-ray of the knee usually shows a delayed skeletal age, with absence of the lower femoral and upper tibial epiphyses. The serum thyroid-stimulating hormone (TSH) level is raised (>10 ml/l) and thyroxine (T_4) is low (<65 mmol/l). In some cases an ileus-like condition develops (p. 251).

Management
Thyroxine should be started using an initial dose of 0.0125 mg daily, increasing after 1 week to 0.025 mg and subsequently to 0.05 mg daily.

Kernicterus

Recognition

The early recognition of kernicterus is important as prompt treatment may prevent permanent brain damage or reduce its severity. The appearance of signs of kernicterus is of course an absolute and urgent indication for exchange transfusion. Unfortunately these symptoms are not very specific, particularly in the small pre-term infant, and the correlation with the level of bilirubin is not exact. Kernicterus should be suspected in any jaundiced infant in whom the following signs and symptoms develop, usually on the third or fourth day in term infants but later in pre-term infants:

1. Hypotonia, poor sucking and decreased activity.
2. Apnoeic attacks.
3. Vomiting.
4. Fits or attacks of rigidity and head retraction.
5. Turning downwards of the eyes.

Phototherapy

Indications

1. Phototherapy should be started at serum bilirubin levels as shown in Table 10.1.
2. Jaundice developing on the first or second day of life, whatever the cause. However, phototherapy will not control jaundice from severe haemolysis where the serum bilirubin level is rising more rapidly than 8.5 μmol/l (0.5 mg%) per hour.
3. After an exchange transfusion in order to make a further transfusion unnecessary or less likely.

Management

1. Both eyes should be shielded, and the reason for this should be explained to the mother. The eyes should be examined at 6-hourly intervals for evidence of infection or trauma to the cornea.

2. The infant's temperature should be recorded every 2 hours.
3. Additional fluids should be given at the rate of 1–2 ml/kg per hour for the term infant and 1–3 ml/kg per hour for pre-term infants. Adequacy of fluid intake should be checked by weighing every 12 hours, and if necessary measuring the osmolality of the urine (this should not exceed 200 mosmol/kg).
4. Phototherapy should not be used for more than 18 hours out of every 24 hours but many units use it continuously over the 24 hours.
5. Serum bilirubin levels should be measured every 12 hours. Attempts to judge the degree of jaundice visually should not be made.
6. Treatment should be stopped when the serum bilirubin has started to fall, but another 12 hours should be allowed before discharging an infant, to see whether the level has started to rise again.
7. If phototherapy has to be used in an infant with a raised level of both unconjugated and conjugated bilirubin (as in severe rhesus isoimmunization), the 'bronze-baby' syndrome may develop, which is alarming but harmless and reversible without treatment.

Conjugated hyperbilirubinaemia

Conjugated hyperbilirubinaemia may be due to:

1. Hepatocellular disease, which results from a variety of disorders (Table 10.3) in which both conjugated and unconjugated fractions of bilirubin are raised. When the level of conjugated bilirubin is high the infant develops a characteristic greenish–yellow colour. Bile-stained urine and pale stools are not always present in hepatocellular disease and, even

Table 10.3 Disorders associated with hepatocellular disease in the neonatal period

Infections	*Disorders*
See Chapter 14	*Metabolic*
Septicaemia (usually Gram-negative organisms)	Galactosaemia (see Chapter 27)
Urinary tract infections (usually Gram-negative organisms)	Fructose intolerance (see Chapter 27)
	Tyrosinaemia
Cytomegalovirus	α_1-Antitrypsin deficiency
Toxoplasmosis	Various storage diseases involving the liver
Rubella	Dubin–Johnson syndrome
Herpes simplex virus	
Coxsackie B viruses	*Endocrine*
Varicella zoster	Hypothyroidism, usually unconjugated hyperbilirubinaemia
Hepatitis B and C	
Listeriosis	Hypopituitarism (may be associated with optic nerve hypoplasia or septo-optic dysplasia (Kaufman *et al.*, 1984)
Malaria	
Chagas' disease	
	Hypoadrenalism, including adrenal hyperplasia
	Miscellaneous
	Chromosomal abnormalities
	Prolonged TPN (p. 335)
	Idiopathic
	50–80% cases (Howard and Mowat, 1983)

Table 10.4 Continued or progressive obstructive jaundice

Disease	*Clinical and other features*
Hepatitis B, C and non-A, non-B	Mother a carrier (mainly of Mediterranean, Asian or Far Eastern origin); also in recipients of repeated transfusions (haemoglobinopathies) and in i.v. drug users
Extrahepatic biliary atresia	Sometimes associated with situs inversus, absence of the inferior vena cava, polysplenia syndrome, ventricular septal defects or intestinal malrotation (Mowat, 1987(i).
Choledochal cyst	Cystic mass in right hypochondrium (p. 113)
Spontaneous perforation of bile duct	Ascites and bile-stained herniae (p. 114)
Intrahepatic biliary hypoplasia	May be familial, associated with chromosomal abnormalities or with biliary atresia. Alagille's syndrome (Alagille *et al.*, 1975) is sometimes familial, with prominent forehead, saddle-shaped or straight nose in same plane, in profile, as the forehead, small pointed chin, systolic murmur
Inspissated bile syndrome	In infants severely affected by Rhesus isoimmunization

when they are present, this does not indicate complete obstruction. Fluctuation in the colour of the stools indicates an incomplete obstruction.

2. Continued or progressive obstructive jaundice. Some of the more common causes of continued progressive obstructive jaundice are shown in Table 10.4.

Recognition

Infants with conjugated hyperbilirubinaemia are rarely jaundiced at birth, with the exception of some infants who are severely affected by rhesus isoimmunization and are developing the inspissated bile syndrome. Hepatosplenomegaly is a non-specific finding.

Jaundice with acute onset

Depending upon the cause, the onset is usually within the first 4 weeks of life; in galactosaemia or fructose intolerance the jaundice may develop quite suddenly, within 1–2 days of the introduction of galactose (as lactose) or fructose (as sucrose) in the feeds. In Gram-negative septicaemias or urinary tract infections (or both combined) the jaundice usually develops rapidly at any time during the neonatal period (and occasionally after the age of 4 weeks), but a more chronic picture may be seen, with evidence of obstructive jaundice.

Haemorrhage

Haemorrhage from liver damage may occur in the acutely ill child, or from malabsorption of vitamin K, or from a combination of both factors.

Bleeding from the umbilicus or from injection sites, or vomiting and fits with a bulging fontanelle may be the first signs of hepatic disease and may occur with a moderate degree of jaundice which has not been taken very seriously.

Continued or progressive obstructive jaundice (Table 10.4)
In this group it is important to distinguish between conditions which cannot be treated surgically (the various forms of hepatitis, α_1-antitrypsin deficiency, intrahepatic biliary hypoplasia) and those that can be relieved by operation (extrahepatic biliary atresia, choledochal cyst, spontaneous perforation of the bile duct). For the diagnosis of progressive obstructive jaundice, ultrasound, the ^{131}I-labelled Rose Bengal faecal excretion test, and liver biopsy are the most useful investigations, usually followed by laparotomy.

Management

The first priority is to identify those conditions that require urgent treatment.

Jaundice with acute onset

1. The management of two important causes, galactosaemia and fructose intolerance, is considered in Chapter 27.
2. Infections, both transplacental and postnatal, are dealt with in Chapter 14.

Haemorrhage
If this is severe and likely to be due to hepatocellular damage, fresh frozen plasma or fresh whole blood should be given immediately. With malabsorption of vitamin K, the prothrombin time returns to normal within 4–6 hours of a parenteral dose of vitamin K, but fresh frozen plasma or fresh whole blood may be required when it is not possible to wait for the effect of vitamin K.

Continued or progressive obstructive jaundice
The investigation and treatment of extrahepatic biliary atresia do not constitute an emergency but it should be noted that the results of anastomotic operations (e.g. the Kasai procedure) are not good if surgery is delayed beyond 8 weeks from birth. However, choledochal cyst and spontaneous perforation of the bile duct may present as emergencies (see below) in the neonatal period.

Some conditions with conjugated hyperbilirubin which require special attention

Choledochal cyst

Recognition The onset may be in the neonatal period and it is important that this diagnosis should be considered at an early stage. Obstructive jaundice develops but is intermittent or varies in intensity. A mass may be palpable in the right hypochondrium. In infants, abdominal distension, fever and vomiting may be additional features. The most helpful initial investigation is ultrasound.

Management The most commonly used operation is a choledochojejunostomy or choledochoduodenostomy.

Spontaneous perforation of the bile duct

Bile peritonitis develops after a leak at the junction of the cystic and common hepatic ducts.

Recognition Initially, there is mild jaundice, failure to gain weight and vomiting. The stools become pale and the urine contains bile. Abdominal distension develops, due to the biliary ascites; hydroceles, umbilical or inguinal herniae may develop and are stained a greenish–yellow colour (Mowat, 1987(ii)).

Management The diagnosis of biliary ascites is confirmed by the aspiration of clear brown fluid. Laparotomy and operative cholangiography will demonstrate the site of the leak. The perforation should be repaired; if there is also an obstruction to the common bile duct a cholecystojejunostomy will be required.

Cholestasis with prolonged total parenteral nutrition

Recognition After prolonged total parenteral nutrition (TPN), a mild conjugated hyperbilirubinaemia develops, with dark urine, but rarely with pale stools. The liver may be moderately enlarged.

Management If possible, TPN should be stopped as soon as jaundice develops. This usually results in the resolution of the jaundice, although the bilirubin level may take some weeks or months to return to normal. Although in most cases the condition appears to be benign, there is a possibility of hepatic cirrhosis and death from liver failure (South, 1987).

Cholestasis associated with hypopituitarism

Recognition The condition may be easily recognized if it accompanies optic nerve hypoplasia or septo-optic dysplasia, with wandering nystagmus (Kaufman *et al.*, 1984). Jaundice, with a moderately raised level of conjugated bilirubin, may develop in the first few weeks of life. The liver is moderately enlarged. Hypoglycaemia is common. The diagnosis of the neurological disorder can usually be made on the clinical features, or a CT scan if there is septo-optic dysplasia with absent septum pellucidum. Investigation shows hypothalamic hypopituitarism.

Management In infancy, treatment with L-thyroxine and cortisone is adequate to abolish the jaundice and prevent hypoglycaemia.

Dubin–Johnson syndrome (probably AR)

Recognition Jaundice may develop shortly after birth or much later. The bilirubin level fluctuates but is usually around 40–90 μmol/l (2.3–5.2 mg%), 50% being conjugated (Mowat, 1985(ii)); the liver is not enlarged. Diagnosis is made on liver biopsy; the liver tissue is black and the histological picture shows characteristic dark granules around the central vein.

Management No treatment is required.

References

Alagille, D., Odièvre, M., Gautier, M. and Dommergues, J.P. (1975) Hepatic ductulate hypoplasia associated with characteristic facies, vertebral malformations, retarded physical, mental and sexual development, and cardiac murmur. *Journal of Pediatrics*, **86**, 63–71

Howard, E.R. and Mowat, A.P. (1983) Hepatobiliary disorders in infancy. In *Recent Advances in Hepatology*, No. 1 (eds H.C. Thomas and R.N.M. Macsween), Churchill Livingstone, Edinburgh, p. 154

Kaufman, F.R., Costin, G., Thomas, D.W., Sinatra, F.R., Roet, F. and Neustein, H.B. (1984) Neonatal cholestasis and hypopituitarism. *Archives of Disease in Childhood*, **59**, 787–789

Mowat, A.P. (1985) Congenital abnormalities of bilirubin metabolism. *Hospital Update*, **11**, (i) pp. 921–923, (ii) p. 928

Mowat, A.P. (1987) *Liver Disorders in Childhood*, 2nd edition, Butterworths, London, (i) p. 74, (ii) pp. 343–344

Olowe, S.A. and Ransome-Kuti, O. (1980) The risk of jaundice in glucose-6-phosphate dehydrogenase deficient babies exposed to menthol. *Acta Paediatrica Scandinavica*, **69**, 341–345

South, M. (1987) Feeding sick babies. *Care of the Critically Ill*, **3**, 67–69

Further reading

Mowat, A.P. (1985) Congenital abnormalities of bilirubin metabolism. *Hospital Update*, **11**, 921–930

Mowat, A.P. (1987) *Liver Disorders in Childhood*, 2nd edition, Butterworths, London

Wennberg, R.D. (1986) Bilirubin physiology. In *Textbook of Neonatology* (ed. N.R.C. Roberton), Churchill Livingstone, Edinburgh, Chapter 18 (Part I), pp. 383–393

Willoughby, M.L.N. (1977) *Paediatric Haematology*, Churchill Livingstone, Edinburgh

Chapter 11

Haemolytic disease, including exchange transfusion

Rhesus incompatibility

Despite a 15% incidence of rhesus negativity in the population, rhesus incompatibility and subsequent rhesus isoimmunization have become rare in the Western World due to the rhesus isoimmunization prevention programme. Despite this, although rhesus isoimmunization is no longer common, it remains a significant risk factor for handicap and requires detailed consideration.

Recognition

Prenatally

All rhesus-negative women should be screened for rhesus antibodies early in pregnancy and from time to time throughout pregnancy. Rhesus-negative women found to have antibodies should be referred to a tertiary perinatal centre because amniocentesis has to be carried out serially during the pregnancy to gauge the degree to which the fetus is affected, to provide optimal prenatal care, possibly including intrauterine transfusion, and to determine the safest time and route of delivery. Rhesus-negative women who do not have antibodies should receive prophylactically passive rhesus anti-D antibody at around 28 weeks and after delivery to prevent the development of active immunization.

The indications for prenatal treatment (p. 26) are as follows:

1. A history of previous severely affected infants.
2. Sonographic evidence of ascites in the fetus, which indicates a haemoglobin level of <40 g/l.

It should be noted that Liley's method of spectrophotometric measurement of the deviation of optical density at 450 nm due to bilirubin in the amniotic fluid is reasonably reliable in the third trimester, less so in the second trimester, and can be misleading between 18 and 25 weeks (Rodeck and Letsky, 1989).

At delivery

The infant may have the following clinical appearances:

1. Apparently normal with hepatosplenomegaly.

2. Jaundice developing in the first 24 hours.
3. Gross hepatosplenomegaly and pallor; such infants may present some resuscitation problems at delivery due to severe anaemia, and may develop very severe jaundice in the first few hours of life.
4. Isoimmune hydrops with severe pallor, generalized oedema, pleural effusion and ascites – these infants are likely to be difficult to resuscitate, requiring emergency abdominal paracentesis and thoracocentesis before they will respond. Intubation is often very difficult because of inability to extend the head due to swelling around the neck and oedema of the airway.

Confirmation of the diagnosis and prediction of severity

Confirmation of the diagnosis of rhesus isoimmunization depends on the results of blood group, bilirubin and Coombs' tests, and haemoglobin and reticulocyte count, carried out preferably on cord blood, as this has specific predictive value. Table 11.1 gives the accepted criteria for management in term infants in whom there are no other contributory factors.

Table 11.1 Classification of infants by means of cord blood results

Rhesus group	*Coombs' test*	*Haemoglobin* (g/l)	*Serum bilirubin* (μmol/l (mg%))	*Category*	*Treatment*
Negative	Negative	Not required	Not required	Unaffected	None
Positive	Negative	Not required	Not required	Unaffected	None
Positive	Positive	>140 and rising	50 (3) or less	Mild	Observe and repeat bilirubin test at 4 hours and at intervals if jaundice develops
Positive	Positive	70–140 and rising	>50 (>3)	Moderate to severe	Exchange transfusion within 4–6 hours
Positive	Positive	<70 or clinically hydropic	>50 (>3)	Very severe	Modified exchange

From Whitfield and Black (1987).

Problems in the interpretation of cord blood results

1. A poor cord sample may give a falsely low haemoglobin reading, due to haemolysis, clotting or the inclusion of Wharton's jelly.
2. A false negative rhesus result and a false negative direct Coombs' test may occur in some severely affected infants and following intrauterine transfusions.
3. If maternal plasmal exchange has been used to control maternal antibody level prenatally, the predictive value of the cord results is not well established, particularly in infants where intrauterine transfusion has been used in addition. In this circumstance, some infants are still severely affected, while others, despite being rhesus positive, appear to have very mild disease. Present evidence suggests that plasmaphaeresis is rarely effective in reducing the risk to the fetus.

Assessment of an affected infant in the absence of a cord blood specimen
The tests indicated above should be carried out on a venous blood sample and sequential bilirubin estimations should be plotted against time to determine the rate of rise and timing of exchange transfusion, if necessary (p. 119).

Management

Supportive treatment
Steps should be taken to reduce the contribution made by other factors likely to add to the severity of hyperbilirubinaemia (p. 103).

Phototherapy (p. 110)
This should never be relied upon to control completely the rise in serum bilirubin level in severe rhesus isoimmunization but may reduce the number of exchange transfusions required and can sometimes avoid the need for exchange transfusion in mild cases.

Exchange transfusion
For exchange transfusion details, see pp. 119–130.

ABO incompatibility

ABO isoimmunization occurs in mother–baby pairs who are ABO incompatible and in whom the mother has anti-A or anti-B haemolysins. These haemolysins are IgG and therefore cross the placenta. The most common situation is where the mother is group O and the baby is group A, although other combinations can occur. In general ABO isoimmunization is not as severe as rhesus isoimmunization; it usually runs a shorter course and rarely causes jaundice in the first 24 hours. Although the degree of jaundice is rarely severe enough to require exchange transfusion, occasionally very severe cases are encountered and exchange transfusion may be required in pre-term infants with ABO incompatibility, and in term infants with other associated factors aggravating the severity of jaundice (p. 103).

Recognition

The infant has a normal haemoglobin or mild anaemia with a mild reticulocytosis. Anti-A or anti-B haemolysins can be detected in maternal serum or coated on to the infant's red cells. The indirect Coombs' test on the baby is usually positive, reflecting free haemolysins in the serum, while the direct Coombs' test is usually negative, but is sometimes positive in severe cases.

Management

1. Phototherapy: This is effective in the majority of cases (p. 110).
2. Exchange transfusion may be required in severe cases and low-birth-weight infants. The blood to be used should be of the same rhesus group

as the baby, but should be of group O washed packed cells resuspended in fresh frozen plasma from AB blood. This eliminates the inclusion of IgM anti-A and -B during the exchange transfusion. Blood used for exchange transfusions should be from donors screened for cytomegalovirus (CMV).

Isoimmunization may also occasionally occur in relation to other rare blood groups, such as rhesus factors other than D (e.g. c̄, Kell, Duffy etc.). These are not discussed further here as the management is the same, except that the fetus suffering from anti-Kell disease has depressed erythropoiesis, rather than haemolysis, and therefore predictions of severity based on bilirubin levels in the amniotic fluid are misleading (Rodeck and Letsky, 1989).

Exchange transfusion (double volume)

Indications

Although exchange transfusion is usually carried out for hyperbilirubinaemia, the technique may also be indicated in acute poisoning, inborn errors of metabolism, septicaemia, sclerema, polycythaemia with hyperviscosity syndrome, and in cases of severe anaemia with heart failure, where the infant is incapable of tolerating any further circulatory volume load.

An exchange transfusion is a potentially dangerous procedure involving major fluid shifts and metabolic disturbance in the infant, and carries a significant morbidity rate, and a 1–2% incidence of sudden unexpected cardiac arrest even in experienced hands.

Indications for exchange transfusion for hyperbilirubinaemia are:

1. Rhesus isoimmunization based on cord blood predictions.
2. Indications from postnatal blood samples based on:
   (a) The serum bilirubin level exceeds an absolute critical value (see below);
   (b) The prediction that the serum bilirubin level will exceed the critical value within 4 hours;
   (c) The rate of rise of serum bilirubin based on three estimations is greater than 8.5 μmol/l (greater than 0.5 mg%) per hour or as below;
   (d) The predictive chart of Allen and Diamond (1958) (Figures 11.1 and 11.2).

One commonly accepted set of critical values at different gestational ages for exchange transfusion (Swyer, 1975) is given in Table 11.2.

Some consider that, even in the smallest infants, there is little point in carrying out exchange transfusion below a bilirubin level of 250 μmol/l (15 mg%). It is generally assumed that pre-term infants and infants who have suffered hypoxia, hypoglycaemia or other serious illnesses are at greater risk for the development of kernicterus. Although the above guidelines are considered safe, they are not based on sound scientific evidence and there is, at present, considerable debate regarding the pathogenesis of kernicterus and what constitutes an appropriate clinical

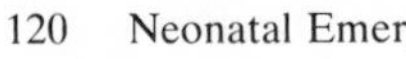

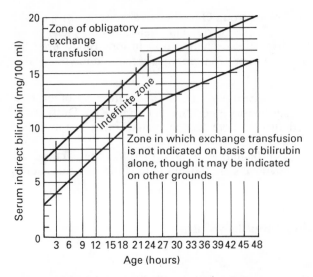

Figure 11.1 Guide to the use of serum indirect bilirubin as the sole criterion for exchange transfusion in mature infants. Note: 20 mg/100 ml = 340 μmol/l. Reproduced from Allen and Diamond (1958) with permission of the authors and publishers

Serum bilirubin (total) (μmol/l)

mg/100 ml	μmol/l
23.4	400
20.5	350
17.6	300
14.6	250
11.7	200
8.8	150
5.9	100
2.9	50
1.8	30
1.5	25
1.2	20
0.9	15
0.6	10
0.3	5
	0

Conversion:

$$\frac{\mu mol/l}{17.1} = mg/100\ ml$$

Figure 11.2 SI unit conversion for serum bilirubin. Reproduced from Bold and Wilding (1975) with the permission of the authors and publishers

Table 11.2 Critical levels of bilirubin indicating exchange transfusion

Gestational age	*Bilirubin level*	
At term	340 μmol/l	(20 mg%)
At 36 weeks	300 μmol/l	(18 mg%)
At 34 weeks	270 μmol/l	(16 mg%)
At 32 weeks	240 μmol/l	(14 mg%)
At 28–32 weeks	200 μmol/l	(12 mg%)

The bilirubin levels given here refer to unconjugated bilirubin only (Swyer 1975).

response to a given serum bilirubin level. Indeed, in North America, possible medicolegal vulnerability may be a more important factor in determing when an exchange transfusion should be carried out than the precision of the data currently available. It must also be recognized that the efficiency in removing bilirubin at exchange transfusion is dependent on the difference in bilirubin level between the donor and the baby's blood. Exchange transfusion below 200 μmol/l (12 mg%) may cause an almost undetectable drop in the bilirubin level over the 6 hours following the exchange transfusion, which may be immediately abolished if there is much haemolysis of the donor blood during the procedure.

Clinical evidence of kernicterus irrespective of the level of serum bilirubin
Worrying signs in a jaundiced infant are lethargy, temperature instability, apnoea, convulsions, opisthotonic posturing and signs which could be confused with infection.

Contraindications to a double-volume exchange transfusion

A double-volume exchange transfusion should not be done initially in hydropic infants or in those who are severely anaemic (cord blood haemoglobin level 70 g/l) with a central venous pressure >12 cm. In such cases a partial (single-volume) exchange should be carried out.

Blood requirements for exchange transfusion

Blood
Most blood banks now provide packed cells from citrate phosphate dextrose (CPD) blood washed and reconstituted with fresh frozen plasma to a haematocrit of around 0.6. This preparation is less hyperosmolar than acid citrate dextrose (ACD) blood and provides a lower acid and potassium load. Blood to be used for an exchange transfusion should have been screened for CMV before use.

Whole concentrated or packed cells
If whole blood is provided, some of the supernatant plasma should be removed before use and the blood should preferably be no more than 48 hours old and certainly less than 5 days old. Using old blood can cause a serious deterioration in the baby's condition; old blood also has a high potassium level, which is potentially dangerous.

Blood group
The blood should be cross-matched against the mother's serum and should be of the same ABO group as the infant and rhesus negative in all cases of rhesus isoimmunization and all rhesus-negative infants requiring exchange transfusion for other reasons. In an emergency, group O rhesus-negative blood can be used irrespective of the infant's ABO group, provided that cross-matching is satisfactory.

Warming of the blood
The blood should be warmed during the exchange transfusion, using a commercial warmer or passed through a heating coil in a water bath at 37°C.

Volume of blood to be exchanged
In infants with hyperbilirubinaemia, normally a double-volume (180 ml/kg body weight) exchange transfusion should be carried out. As exchange transfusion is an exponential washout procedure, however, the first half of the exchange transfusion achieves most of the intended beneficial effects and in infants who do not tolerate the procedure well, a decision may have to be made to stop it after 85–100 ml/kg to minimize the risk to the infant.

Albumin loading
Although there is some theoretical benefit in loading a jaundiced baby with albumin before exchange transfusion in order to attempt to bind more bilirubin, a number of studies have shown no apparent benefit.

Preparation

Equipment
A complete list of the equipment is given in Table 11.3. It is important that the infant is nursed in a good light, preferably under a radiant overhead warmer, unless of extremely low birth weight and connected to a cardiorespiratory monitor.

Infant's condition
The condition of the infant should be improved as much as possible before the exchange transfusion, particularly by the correction of any blood gas abnormalities by ventilatory support; if it is anticipated that the infant will deteriorate with the handling necessary to carry out the exchange transfusion, prophylactic ventilation before the start of the transfusion should be considered. Feeding should be stopped 4 hours before the exchange transfusion and the stomach should be emptied by nasogastric aspiration.

Assistance
At least one assistant should be present to record the progress of the exchange transfusion and to confirm the cumulative blood volumes removed and transfused and to monitor the infant's response. Both operators should be aware of the possibility of unexpected cardiac arrest and should have resuscitation equipment readily at hand.

Table 11.3 Equipment for exchange transfusion

Equipment	*Drugs/intravenous fluids/ containers*	*Sterile equipment*	*Sterile instruments*
1. Resuscitation equipment	1. Blood; one or two units of semipacked cells of appropriately cross-matched blood	1. Two 20 ml syringes*	1. Four pairs mosquito forceps
2. Suitable environment for the infant: incubator/operating table/radiant heated intensive care cot	2. Heparinized saline (1 unit per ml 0.9% NaCl)	2. One four-way stopcock, or two three-way stopcocks*	2. One pair of dissecting forceps (fine, untoothed)
3. Intravenous stand with space for two bottles	3. Sodium bicarbonate 8.4% or 5%, 10 ml ampoules	3. Two adult blood giving sets*	3. One pair stitch holding forceps
4. Cardiorespiratory monitor electrodes and leads	4. Lignocaine 1% (if umbilical cutdown is required)	4. One extension tubing for waste*	4. One umbilical probe
5. Adequate light	5. Haematology blood tubes	5. Two umbilical catheters, 5 and 8 FG*	5. Four towel clips
6. Electronic thermometer with rectal and skin probe	6. Serum blood tubes	6. Sterile towels with central hole and gauze swabs *	6. One scalpel and blade
7. Clock	7. Sterile universal container (for catheter tip)	7. Two sterile antiseptic containers*	7. One pair of fine scissors
8. Blood heater or water bath at 37°C	8. Antiseptic	8. Two gowns	8. 2-o silk suture on fine cutting needle (for purse string suture)
9. Adult urine collection bag or other receptacle for blood waste*		9. Gloves, sizes $6^{1/2}$–8	9. One ruler with centimetre graduations*

*These items are contained in the usual disposable exchange transfusion packs.

Immobilization
The infant's limbs should be gently restrained to prevent dislodgement of the umbilical catheter.

Apparatus
Disposable exchange transfusion sets are the safest and most convenient to use. A supply of heparinized saline (0.9% NaCl) should be available for rinsing out the tubing and syringes to prevent clotting (1 unit of heparin per ml in saline).

Technique

Standard method: umbilical vein catheterization (see also p. 310 for other indications)

Preparation of the infant

1. The infant should be immobilized gently by all four limbs, with the hips abducted at 45°. The infant should then be connected to a cardiorespiratory monitor, and intubated if respiratory problems are anticipated. All this can be done in an incubator, but is easier under a radiant overhead heater.
2. The operator should scrub up, put on gown and gloves. The syringe should be connected to the flushing solution (saline with 1.0 unit of heparin/ml), to the three-way stopcock and catheter, and flushed through with the heparinized saline to exclude air bubbles.

Insertion of the catheter

1. A piece of cord tape is loosely knotted around the base of the cord and the umbilical cord divided about 2.5 cm above its junction with the abdominal wall. A 5, 6 or 8 FG (French gauge) catheter with an end hole is connected to a three-way stopcock and a 10 ml syringe filled with heparinized saline and rinsed through to eliminate all air bubbles. The umbilical vein is identified and the catheter advanced a predetermined distance up the umbilical vein to bring the tip into the region of the inferior vena cava above the diaphragm (Figure 11.3). If the catheter goes the full distance it is likely that the tip is in the inferior vena cava above the diaphragm or is just into the right atrium; this is the ideal position ('high position'). If the catheter will not go the required distance but blood comes back, the catheter is probably in one of the veins of the liver. It is sometimes possible to withdraw the catheter a little and to manipulate it into the inferior vena cava, but this is not usually possible. Once a free flow of blood is obtained the position of the catheter should be confirmed by X-ray or ultrasound. The catheter should then be tied in using tape. It is important to realize that with the tip of the catheter above the diaphragm a sudden inspiratory effort by the infant will lead to a sizable venous air embolism if the catheter is permitted to be open to air at atmospheric pressure at any of its connections. It is possible to measure central venous pressure during the procedure using the umbilical vein catheter, but the risk of air

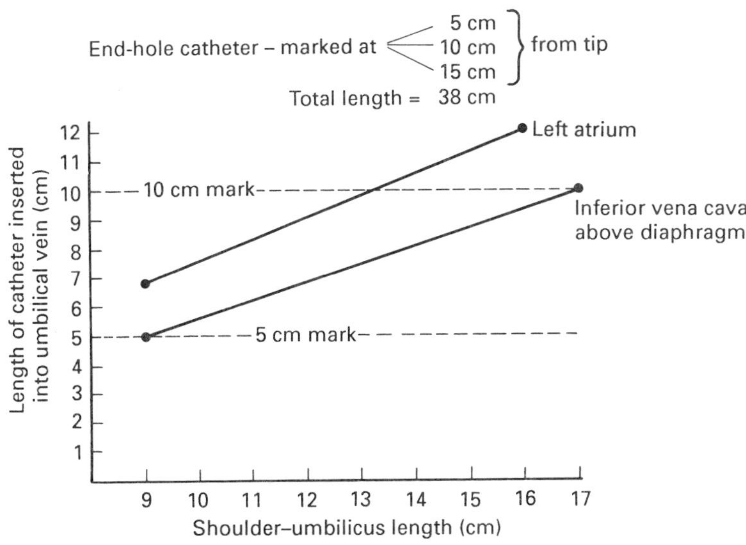

Figure 11.3 An umbilical vein catheterization guide. Modified from Swyer (1975) with the permission of the author and publishers

embolism must be carefully weighed. Central venous pressure should be within 5–8 cm. If the pressure is much higher than this, a partial exchange transfusion may be indicated. It may not be possible to get the tip of the catheter into the inferior vena cava because, as the catheter is advanced, it tends to go into the liver every time. In this situation a low catheter position may have to be accepted. The best low catheter position is about 2 cm further in than the point at which blood is easily obtained during insertion of the umbilical venous catheter.

2. A 10 ml rather than 20 ml syringe is preferable because the volume and pressure variation in the right atrium and the consequent fluctuations in blood pressure are less. The use of a smaller syringe reduces the temptation to proceed too fast. However, using a small syringe makes the dead space of the catheter and stopcock more significant.
3. An initial blood sample should be retained for haemoglobin, bilirubin and any other investigations which may be required, particularly if the reason for the severe jaundice is not yet established.
4. Blood pH: if washed resuspended red cells made up with fresh frozen plasma is the blood source used for the exchange transfusion, it is likely that no manipulation of pH will be required. If the initial pH, however, is less than 7.20, the acidaemia should be partly corrected by injecting 5 mmol $NaHCO_3$ into the blood bag.
5. Calcium gluconate is contraindicated because it is a potentially dangerous drug which has no lasting effect on the infant's ionized

calcium level. There is little excursion in the baby's serum calcium level if citrate phosphate dextrose blood is used. Boluses of calcium gluconate up the umbilical vein may produce a frightening bradycardia. There is no indication for giving digoxin, but frusemide 1 mg/kg i.v. may be used in hydropic infants or those with a high central venous pressure. Infants receiving antibiotics should have the appropriate amount added to the donor blood, to produce the desired blood level in the baby, otherwise the antibiotics will be washed out of the circulation during the exchange transfusion.

6. Duration of the procedure: an exchange transfusion should not be completed in less than 1–1.5 hours in order to produce the maximum removal of bilirubin. An infant will tolerate a slow gentle procedure which produces slower and less marked fluid shifts and fluctuations in body chemistry rather than a more rapid procedure.
7. At the end of the transfusion, the umbilical vein catheter should be removed and the vein occluded by a purse string suture around the base of the cord unless another transfusion is anticipated within the next 6 hours. The tip of the catheter should be sent for culture.

Alternative techniques for access to the venous system

1. If there is difficulty passing the catheter past the umbilical ring, this may be due to clots in the vein which can sometimes be sucked out by the syringe on the end of the catheter. Difficulty may also be encountered because of folding or narrowing of the vein. If this is so, the vein can usually be entered above the umbilical stump, just before it passes upwards towards the liver. There are two approaches:
   (a) A vertical incision is made at 12 o'clock in the funnel of fibrous tissue at the base of the cord and the cut extended upwards for 2–3 cm into the skin of the abdomen. With gentle traction on the cord the vein in its upward course usually becomes obvious. The vein is dissected free at its uppermost part and a 45° incision is made with fine pointed scissors. The catheter can usually be passed upwards through the opening without any difficulty; or
   (b) A crescentic incision is made 1–2 cm above the umbilicus and the underlying fascia dissected until the vein is identified. This dissection is not easy, since the peritoneum lies immediately beneath the vein and may be opened inadvertently. If a small opening is inadvertently made in the peritoneum, however, it can be easily sutured without appealing for surgical aid.
2. Use of the saphenous vein. This should only be used when all other approaches to the umbilical vessels have failed or in an older child in whom the umbilical vessels are not available and the arteriovenous exchange transfusion route has proved impossible. A horizontal incision is made parallel to, but about 1 cm below, the inguinal fold, medial to the femoral artery. The vein passes through the fascia at this point and joins the femoral vein. The saphenous vein is very small and a smaller than usual size of catheter may be required. The catheter should be passed up into the inferior vena cava in the usual way. Swelling of the leg is not uncommon after this procedure but appears to resolve without

any evidence of permanent venous obstruction. The main danger of the saphenous vein approach is of uncontrollable venous oozing due to damage to the vein inside the fascia.

Arteriovenous exchange transfusion

With this method blood is withdrawn from an artery and returned to a major vein. The advantage of this procedure is that the umbilical vein is not used and, if the blood is withdrawn from the artery at the same rate as it is injected into the vein, there is no net circulating blood volume change and less fluctuation in central venous pressure and blood pressure. This may be of particular importance in low-birth-weight infants where blood pressure fluctuations are directly transmitted to the brain due to lack of autoregulation of cerebral blood flow, and may increase the risk of intraventricular haemorrhage and periventricular leucomalacia.

The site for arterial blood withdrawal may be the umbilical artery if there is already an umbilical arterial catheter in place, or may be a radial or posterior tibial artery. This may be cannulated using transillumination by someone experienced in this procedure (Chapter 29). It is usually possible to insert a 21 or 22 FG Teflon venous catheter (e.g. Jelco or Abbcath) into a suitable vein on the back of the hand or into the long saphenous vein at the ankle. Withdrawals and infusions are carried out by two separate operators who synchronize their actions. Care must be taken to rinse out the arterial line with heparinized saline periodically to prevent clotting. If venous and arterial access can be achieved, this technique is a satisfactory alternative to central exchange transfusion by the standard method, and is more desirable than the use of the alternative routes described above. With the arteriovenous exchange transfusion method, care must be taken not to carry out the procedures too fast, because this may diminish the efficacy in removing bilirubin and increase the amount of haemolysis. There are no clear data in the literature comparing the relative risks of necrotizing enterocolitis using the standard or arteriovenous methods.

Complications of exchange transfusion

Insertion of the umbilical venous catheter

1. Bleeding from accidental disconnection.
2. Air embolism (see p. 125).
3. Perforation of the left atrium (through the foramen ovale) causing cardiac tamponade.
4. Perforation through the vein into the peritoneum, causing shock and haemoperitoneum. No blood can be obtained from the catheter, the position of which should be checked by a lateral X-ray of the abdomen.

Potential problems during exchange transfusion

1. Arrhythmias are not uncommon during exchange transfusions, more commonly if the catheter tip is in the right atrium. Transfusion with

inadequately warmed or old blood with a low pH or a high potassium level close to the sinoatrial node frequently causes worrying arrhythmias. In addition, even in the best circumstances, there is a 1–2% risk of sudden unexpected cardiac arrest during exchange transfusion. It is important that staff involved in doing exchange transfusions are aware of this and that all appropriate resuscitatory equipment is immediately available.
2. If the umbilical venous catheter tip is above the diaphragm, it is potentially hazardous to measure central venous pressure without a closed system. If the Luer end of the catheter is disconnected and held up to gauge central venous pressure and the baby gasps, air will be sucked up the umbilical catheter resulting in a massive and potentially fatal air embolism.

Care after exchange transfusion

1. The baby's cardiorespiratory status must be monitored for 2–4 hours after the exchange transfusion, and, if an umbilical catheter has been used, the catheter site must be observed for bleeding.
2. A post-exchange blood sample for measurement of bilirubin and haemoglobin level or haematocrit should be sent 1 hour after the end of the exchange transfusion.
3. The clinical condition leading to exchange transfusion must be followed to assess the effect of the procedure and to obtain an early indication if the procedure will need to be repeated. Most frequently this involves monitoring of bilirubin and haematocrit levels. Repeated exchange transfusions may be required if there is a rapid rise in bilirubin level post-exchange. If the exchange transfusion was required for jaundice, maximal phototherapy should be continued.
4. The baby should be fed within 2 hours of the end of the exchange transfusion, unless there are contraindications to feeding, as this will encourage maintenance of a normal blood glucose level and passage of stool. In difficult cases of severe jaundice, consideration should be given to changing to a bottle feed for 48 hours in babies who are breast fed.
5. Exchange transfusion produces a major and acute disturbance in the cardiovascular and biochemical status of the infant in addition to the desired effects. The clinically more important of these complications are considered below.
6. In cases of rhesus isoimmunization, follow up should include weekly haemoglobin or haematocrit measurement till 8 weeks of age. These infants should be started on folic acid supplements before discharge.

Early complications of exchange transfusion

1. Hypoglycaemia is a significant risk in the first hours after exchange transfusion. There is a high concentration of glucose in fresh blood bank blood, and the baby's blood glucose increases during the exchange transfusion resulting in insulin production. When the

exchange transfusion ends, the glucose infusion rate drops precipitously but insulin production falls more slowly, resulting in a tendency to hypoglycaemia. Infants with rhesus isoimmunization have pancreatic islet cell hyperplasia. So also do infants of diabetic mothers who are more likely to have exchange transfusions because they tend to develop jaundice and are likely to get hyperviscosity syndrome. In these infants therefore there is a risk of significant sustained hypoglycaemia, and a close watch must be kept on the blood glucose, and such infants should usually have intravenous access maintained until at least 6 hours after the exchange transfusion.

2. Exchange transfusion induces considerable fluid and electrolyte shifts in the baby. The baby's sodium, potassium, chloride, calcium and phosphate levels may be greatly altered by exchange transfusion, depending on the level of these substances in the blood used for the exchange transfusion. In particular if the blood is not very fresh, and if washed resuspended red cells reconstituted with fresh frozen plasma (which is the preparation most commonly used) is not available the potassium level may be dangerously high. It is possible to convert a previously healthy baby into a very ill one by using blood which is not fresh and of good quality. Nowadays, with the high quality refined product supplied by most blood transfusion services, the electrolytes are little affected by exchange transfusion, and infants requiring multiple exchange transfusions may even become potassium depleted.

   Bank blood is hyperosmolar and pulls fluid into the circulating compartment. In a term baby it has been estimated that the circulating blood volume may increase by as much as 60–80 ml after a double-volume exchange transfusion in which the same amount of blood was replaced as was removed. An infant with a cardiorespiratory problem may go into overt cardiac failure due to fluid overload even though the volume transfused equals the volume removed. Rhesus babies with incipient hydrops are particularly at risk. For this reason, most operators leave a cumulative deficit during exchange transfusion of 20–40 ml, and careful consideration should be given to giving a dose of frusemide at the end of the exchange transfusion in infants particularly at risk. Most normal infants can cope with this easily, however, the only clinical evidence of the increase in circulating volume being an increased urine output in the 12 hours after the exchange transfusion.

3. If the donor blood contains significant amounts of citrate (ACD blood), the baby may become alkalotic some hours after the exchange transfusion as the citrate is metabolized to bicarbonate.

4. Blood samples taken from the last syringeful of blood at the end of an exchange transfusion do not truly reflect the degree of change in bilirubin or haematocrit induced by the exchange transfusion, as it takes some considerable time for equilibration throughout the baby's body compartments to take place. For this reason it is suggested above that the post-exchange blood measurements should be taken 1 hour after completion of the procedure.

5. Another potentially important factor affecting bilirubin and haematocrit levels post-exchange is the possibility of exchange transfusion with

mismatched blood. Many of the infants needing exchange transfusion because of isoimmunization have not only the antibody causing the isoimmunization but multiple other blood group antibodies which may make finding a suitable blood donation extremely difficult. There is, therefore, despite the greatest care with blood cross-matching, a significant possibility of incompatible donor blood being used unwittingly for an exchange transfusion.

The baby may develop pyrexia, lethargy, apnoea, hypotension, signs of respiratory distress, a blotchy skin rash or no symptoms. The baby should receive appropriate supportive care. Much more of a problem is the catastrophic rise in the bilirubin level, and fall in haematocrit. A baby with a slowly rising bilirubin level before the exchange transfusion may suddenly become severely jaundiced and anaemic within 6 hours of the end of an exchange transfusion that was thought to have corrected the problem. For this reason, in all cases of exchange transfusion, bilirubin and haematocrit must be checked 3–4 hours after the end of the exchange transfusion even though this is only 2 or 3 hours after the measurement of post-exchange levels 1 hour after the end of the exchange transfusion.

6. Repeated exchange transfusion may also affect coagulation and haematological values. If fresh frozen plasma is used to reconstitute the packed cells, there are rarely induced coagulation problems in the baby, as coagulation factors are being replaced at the same time as they are being washed out. The platelet count may fall very low with risk of bleeding from the umbilicus and elsewhere. After a second or subsequent exchange transfusion it is advisable to give a platelet transfusion.
7. All of the feedback mechanisms in the body, such as most aspects of endocrine control, are upset by exchange transfusion but these are not usually of clinical significance.
8. Other acute complications include complications of transfusions in general such as accidental infection with cytomegalovirus, hepatitis B and human immunodeficiency virus (HIV).
9. Sepsis. This is more likely to occur as a result of prolonged retention of an umbilical arterial catheter in the vein than from the exchange transfusion itself. Repeated exchanges increase the risk of infection and some units use prophylactic antibiotics when repeated exchange transfusions are required. Evidence of infection usually appears 12–24 hours after the exchange transfusion.
10. Portal thrombosis. This may be a complication of septic thrombophlebitis of the portal vein or it may occur without obvious infection, presenting as gastrointestinal bleeding from oesophageal varices in mid-childhood. In the acute situation the infant has gross splenomegaly accompanied by prolonged obstructive jaundice and moderate hepatomegaly. It is usually advisable to treat with antibiotics because of the risk of an infective element.
11. Necrotizing enterocolitis (pp. 255–259). The involvement of exchange transfusion in the aetiology of necrotizing enterocolitis is not clearly defined, but the two are frequently associated. The first sign is usually the passage of blood per rectum and failure to tolerate oral feeds, with green or blood-stained nasogastric aspirates.

Partial exchange transfusion (single-volume exchange transfusion)

Indications

1. Hydrops in a severely ill infant with chronic anaemia from any cause, with a high central venous pressure.
2. Polycythaemia (p. 216).
3. Septicaemia (p. 194).

Management

Hydropic and anaemic infants
Concentrated or packed red cells should be used of the same ABO group as the infant and considerations of rhesus group are the same as for a double-volume exchange transfusion (see above). If the central venous pressure (CVP) is greater than 12 cm, the initial pressure should be recorded and frusemide given intravenously or intramuscularly. Transfusion is then started by the removal of 20 ml blood and its replacement by 10 ml of donor blood. The CVP is measured again. After each cycle of the exchange transfusion, a 10 ml deficit is left until the CVP recorded is between 5 and 8 cm, by which time a cumulative deficit of 40–80 ml of blood will have been achieved. This procedure alleviates the infant's heart failure while treating the anaemia. This procedure should be carried out slowly and the infant should be allowed time to adapt. Conventional exchange transfusion using the double-volume technique will have to be carried out subsequently, based on the rate of bilirubin rise. If the CVP pressure is less than 5 cm, the circulating volume should be expanded by an incremental transfusion, taking 10 ml out and replacing with 20 ml of donor blood. This is continued until the CVP is between 5 and 8 cm. If shock develops, the use of dopamine (p. 170) should be considered.

Septicaemia
There is inconclusive evidence that exchange transfusion may improve the survival rate in infants with fulminating septicaemia, presumably by removing endotoxins, replenishing opsonin and complement levels, and correcting coagulation abnormalities due to disseminated intravascular coagulation. Infants with severe respiratory problems may also be benefited by the more favourable oxygen dissociation curve of adult haemoglobin compared with fetal haemoglobin. Under these circumstances a single-volume exchange may be carried out using fresh whole blood, if at all possible. Consideration should also be given to 'topping up' the infant with fresh frozen plasma, platelets and perhaps maternal white cells, at the end of the exchange. Such patients do not tolerate exchange transfusion well and extreme caution is necessary.

Polycythaemia
Polycythaemia (a venous haematocrit greater than 0.7) may be a serious problem due to the increase in blood viscosity as the haematocrit rises above this value. Such infants appear cyanosed and may develop symptoms and disorders related to poor perfusion and cardiac decompensation.

These include lethargy, irritability, fits, poor peripheral perfusion, heart failure and oliguria. At autopsy, clotted blood (or 'sludge') may be found in the cerebral sinuses, and sinus thrombosis; there is an increased risk of necrotizing enterocolitis. Polycythaemia, thrombocytopenia and hypoglycaemia tend to occur together, so that the infant with polycythaemia should be investigated for the other two disorders as soon as the disorder is recognized.

A controlled trial of treatment with exchange transfusion for infants with polycythaemia was carried out by Black and Lubchenko (1982). In the first year of life, infants who received dilutional exchange transfusions in the newborn period showed some improvement in behaviour and development over those with polycythaemia who did not receive this treatment. However, there was an increased incidence of neonatal necrotizing enterocolitis in the group who had the dilutional exchanges.

Subsequent follow up in this study failed to show any long-term benefit from dilutional exchanges for neonatal polycythaemia but did show differences in neurodevelopmental parameters between children with untreated neonatal polycythaemia and true non-polycythaemic controls.

The role of dilutional exchange transfusion in infants with neonatal polycythaemia is still unclear, but may be considered in infants with severe symptoms, possibly attributable to hyperviscosity, with very high haematocrits (>0.8).

Recognition Polycythaemia and hyperviscosity are most likely to occur in:

1. The infant of a diabetic mother.
2. The small-for-gestational-age (SGA) infant or postmature infant.
3. An identical twin, the recipient of a twin-to-twin transfusion.
4. Delayed cord clamping with the infant lower than the placenta may be a factor aggravating polycythaemia in some cases.

A capillary haematocrit should be measured in all infants at risk, and, if this is found to be greater than 0.65, an adequate fluid intake should be ensured to prevent dehydration and further increase in the haematocrit. A further venous haematocrit (this is more accurate than a capillary haematocrit) should be measured, and, if this is greater than 0.8, serious consideration may be given to carrying out a dilutional exchange.

Religious objections to transfusion and refusal of consent

Depending on the unit, a formal signed consent form may be required for exchange transfusion. At the least, verbal consent must be obtained and the indications for the exchange transfusion outlined to the parents, emphasizing the fact that the procedure is considered to be less hazardous than the anticipated complications of the problem for which the procedure is to be carried out. On rare occasions this may be refused due to the parents' beliefs. This situation can usually be foreseen and parental rights may have to be overruled by the social work department in favour of the infant. This is enacted by obtaining a Place of Safety Order under the

Children and Young Persons Act 1969 in England, as for children who are neglected or injured by their parents; or the infant may be made a Ward of Court. Under these circumstances it is important to obtain a written statement in the infant's chart that the exchange transfusion is necessary and is a life-saving procedure to be carried out as an emergency, signed by the consultant in charge and also by another consultant who is not involved in the care of the child, who has reviewed the patient and the situation. The hospital administration should be informed and the doctor may wish to discuss the situation with a Medical Defence Association.

References

Allen, F.H. and Diamond, L.K. (1958) *Erythroblastosis Fetalis, Including Exchange Transfusion Technique*, Little, Brown, Boston

Black, V.D. and Lubchenko, L.O. (1982) Neonatal polycythemia and hyperviscosity. *Pediatric Clinics of North America*, **29**, 1137–1147

Bold, A.M. and Wilding, A. (1975) *Clinical Chemistry; Conversion Scales for SI Units*, Blackwell Scientific Publications, Oxford

Rodeck, C.H. and Letsky, E. (1989) How the management of erythroblastosis fetalis has changed. *British Journal of Obstetrics and Gynaecology*, **96**, 759–763

Swyer, P.R. (1975) *Intensive Care of the Newly Born*, Karger, Basel, p. 147

Whitfield, M.F. and Black, J.A. (1987) Rhesus and other forms of immunisation. In *Pediatric Emergencies*, 2nd edn (ed. J.A. Black), Butterworths, London, p. 689

Further reading

Bowman, J.M. (1986) Haemolytic disease of the newborn. In *Textbook of Neonatology* (ed. N.R.C. Roberton), Churchill Livingstone, Edinburgh, Chapter 19 (Part IV), pp. 469–483

Levine, R.L., Fredericks, W.R. and Rappoport, S.I. (1982) Entry of bilirubin into the brain due to opening of the blood brain barrier. *Pediatrics*, **69**, 255–259

Maisels, M.J. (1972) Bilirubin: on understanding and influencing its metabolism in the newborn infant. *Pediatric Clinics of North America*, **19**, 447–501

Maisels, M.J. (1981) Neonatal jaundice. In *Neonatology* (ed. G.B. Avery), Lippincott, Philadelphia, pp. 474–544

Maisels, M.J. (ed.) (1990) Neonatal jaundice. *Clinics in Perinatology*, **17**, 245–507

Perlman, M. and Frank, J.W. (1988) Bilirubin beyond the blood brain barrier. *Pediatrics*, **81**, 304–315

Ritter, D.A., Kenny, J.D., Norton, H.J. and Rudolph, A.J. (1982) A prospective study of free bilirubin and other risk factors in the development of kernicterus in premature infants. *Pediatrics*, **69**, 260–266

Schreiner, R.L. and Glick, R. (1982) Interlaboratory bilirubin variability. *Pediatrics*, **69**, 381–382

Swyer, P.R. (1975) *Intensive Care of the Newly Born*. Karger, Basel, p. 188

Turkel, S.B., Miller, C.A., Guttenberg, M.E., Moynes, D.R. and Hodgmen, J.E. (1982) A clinical pathological reappraisal of kernicterus. *Pediatrics*, **69**, 267–272

Chapter 12

Acute respiratory disorders, including stridor

General considerations

Respiratory problems are a major cause of life-threatening illness in the newborn. The improvement in neonatal survival and morbidity in the last 15 years is due to the availability of effective management of respiratory problems. The majority of pre-term infants with respiratory problems suffer from respiratory distress syndrome (RDS). The term infant with respiratory distress constitutes a separate problem and presents greater difficulties in diagnosis.

Recognition

Infants with breathing difficulties usually have signs of 'respiratory distress', which are:

Tachypnoea
Tachycardia
Chest/subcostal recession
Nostril flaring
Grunting
Cyanosis

These signs are non-specific and may be caused by a variety of different respiratory or non-respiratory disorders (Table 12.1).

Infants with diminished respiratory drive, muscular exhaustion or muscular weakness may not have these signs but may still have severe alveolar hypoventilation (Table 12.2). Signs of respiratory distress indicate that ventilatory failure may develop, or it may be a significant problem already, whatever the primary cause. An evaluation of the infant requires:

1. A full history and clinical examination.
2. A chest X-ray.
3. Assessment of arterial blood gas status.

Careful review of the obstetric history provides important diagnostic information. Prenatal ultrasound examination may have identified possible anomalies (e.g. pulmonary hypoplasia, diaphragmatic hernia, congenital

le 12.1 Differential diagnosis of respiratory distress

n-respiratory

ticaemia*
t failure (e.g. congenital heart disease, patent ductus arteriosus, transient myocardial
emia (Chapter 13)
olic acidosis (Chapter 27)*
ral irritation
e anaemia (Chapter 7)
heating in an incubator (Chapter 21)

atory

Upper
Airway obstruction due to mucus
Obstructive malformations of the nose, pharynx, larynx, trachea or bronchi
Malformations compressing the trachea

Lower
Space-occupying lesions in the thorax
Diaphragmatic hernia
Pleural effusion, chylothorax, haemothorax (p. 158)
Pneumothorax,* pneumomediastinum,* pneumopericardium,* pneumoperitoneum* (p. 151)
Large space-occupying malformation in the thorax

Lung disease
RDS and its complications *
Neonatal pulmonary oedema ('wet lung')*
Meconium aspiration syndrome
Persistent fetal circulation *
'Immature lung'*
Atelectasis*
Pneumonia*
Haemorrhagic pulmonary oedema* (pulmonary haemorrhage)
Pulmonary hypoplasia

*More commonly seen in pre-term infants.

Table 12.2 Causes of ventilatory failure which may or may not have signs of respiratory distress

Apnoeic attacks of prematurity (p. 55)
Phrenic nerve palsy (p. 51)
Neurological abnormalities such as myotonic dystrophy (p. 23)
Muscular dystrophy
Drug effects (magnesium toxicity, sedatives, anaesthetics, anticonvulsants)

heart disease, hydrops), and obstetric dates and early ultrasound assessment of maturity should be correlated with the clinical findings in establishing the gestational age of the infant. Diabetes during the pregnancy, rhesus isoimmunization and prenatal amniotic fluid surfactant measurements all influence the probability of the infant developing surfactant-deficient RDS. Delivery and resuscitation details may be relevant in anticipating the severity of RDS and the possible impact of hypoxia on the infant's prognosis. Clinical examination should identify any significant abnormalities such as displacement of the mediastinum, severity of symptoms and the degree of oxygen dependency. Because of the wide differential diagnosis and the limitations of clinical evaluation, a chest X-ray is essential in any newborn with respiratory distress at the time of the first assessment, because the principal aim of management is to reach an accurate diagnosis as soon as possible, and to anticipate the rate and degree of possible deterioration. The arterial blood gas status of the infant is also essential to an accurate first assessment. It should then be possible to predict the facilities and management likely to be required in the next few days.

Management

General considerations

The management of an infant with a serious respiratory problem requires a considerable commitment of equipment, and medical, nursing and ancillary staff. Intensive nursing care must be provided by an experienced neonatal nurse who is responsible for two or at the most three infants; if the infant becomes unstable, requires paralysis, or has repeated problems with pneumothorax, one nurse may be required for that infant alone. This level of nursing must be maintained for 24 hours a day and, in neonatal intensive care units (NICUs), for 365 days a year. Competent trained medical staff have to be immediately available in the hospital when ventilatory assistance may be required.

These staffing requirements make management of infants with respiratory problems for more than 24 hours possible only in a specially designated NICU where the outcome for infants needing management is much better than in small local neonatal units; the results are improved if patients likely to require ventilatory support are delivered in a high-risk perinatal unit combining the necessary obstetric and neonatal expertise (Usher, 1974).

Intensive respiratory management requires much equipment. Within a few hours of birth an infant may require an incubator, three infusion pumps, a heart rate/respiratory rate/blood pressure monitor, oxygen analyser, head box, neonatal ventilator, intravascular oxygen monitor, access to transcutaneous oxygen and carbon dioxide monitors and fully miniaturized neonatal laboratory facilities. Each incubator area requires at least 12 electrical sockets, piped oxygen and air with two outlets each per incubator, and piped vacuum. A unit not purpose-built and equipped for full-scale neonatal intensive care cannot cope with these demands for more than 24 hours but must be able to stabilize the infant before transfer to an NICU.

Early diagnosis

Every attempt should be made to make an early accurate diagnosis. Failure to establish a diagnosis, however, must not delay supportive treatment.

Arrangements must be made to provide adequate nursing cover (see above).

Cardiorespiratory monitoring

An infant with a developing respiratory problem may deteriorate quickly in the few hours after birth. Minimal handling is important. For these reasons, an ECG and respiratory monitor are necessary to follow the infant's condition minute by minute.

Oxygen therapy and blood gas monitoring

Oxygen is a dangerous drug and oxygen therapy must be prescribed in terms of concentration measured by an oxygen analyser, not in litres per minute. Arterial blood gases must be monitored repeatedly (at least 6-hourly) in infants with respiratory difficulties to assess adequacy of oxygen therapy, metabolic acidosis and the effectiveness of the infant's spontaneous breathing. Blood gases should be usually maintained within the following limits:

Arterial Po_2	8.0–11.0 kPa (60–80 mmHg;torr)
pH	>7.3
Arterial Pco_2	4.0–8.0 kPa (30–60 mmHg;torr)

Initially humidified oxygen should be given using a head box at a concentration which just abolishes cyanosis. Infants with mild transient respiratory difficulties who need less than a fractional concentration (FiO_2) of inspired oxygen of 0.30 (30%) to maintain adequate oxygenation in the first 6 hours of life can usually be managed without an umbilical arterial catheter and monitored by intermittent arterial sampling or by capillary sampling (for pH), combined with a transcutaneous oxygen and carbon dioxide electrode or pulse oximeter. Infants needing more than a fractional concentration inspired oxygen of 0.30 (30%) in the first 6 hours should have an arterial line inserted. Umbilical arterial catheters provide arterial samples and continuous arterial Po_2 monitoring, using the Searle intravascular oxygen electrode, and also give access for fluid infusion. The infant's respiratory progress is then followed by serial blood gas measurements every 4–6 hours, or more frequently if indicated. Arterial Po_2 can be regulated by adjustment of inspired oxygen concentration. Acidosis can be corrected by cautious bicarbonate administration if the base deficit is more than 6 mmol/l. Sodium bicarbonate 4.2% contains 0.5 mmol $NaHCO_3$ per ml (5% $NaHCO_3$ contains 0.6 mmol/ml); the dose for half correction of the metabolic acidosis is calculated by 1/3 × base deficit × body weight (kg) which gives the volume (in ml) of 4.2% $NaHCO_3$ required. Bicarbonate should be given slowly over 10–15 minutes and the blood gas measurement repeated 30 minutes later. If an unventilated infant has a combined respiratory and metabolic acidosis with the arterial Pco_2 greater than 8 kPa (>60 mmHg;torr) bicarbonate **must not** be given because, in neutralizing the hydrogen ions, further carbon dioxide will be generated which cannot be excreted through the lungs in an infant with incipient ventilatory failure. The result is carbon dioxide narcosis and apnoea precipitated by bicarbonate administration. THAM (tris-hydroxyaminomethane) is a buffer containing no sodium and is less hyperosmolar than 4.2% or 8.4% $NaHCO_3$, which can be given to correct a metabolic acidosis in the presence of a raised $P\text{CO}_2$. THAM is used as a 7% solution; 1 ml of a 7% solution is approximately equivalent to 1 ml of 4.2% of $NaHCO_3$ or 0.5 ml of the 8.4% solution. THAM may cause apnoea (a 3.5% solution is less likely to cause apnoea) and should only be used in situations where respiratory assistance is already being provided or is immediately available. A rising arterial $P\text{CO}_2$ indicates progressive failure to breathe adequately and can only be corrected by ventilatory assistance.

Fluid and electrolytes

Infants with significant respiratory problems have ileus for the first 24–48 hours or longer. A tachypnoeic infant (over 60 per minute) requiring an inspired oxygen concentration greater than 0.30 (30%) by 3 hours of age should not be fed until there are indications that the respiratory problem is improving. An intravenous infusion of glucose 10% at 60 ml/kg per 24 hours should be started to maintain hydration, to provide calories and to prevent hypoglycaemia. This can be given by the umbilical arterial line. Electrolyte supplements should be added to the infusion to provide maintenance electrolytes after 24 hours (sodium 25 mmol/l, potassium 20 mmol/l, calcium 40 mmol/l).

Possible infection

Infection may be contributory to the infant's respiratory difficulties, and antibiotic treatment should be started if indicated. Prolonged ruptured membranes (more than 48 hours), genital tract infection in the mother, a chest X-ray compatible with aspiration pneumonia, or other evidence such as a low neutrophil count indicate a full infection screen, and appropriate antibiotics should be started (e.g. ampicillin and gentamicin, see Chapter 14).

Group B streptoccocal pneumonia and septicaemia may be so difficult to differentiate from other causes of early respiratory distress that many nurseries give ampicillin prophylactically (after a neutrophil count, throat swab and blood culture have been sent) to all infants with respiratory distress (p. 195).

Ventilatory assistance

Indications for ventilatory assistance in infants with deteriorating respiratory status are:

1. Hypoxaemia; (arterial $P\text{O}_2 < 8.0$ kPa or 60 mmHg;torr) despite an $\text{FiO}_2 > 0.70$ (70%) or an arterial oxygen saturation ($S\text{O}_2$) <87%.
2. Ventilatory failure, arterial $P\text{CO}_2$ greater than 8.0 kPa (60 mmHg;torr).
3. Severe acidaemia (pH <7.20) due to combined metabolic and respiratory components (see above).

4. Deteriorating clinical state of an uncomfortable struggling infant (a clinical decision).
5. Infants with respiratory difficulties who need surgery usually need ventilation postoperatively.
6. Infants with combined respiratory and cardiac problems often need ventilation for heart failure as a temporary measure.

In some infants, particularly those of more than 30 weeks' gestation and more than 1.5 kg, endotracheal intubation and ventilation can be avoided by using continuous positive airway pressure (CPAP) (for complications, see pp. 326–327). This is useful only when oxygenation is the major problem and pH and arterial $P\text{CO}_2$ are well maintained. An >0.30–>0.60 (30–60%) has been used as an indication for initiating CPAP, using nasal catheters at 5–8 cmH$_2$O. The response of arterial $P\text{CO}_2$ and pH after application of CPAP is unpredictable, particularly if the infant needs an inspired oxygen concentration of 0.6 (60%) or more. The infant's subsequent clinical and blood gas status may necessitate intubation and ventilation soon after beginning CPAP. Large infants (more than 36 weeks) usually dislike nasal catheters and are not good candidates for CPAP. Infants requiring an inspired oxygen concentration greater than 0.85 (85%) on CPAP of 8 cmH$_2$O should be intubated and ventilated. In many units nasal CPAP is rarely used in infants with significant respiratory problems; this is because of the small number of infants who require CPAP but who do not need ventilation later, problems with restlessness in larger infants, difficulty with gas escape through the mouth, damage to the nasal septum from nasal catheters and the more precise degree of respiratory control offered by intermittent positive pressure ventilation (IPPV). In the majority of infants ventilatory assistance involves endotracheal intubation and IPPV (Chapter 2). Reasonable starting settings for IPPV for infants with respiratory problems ventilated on the above criteria would be:

FiO$_2$	1.00 (100%)
Peak inspiratory pressure (PIP)	
>34 weeks	20 cmH$_2$O
<34 weeks	15 cmH$_2$O
Prolonged end-expiratory pressure (PEEP)	5 cmH$_2$O
Inspiratory time	0.5–0.8 seconds
Rate	40/minute

Adjustments would then be made in accordance with blood gas results.

Sedation or paralysis

Infants often breathe against the ventilator. This is undesirable and increases the risk of pneumothorax, and cerebral haemorrhage or ischaemia and causes oscillations in arterial $P\text{O}_2$, frequently down to low levels. Sedation with morphine 0.1–0.2 mg/kg per dose as often as required, up to 3-hourly, or as an infusion (0.05 mg/kg loading dose, then 0.015 mg/kg per hour), may be tried and rarely causes a significant drop in blood pressure. If morphine is ineffective, muscle paralysis with pancuronium 0.1–0.2 mg/kg per dose i.v. may be required, repeated about

4-hourly as signs of muscular activity return (Pollitzer *et al.*, 1981). Paralysis is an indication for one-to-one nursing because of the danger of accidental extubation in a paralysed infant. Chloral hydrate, given orally to infants in the first few days of life, is extremely unpredictable in its effect because of variable absorption. It is easy to produce an overdose with oral chloral hydrate, which may be absorbed only when recovery starts, with the result that the infant is floppy and unresponsive for the remainder of the first week.

Persistent hypoxaemia

An infant needing IPPV with an inspired oxygen concentration of 1.00 (100%) with optimal PIP to obtain good inflation PEEP of 5, and an appropriate ventilator rate, who then begins to have persistently borderline arterial Po_2 levels presents a major problem in ventilator management. Usually by this stage the infant is paralysed to eliminate muscular activity which causes intermittent drops in arterial Po_2. In such infants there is usually some persistent fetal circulation with right-to-left shunting and pulmonary hypertension. Tolazoline is an α-adrenergic blocker and pulmonary vasodilator which affects cardiac afterload and may improve oxygenation, sometimes dramatically (Goetzman *et al.*, 1976). Its effect on systemic blood pressure is unpredictable and it should not be used without effective monitoring and support of arterial blood pressure.

Any metabolic acidosis should be corrected with bicarbonate before administration of tolazoline. The response in arterial Po_2 to a bolus test dose of 1 mg/kg given intravenously is best observed using a continuous oxygen monitor (Searle intravascular or transcutaneous Po_2). If there is no effect on Po_2, a further test dose of 2 mg/kg should be given. If this does not increase Po_2, a test dose of 4 mg/kg can be given but this rarely produces a benefit if 2 mg/kg has been unsuccessful. If a response is observed, a continuous infusion of tolazoline is started immediately after the bolus to give the dose of the successful bolus (1–4 mg/kg) per hour. The blood pressure must be supported with infusions of fresh frozen plasma (FFP), 10–20 ml/kg over 15–60 minutes if there is a significant drop following tolazoline.

Failure of FFP to return the blood pressure to pre-tolazoline levels should be treated with a continuous infusion of dopamine at 2–5 μg/kg per minute. Support of blood pressure and cerebral perfusion is important and blood pressure surges should be avoided because of their potential effect on the brain.

Complications

A careful watch must be kept for complications related to the primary respiratory pathology in ventilated infants (Table 12.3).

Respiratory distress syndrome (idiopathic respiratory distress syndrome, hyaline membrane disease)

RDS is a disorder of the pre-term lung in which the primary defect appears to be lack of surfactant, which is important in stabilizing alveolar size and

Table 12.3 Deterioration in a ventilated infant

Symptom	*Problem*	*Action*
1. Ventilator stops generating set pressure, and colour and heart rate deteriorate	ETT dislodged ETT disconnected Ventilator malfunction Piped gas supply failure (unlikely)	Reintubate Reconnect Hand bag infant and investigate Obtain emergency gas cylinder
2. Ventilator pressure does not drop during expiration; infant's condition deteriorates	Ventilator expiratory tube kinked Ventilator expiratory valve sticking	Unkink Hand bag infant and investigate
3. Sudden deterioration in infant's colour, heart rate and BP, but ventilator still generates pressure	*Respiratory* ETT kinked ETT blocked Pneumothorax	 Unkink Suction, reintubate Heart displaced? Transilluminate/chest X-ray. Insert pleural drain (p. 314)
	Pneumopericardium	Head blue, body white. Transilluminate. Insert pericardial drain (p. 317)
	Collapsed lung or major lobe	Chest X-ray. Physiotherapy and suction, bronchial lavage
	Haemorrhagic pulmonary oedema	Blood-stained frothy fluid up ETT. Chest X-ray. Suction, increase ventilation (p. 144)
	Massive pulmonary interstitial emphysema	Chest X-ray. Manipulate ventilatory settings (p. 153)
	Non-respiratory Tension pneumoperitoneum	 Abdominal X-ray. Drain
	Massive intracranial haemorrhage	Cranial ultrasound. Circulatory support. Transfusion
	Patent ductus arteriosus opened up	Chest X-ray. Echocardiogram, increase ventilation, particularly mean airway pressure
	Necrotizing enterocolitis	Abdominal X-ray. Support (p. 257)
	Septicaemia	Infection screen. Antibiotics (p. 193)
	Hyperkalaemia with arrhythmias	Measure electrolytes, ion exchange/resin, calcium, glucose and insulin
	Hypoglycaemia	Blood glucose, increase glucose infusion rate

ETT, endotracheal tube; BP, blood pressure.

retaining end-expiratory alveolar air (Avery and Mead, 1959). Deficiency leads to diminished lung volume, reduced lung compliance and increased physical work in breathing. There is progressive alveolar protein leak and an influx of inflammatory cells into the lungs. Intrapulmonary shunting and ventilation/perfusion mismatch lead to cyanosis. Hypoxaemia and acidosis cause pulmonary arteriolar constriction and continuance of the fetal state of high pulmonary vascular resistance. This in turn results in more right-to-left shunting and more cyanosis. Failure to correct this vicious cycle leads to progressive acidaemia, ventilatory and circulatory failure and death.

RDS occurs in pre-term infants, usually of less than 35 weeks' gestation, and occasionally in infants over 35 weeks, mainly in infants of diabetic mothers. The likelihood of RDS can be predicted prenatally by an amniotic fluid lecithin/sphingomyelin ratio of less than 2:1 and the absence of phosphatidylglycerol. It is more common and severe in infants who have been hypoxic and in those delivered by caesarean section without a preceding period of labour. Betamethasone or dexamethasone given to the mother 24 hours or more before delivery is thought to reduce the incidence of this condition. Male infants are more often and more severely affected.

Recognition

1. The pre-term infant develops signs of respiratory distress (see above) within the first few hours of life and by 6 hours the signs are well established and getting worse. The natural history is of progressive deterioration till about 48 hours after which there is improvement. Ventilation may be required from the first few hours, or when the infant becomes exhausted after 48 hours.
2. Chest X-ray shows diminished lung volume, 'ground glass' opacification of the lung-fields and air-filled bronchi, contrasting with the rather solid lung-fields, the 'air bronchogram'. The ground glass appearance is due to microscopic areas of collapse adjacent to dilated terminal bronchioles.
3. The differential diagnoses are coincidental cardiac disease, and incipient group B streptococcal septicaemia and pneumonia.

Management

Management follows the outline given previously for the infant with respiratory difficulties. The principal complications are pneumothorax and other manifestations of displaced air (pp. 151–154), haemorrhagic pulmonary oedema (pp. 155–156) and the complications of ventilator management and prematurity. Infants with severe lung immaturity who require very aggressive ventilation in the first few days are likely to develop bronchopulmonary dysplasia.

It is important to avoid interstitial emphysema and pneumothorax by cautious use of high mean airway pressures and high peak pressures because these complications make management of the primary disorder much more difficult, and increases the mortality and morbidity.

The outcome for infants with RDS is usually good. Very few infants over 1.0 kg now die of ventilatory problems even though it is these who have the classic form of the disease. Despite aggressive ventilation and resulting bronchopulmonary dysplasia, few infants have long-term respiratory sequelae. The prognosis will be improved by the use of exogenous surfactant (p. 161).

‘Immature lung’ (‘chronic pulmonary insufficiency of prematurity’)

In recent years as increasing numbers of infants below 1.0 kg birth weight and 26 weeks’ gestation have survived, a separate clinical syndrome of ‘pulmonary immaturity’ has been identified. The primary problem appears to be structural immaturity rather than the biochemical problem seen in RDS which is more common in infants of 28 weeks or more.

Recognition

The infant is usually extremely immature and may require energetic resuscitation and ventilatory support initially; but within 24 hours of delivery, the chest X-ray is virtually normal or has a slightly hazy appearance, and minimal ventilation and little oxygen (fractional concentration of inspired oxygen of 0.25 (25%). However, because of immaturity the infant cannot breathe adequately and so cannot be weaned from the ventilator.

Within the next 3 weeks, the lung-fields become hazy on the chest X-ray, the ventilation and oxygen requirement increase, and the infant develops bronchopulmonary dysplasia. Pneumothorax is rare and consequently there is a lower incidence of intracranial haemorrhage or ischaemia than in more mature infants with classic RDS requiring high ventilation pressures in the acute phase.

Management

Management follows the plan given above and that given in Chapter 4 for the very low birthweight infant.

Atelectasis

Some infants with mild surfactant deficiency or retained secretions in the airways have difficulty in expanding their lungs at delivery and in keeping them expanded during the first few days of life. These infants have generalized or lobar atelectasis as the primary problem, which resolves during the first 3 days of life.

Recognition

1. The infant is usually over 34 weeks’ gestation and has signs of respiratory distress and increased oxygen requirement.
2. The chest X-ray shows scattered areas of atelectasis or one or more collapsed lobes.
3. Differential diagnosis includes RDS, pulmonary aspiration, congenital pneumonia or group B streptococcal pneumonia.

Management

1. Management follows the general outline given above.
2. Blood culture and antibiotics are usually advisable because infection may be contributing to the problem.
3. Physiotherapy and suction are an important part of treatment, to try to expand the atelectatic areas of lung.
4. Short-term intubation and ventilation may be required if the infant's condition is unsatisfactory, providing inflation of the lungs and the opportunity to suck out the trachea directly. Ventilation is rarely required beyond 3 days.
5. Complications are those of the treatment required to keep the lungs expanded; the prognosis is usually extremely good.

Neonatal pulmonary oedema

This is also called wet lung, transient tachypnoea of the newborn (TTN), and respiratory distress syndrome type II.

Neonatal pulmonary oedema is a transient disorder of lung function caused by abnormally large amounts of fluid in the interstitium of the lung, usually resulting in mild difficulties with gas exchange but a considerable reduction in compliance and increase in the work of breathing. The chest X-ray shows some haziness of the lung-fields but well-expanded lungs and good lung volume. Often, fluid is visible in the fissures, and sometimes the lymphatic channels in the lungs can be seen as linear streaks radiating towards the hilum. This syndrome is most commonly seen in infants over 34 weeks' gestation who have been delivered by caesarean section and have not cleared their lung fluid at the time of delivery. Neonatal pulmonary oedema may also occur in infants who have been hypoxic, have received an excessive fluid intake or have cardiac failure.

Recognition

1. The predisposing causes described above are important in reaching a diagnosis.
2. Chest X-ray findings are as outlined above.
3. Respiratory distress with minor oxygen requirements.

An infant shown to need greater than an inspired oxygen concentration of 0.40 (40%) is likely to have more than pure neonatal pulmonary oedema; group B streptococcal pneumonia is a likely diagnosis.

Management

1. Management follows the general outline given above.
2. If the infant has been hypoxic, complications of hypoxia need to be anticipated.
3. If fluid intake has been excessive this should be reduced and consideration given to the use of one dose of frusemide 1–2 mg/kg.

4. Occasionally an infant with neonatal pulmonary oedema may need ventilation because of poor lung compliance and ventilatory failure. This is usually required for no more than 36 hours.
5. Differential diagnoses include RDS, pulmonary infection and cardiac lesions such as the hypoplastic left heart syndrome where cyanosis may not be obvious early in the illness. A moderate-to-severe metabolic acidosis on an arterial blood gas sample (base deficit >8 mmol/l) makes uncomplicated pulmonary oedema unlikely.

Meconium aspiration syndrome

Meconium aspiration is usually due to intrauterine hypoxia, causing gasping *in utero*, with inhalation of meconium, amniotic fluid and vernix. Significant meconium aspiration syndrome, however, is an unusual sequel to meconium staining of the amniotic fluid. Thick meconium in the bronchial tree causes air trapping and gaseous overdistension of the lungs. Squames in the alveoli may cause a diffusion block, and bile salts and enzymes cause chemical pneumonitis and a tissue reaction within 48 hours. Some infants with meconium aspiration develop severe persistent fetal circulation (PFC) (p. 172) and require very energetic management while others avoid this complication and have a relatively mild course, without requiring ventilation. Fetal distress in a pre-term infant rarely causes the passage of meconium, and when meconium staining does occur in the pre-term infant, it is more likely to be due to an intrauterine infection.

Recognition

1. Meconium aspiration syndrome is usually a disease of term and post-term infants. Those with intrauterine growth retardation and fetal distress are at highest risk. In postmature infants there is often green staining of the nails and umbilicus, as well as other signs of postmaturity.
2. There is thick meconium staining of the amniotic fluid at delivery and meconium visible in the airway on laryngoscopy.
3. The infant has signs of respiratory distress, with widespread crepitations in both lung-fields, and the chest may appear over-expanded and the infant very breathless.
4. Chest X-ray shows an aspiration pattern usually affecting the right side more than the left, with areas of collapse and adjacent areas of overdistension. The chest X-ray may appear almost normal yet the baby subsequently develops severe PFC.
5. Infants who develop PFC may not look particularly ill in the first few hours. Any infant with meconium aspiration syndrome who needs more than an inspired oxygen concentration of 0.30 (30%) has significant right-to-left shunting and is likely to decompensate suddenly, with severe hypyoxia due to PFC, and become critically ill in the next 12–24 hours. Such infants should be cared for in a fully equipped NICU.
6. Infants with meconium aspiration syndrome may have signs of hypoxic ischaemic encephalopathy and evidence of hypoxic ischaemic injury to

other body systems (heart, kidneys, gastrointestinal tract, coagulopathy).

7. The differential diagnosis includes cyanotic heart disease, aspiration pneumonia from other causes, and group B streptococcal pneumonia and septicaemia.

Management

1. Deep suction of the trachea is recommended before the first breath (if possible) at the time of delivery in infants with thick meconium in the amniotic fluid, and when meconium is seen below the cords at laryngoscopy during resuscitation (p. 35). Bulb aspirators are completely inadequate for sucking out meconium; piped wall suction should be used, with an 8 FG, or larger, catheter.
2. Intermittent positive pressure ventilation may be required (see below), and external cardiac massage if the apex beat is less than 50 beats per minute.
3. Oxygen should be given by head box to maintain arterial Po_2 above 12.0 kPa (90 mmHg;torr). A high arterial Po_2 is desirable because of the low risk of retinopathy of prematurity in term infants and the considerable risk of sudden severe hypoxaemia due to unstable PFC.
4. If the membranes have been ruptured for more than 48 hours, the amniotic fluid is smelly, or the mother has evidence of chorioamnionitis, such as pyrexia or leucocytosis, a 5-day course of antibiotics should be given to the infant, after a full infection screen.
5. Many infants with meconium aspiration syndrome have a significant metabolic acidosis because of hypoxia and this should be corrected with bicarbonate.
6. Chest physiotherapy and suction are required during the first few days of life to remove respiratory secretions and meconium.
7. Pneumothorax (p. 151) is a common complication of meconium aspiration syndrome.
8. The infant should not be fed in the first 24 hours, unless there is no significant respiratory problem. The stomach should be washed out with saline before feeding, to remove meconium.
9. Glucose 10% should be given intravenously with added calcium 40 mmol/l at 60 ml/kg per 24 hours. Excessive fluid intake must be avoided because hypoxic infants often have transient renal failure, and cerebral oedema may be exacerbated by an excessive fluid intake. No potassium should be added until there is an adequate urine output (more than 2 ml/kg per hour).
10. Blood glucose and calcium levels should be checked 6-hourly in the first 24 hours and thereafter as required; calcium and glucose intake in the infusion are regulated accordingly.
11. Infants needing an inspired oxygen concentration greater than 0.30 (30%) should have an umbilical arterial catheter inserted and blood gases estimated 4-hourly in the first 24 hours.
12. The decision to ventilate an infant with meconium aspiration syndrome should not be delayed too long. Suggested indications for ventilation are: an FiO_2 of greater than 0.6 (60 per cent) to maintain

an arterial Po_2 of approximately 12 kPa (90 mmHg;torr), or a struggling infant with rising arterial Pco_2 and falling arterial Po_2. There is no place for CPAP with meconium aspiration syndrome because pulmonary overdistension is a major problem. The infant with meconium aspiration syndrome and persistent fetal circulation usually needs:

(a) High fiO_2 (near 1.0) (100%);
(b) High PIP 25 cmH_2O and above (sometimes up to 50 or 60 cmH_2O);
(c) Short inspiratory time 0.2–0.4 second;
(d) Fast rate 80–120 per minute;
(e) Minimal PEEP 0–2.

These settings are at the upper limit of performance for most currently available infant ventilators. The difficulty is in obtaining high PIP but short inspiratory time and zero PEEP. Short inspiratory time and zero PEEP are important in limiting further air trapping and pulmonary overdistension. A volume ventilator such as the Siemens servo-ventilator may be required. The infant should also be paralysed with pancuronium 0.1–0.2 mg/kg per dose.

13. For further management of PFC, see pages 174–175. Typically, infants with meconium aspiration and PFC need aggressive ventilation, and paralysis for 5–7 days before weaning from ventilation can occur. For extracorporeal membrane oxygenation see pp. 161 and 175.

Complications
Pneumothorax is a frequent complication of meconium aspiration syndrome in both ventilated and non-ventilated infants. Bronchopulmonary dysplasia is likely after prolonged aggressive ventilation. The neurological prognosis depends on the severity of brain injury from hypoxia. The majority of infants with severe meconium aspiration syndrome survive. Of those who die, a few die of ventilatory failure, most dying of complications of hypoxia (hypoxic-ischaemic encephalopathy, heart failure, renal failure, disseminated intravascular coagulation and necrotizing enterocolitis).

Aspiration pneumonia

Aspiration pneumonia in the newborn may be sterile if due to prenatal aspiration of amniotic fluid or milk aspiration in the newborn period; or it may be potentially infected if due to aspiration of infected amniotic fluid or secretions in the birth canal. It is most frequently seen in term infants.

Recognition

1. The infant develops signs of respiratory distress and requires oxygen.
2. Chest X-ray shows patchy opacification of both lung-fields with the bases and right side being more affected.
3. Differential diagnosis usually includes meconium aspiration syndrome, group B streptococcal septicaemia and pneumonia, and congenital heart disease.

Management

1. Management follows the guidelines for respiratory management given above.
2. Antibiotics should normally be started after a blood culture, throat swab and urine have been sent for group B streptococcal coagglutination test, because of the difficulty in excluding this infection.
3. Chest physiotherapy, oxygen with monitoring and suction should be given to help clear the bronchial tree.
4. In term infants, only those with massive aspiration are likely to need ventilation.
5. The prognosis is good; complications are those of the treatment required (see above).

Intrauterine pneumonia

Intrauterine pneumonia may develop after the aspiration of infected amniotic fluid when there has been premature rupture of the membranes for some time and may occur with chorioamnionitis with intact membranes on occasion. This complication of premature rupture of the membranes is surprisingly rare even when there are signs in the mother of active chorioamnionitis. Lobar pneumonia may also occur *in utero* with intact membranes and is usually caused by infection of the mother with influenza or para-influenza virus, with transplacental infection of the infant.

Recognition

1. The infant may have signs of respiratory distress or may be asymptomatic.
2. There is often a history of viral infection of the mother in the 3 weeks before delivery.
3. Chest X-ray may show obvious lobar consolidation.

Management

1. This follows the guidelines for respiratory management given above.
2. Blood from mother and infant should be sent for serological studies for currently infecting respiratory viruses, and for virus culture from the infant's throat or tracheal secretions.
3. Consideration may be given to treatment with antibiotics if a bacterial cause is suspected or cannot be excluded.

Tracheo-oesophageal fistula and oesophageal atresia

Although not a respiratory malformation, the emergency aspects of tracheo-oesophageal fistula concern the respiratory tract, and produce respiratory difficulties in most infants. The majority have a blind upper oesophageal pouch and a communication between the lower segment of the oesophagus and the trachea or main bronchi. The respiratory consequences are:

1. Aspiration of swallowed saliva into the lungs from above.
2. Aspiration of gastric contents into the lungs from below.
3. Ventilation, if required, leads to progressive gaseous distension of the abdomen due to air tracking from the main airway into the gastrointestinal tract through the fistula, and further respiratory compromise. The results of surgical repair are generally good except where there is a long oesophageal defect, or multiple associated malformations. The most important threat to survival is repeated aspiration of gastrointestinal secretions into the lungs before surgery.

Recognition

1. The mother usually has polyhydramnios and the anomaly is suspected before delivery, on the basis of a prenatal ultrasound examination.
2. The infant is 'mucusy' and develops signs of respiratory distress with episodes of choking and cyanosis. Feeding must be avoided because it will produce cyanosis, aspiration and collapse.
3. On the chest X-ray a widening of the upper mediastinal shadow may be seen; this is the distended upper pouch.
4. A stiff PVC tube (8 FG) with a radio-opaque tracer should be passed through the nose, and characteristically sticks at 10 cm in term infants; a lateral and anteroposterior X-ray should then be taken. If there is difficulty in interpreting the X-ray, the advice of a radiologist should be sought before dye is introduced into the upper pouch, because of the risk of aspiration.
5. Tracheo-oesophageal fistula often coexists with other anomalies particularly the VATER (vertebral anomalies, anal atresia, tracheo-oesophageal fistula, cardiac defects, radial dysplasia), and Trisomy 18; therefore a careful search for other anomalies must be made.

Management

1. Once the diagnosis is made, the surgical correction of the defect by a paediatric surgeon experienced in neonatal surgery is an urgent priority. The infant must **not** be fed enterally.
2. A Replogle tube should be placed in the upper pouch and connected to continuous suction; the mouth should be sucked out hourly.
3. The infant should be nursed slightly head up to try to prevent aspiration into the lungs from below, and prone to assist clearing of oral secretions.
4. General respiratory management should be as indicated above.
5. The combination, in a pre-term infant, of RDS and tracheo-oesophageal fistula presents a difficult challenge for both neonatologist and surgeon. Depending on the condition of the infant, it may be possible to carry out a full repair of the fistula during the first hours of life before the RDS has developed to its full severity; however, a compromise and less traumatic approach is to tie off the fistula and carry out a gastrostomy, with delayed repair of the atresia. If high

ventilation pressures are required, some type of surgical procedure will become necessary because of the abdominal distension.

6. Pulmonary complications are dependent on the degree of pulmonary damage from aspiration.

Group B streptococcal pneumonia and septicaemia

This is a common cause of severe respiratory distress complicated by PFC in term and pre-term infants (p. 195 for group B streptococcal septicaemia and p. 172 for PFC).

'Displaced air syndrome' (pneumothorax and related conditions)

Pneumothorax and other forms of displaced air are common complications in the newborn period. Pneumothorax itself is the most common, but pneumomediastinum, pneumopericardium, pneumoperitoneum and pulmonary interstitial emphysema may be regarded as variants or extensions of the same process – ectopic dissection of respiratory gases into the lymphatic system and communication of this with the serous body cavities. Displaced air and particularly pneumothorax occur in four groups of patients:

1. Normal infants around the time of birth. This is a reflection of the high negative intrapleural pressures generated by lusty term infants in the first few breaths. The incidence is increased by intubation. Pneumothoraces in this group of infants usually resolve spontaneously and rapidly without intervention and are often unrecognized.
2. Meconium aspiration syndrome (p. 145). Meconium aspiration syndrome is the major cause of significant pneumothorax in term infants.
3. RDS. Pneumothorax is a complication of the disorder and of its treatment, particularly with high pressure ventilation, and frequently coexists with pulmonary interstitial emphysema.
4. Other infants needing high pressure ventilation (e.g. pulmonary hypoplasia, hydrops).

In infants with terminal ventilatory failure, pneumothorax is often the cause of death because progressive increases in ventilation pressures are made in an attempt to achieve better blood gas results. Air embolism occurs when the displaced air bursts into the circulatory system and at times even into the cerebrospinal fluid. Tension pneumothorax and tension pneumopericardium have marked effects on the venous and arterial pressure in the brain, leading to intraventricular haemorrhage and periventricular leucomalacia (Hill, Perlman and Volpe, 1982) (p. 62). The development of a bronchopleural fistula makes respiratory management extremely difficult. For these reasons great efforts must be made to prevent the development of displaced air.

Prevention

1. Excessive pressures should not be used for resuscitation of the newborn, and endotracheal intubation should be used with care, recognizing its potential for causing pneumothorax.
2. CPAP or ventilation should not be used unless the infant's condition justifies it.
3. The benefits and risks of upward adjustments in mean airway pressure and PIP need to be carefully weighed up in managing ventilated infants (Primhak, 1983).
4. Infants should not be permitted to breathe against or fight the ventilator because this increases the risk of pneumothorax; sedation or paralysis should be used to prevent this in the first weeks of life when the risks of pneumothorax and intraventricular haemorrhage are highest (Greenough, Morley and Davis, 1983; Greenough *et al.*, 1984).

Pneumothorax

Recognition

1. The infant has one of the predisposing causes and develops, often suddenly, signs of respiratory distress, or the respiratory status suddenly deteriorates.
2. With tension pneumothorax the mediastinum is usually obviously shifted, with a change in the position of greatest intensity of the heart sounds and a change in the ECG tracing on the oscilloscope. Air entry over the affected lung-field may be diminished (because of an inadequate expansion of the lung) or may be louder and have a breathy amphoric quality. The abdomen may appear distended due to eversion of the diaphragm on the affected side, and if the tension pneumothorax is on the right side the liver will be pushed down so that its edge can be easily felt in the epigastrium and right hypochondrium.
3. When the pneumothorax is smaller, clinical signs may not be at all obvious and the diagnosis can easily be missed.
4. Transillumination of the chest using a cold fibreoptic light source at the bedside can rapidly confirm the presence and position of a pneumothorax, but is unreliable in infants above 2.0 kg body weight. Anteroposterior and lateral chest X-ray, as an emergency, takes longer but gives more accurate information and provides a record of the findings.
5. Timing of the development of the pneumothorax is an important clue to clinical deterioration of the infant. Although the pneumothorax may occur at the time of maximum ventilation pressure, it also occurs in infants who are doing well at around 3 or 4 days, at a time when lung compliance suddenly improves.

Management

1. Conservative: a pneumothorax is in a state of dynamic equilibrium, with its size determined by the relative rates of absorption and reaccumulation of air. In the majority of term infants who develop a pneumothorax

at the time of first lung expansion (in the first category of recognition above) the pneumothorax resolves spontaneously in the first 30–40 minutes without the diagnosis ever being made. If the pneumothorax is small and not progressive, the infant stable, and in a controlled environment with adequate trained medical and nursing staff, conservative treatment is often successful. The infant is nursed in an incubator and carefully observed. Feeds are withheld, fluid balance maintained by glucose 10%, and a high concentration of oxygen is given to help to wash out nitrogen from a pneumothorax space and to hasten absorption. In pre-term infants the potential risk of retinopathy of prematurity limits the maximum oxygen concentration which can be used and the arterial $P\text{O}_2$ should be kept no higher than 12.0 kPa (90 mmHg;torr). If the infant's condition deteriorates or a significant pneumothorax persists after 24 hours of conservative treatment, a chest tube should be inserted. If shock develops, fresh frozen plasma (FFP) may be given, and dopamine (p. 170) if the response to FFP is poor.
2. Pleural drainage: a chest tube is inserted and connected to an underwater seal drain with a negative pressure of $-5\,\text{cmH}_2\text{O}$ (p. 314).

Pneumomediastinum

Pneumomediastinum may occur in the presence of pneumothorax, or alone.

Recognition

1. The infant is markedly breathless with signs of respiratory distress.
2. Chest X-ray shows upward displacement of the thymic lobes by air in the upper mediastinum and air may be seen lateral to the heart on both sides, and anterior to the heart on the lateral chest X-ray.

Management

1. Conservative treatment as above. The air is multilocular and cannot be effectively drained.
2. A subsequent pneumothorax may develop, needing drainage; therefore the infant should be observed carefully.

Pneumopericardium

Small air leaks into the pericardium are an unusual complication of RDS, and tension pneumopericardium is rare.

Recognition

1. Small amounts of air may be seen as a chance finding on the chest X-ray of an infant with RDS or other severe respiratory problem needing energetic ventilation.

2. A tension pneumopericardium produces cardiac tamponade with circulatory collapse. The head is often deep blue and plethoric, and the rest of the infant is pasty white. There is apparent incompatibility between the collapsed pulseless state of the patient, and the continuing, apparently normal, ECG activity seen on the monitor.
3. Transillumination of the left precordium in infants weighing less than 2.0 kg shows a circle of light with the dark heart seen beating within it.
4. Chest X-ray has a characteristic appearance which may be difficult to differentiate from pneumomediastinum if the two coexist.

Management

1. A pericardial catheter should be rapidly inserted and connected to an underwater sealed drain with 5 cmH_2O suction in cases of tension pneumopericardium (p. 317).
2. Where small amounts of air are identified in the pericardial sac on routine chest X-ray, a conservative approach may be taken but the patient must be observed carefully and X-rays taken 12-hourly until the air disappears.

Pneumoperitoneum

Pneumoperitoneum can develop as a complication of pneumothorax in infants with a patent pleuroperitoneal canal, without any pathology in the abdomen. Gastric perforation or perforation due to necrotizing enterocolitis may also cause a pneumoperitoneum.

Recognition

1. An infant, usually ventilated, with RDS or meconium aspiration, suddenly deteriorates with pneumothorax and abdominal distension.
2. Chest X-ray shows a pneumothorax and free gas in the abdomen.
3. In the absence of a pneumothorax acute gastric perforation and necrotizing enterocolitis are the most likely causes, both of which can produce sudden massive pneumoperitoneum in a sick infant.

Management

1. When a complication of a pneumothorax a pneumoperitoneum responds to drainage of the pneumothorax.
2. Occasionally a peritoneal drain has to be inserted (p. 000).

Pulmonary interstitial emphysema

Pulmonary interstitial emphysema (PIE) is a common complication in ventilated infants with severe RDS in which respiratory gases dissect into the pulmonary lymphatics and lung parenchyma (Plenat *et al.*, 1978). Two anatomical variants are described:

1. Subpleural PIE where there are a few largish subpleural blebs which take up space in the thorax but have little effect on lung function. A pneumothorax will result if one of these blebs bursts into the pleural cavity.
2. Diffuse parenchymal PIE where small bubbles of gas are scattered throughout the lung parenchyma and lymphatics, and cause widespread disruption of the lung architecture and function. The pulmonary vascular resistance rises, the airway becomes distorted, there is increased ventilation–perfusion mismatch and the lungs become extremely stiff; ventilation management becomes extremely difficult. Infants who survive diffuse parenchymal PIE usually develop severe bronchopulmonary dysplasia.

Most cases of PIE are a mixture of both of the above.

Recognition

1. A ventilated infant with RDS or immature lung suddenly develops increasing requirements for ventilation and oxygen.
2. Chest X-ray shows a characteristic appearance, with the lungs becoming more translucent; this is due to numerous small gas-filled cysts scattered throughout the lung, some larger than others and some situated at the pleural surface of the lung.

Management

1. There is no satisfactory treatment and most pre-term infants who die of lung immaturity or RDS in the first few days die from this complication.
2. Despite the desire to reduce ventilation pressures because of reduced lung compliance, increases have to be made to keep the infant alive. This in turn further exacerbates the interstitial emphysema.
3. A rapid ventilatory rate with a short inspiration time is thought to reduce further deterioration in lung function. New forms of infant ventilation such as high-frequency oscillation may reduce the incidence of PIE and severe bronchopulmonary dysplasia, but this form of management still needs evaluation.

Bronchopulmonary dysplasia

Bronchopulmonary dysplasia (BPD) is included here for completeness, but is a chronic rather than an acute problem. The incidence of BPD has risen as mortality rates from respiratory causes have fallen because of better respiratory equipment and management. It is usually the result of prolonged high pressure ventilation using high inspired oxygen concentration, but the original lung pathology and immaturity of the infant also contribute. The disease is more common, more severe and more protracted, and the prognosis worse, in small male infants.

Recognition

1. The infant has a predisposing reason for ventilator management but has persistent lung disease with requirement for oxygen, and sometimes ventilation, beyond 28 days of life.
2. The chest X-ray at 2 weeks may show predominantly solid X-ray-dense lung-fields, but as the disease progresses multiple lung cysts coexist with patchy atelectasis. Later there may be extensive fibrosis with gross distortion of the lung parenchyma.
3. Progressively increasing oxygen and ventilation requirement due to extensive ventilation–perfusion mismatching, cor pulmonale, intolerance of fluid and wheezing are late features.

Management

1. Although ventilator management may have been the major predisposing cause for the BPD, there may be no choice but to continue ventilation because of the state of the patient. Frequently high pressures and inspired oxygen concentration are required for prolonged periods.
2. Fluid intake should be restricted to 120–150 ml/kg per 24 hours, and intermittent diuretic treatment may help the ventilatory difficulties (hydrochlorothiazide 2–4 mg/kg per 24 hours in two divided doses; frusemide 2 mg/kg per dose).
3. Bronchodilators (salbutamol by nebulizer; 0.25–0.5 ml of 5 mg/ml solution per dose, or aminophylline, loading dose 6.25 mg/kg followed by 5–7.5 mg maintenance 12 hourly) may help in wheezy infants.
4. The role of corticosteroid treatment for BPD is not well defined. Although steroids may reduce oxygen and ventilation requirements in the short term, weaning from the steroid is accompanied by reappearance of the same problems, and there are significant risks of long-term steroid treatment in small sick neonates (infection, growth retardation, exacerbation of cor pulmonale).

Complications

Emergency complications occurring in infants with BPD are:

1. Pneumothorax in a previously stable baby caused by rupture of a lung cyst.
2. Sudden cardiac decompensation due to cor pulmonale and fluid accumulation.
3. Acute respiratory infection causing a dramatic sudden deterioration in the baby's condition out of proportion to the apparent severity of the illness.
4. The onset of mild diarrhoea in a fluid-restricted infant on diuretics for BPD may be associated with rapid decompensation due to fluid and electrolyte imbalance.

Haemorrhagic pulmonary oedema ('pulmonary haemorrhage')

The cause of haemorrhagic pulmonary oedema is not known. There is a sudden out-pouring from the lungs of large amounts of bright-red frothy fluid which obstructs the airway and makes ventilation difficult. The rate of production is such that no sooner is the airway cleared by suction, than it refills with fluid. The fluid is not pure blood; it comes from the alveoli and has a haematocrit of around 20% so the term 'haemorrhagic pulmonary oedema' is more correct than 'pulmonary haemorrhage'. Haemorrhagic pulmonary oedema occurs in two groups of infants:

1. Hypoxic term infants in whom initial resuscitation at delivery is complicated by large amounts of haemorrhagic pulmonary oedema fluid.
2. Pre-term infants being ventilated for RDS in whom there is a sudden deterioration, with blood-stained fluid coming up the endotracheal tube.

Recognition

1. The infant belongs to one of the above two groups.
2. Blood-stained frothy fluid is sucked from the trachea.
3. Chest X-ray shows opaque lung-fields ('white out').

Management

1. Every attempt is made to secure and maintain a clear airway by frequent suction.
2. Very high ventilation pressures are needed to obtain gas exchange in the first 2 hours after the onset when the lungs are very stiff.
3. Circulatory support should be given with packed cells, fresh frozen plasma, and dopamine if the blood pressure falls.
4. A platelet count should be performed and platelets given if the count is low. Fibrinogen levels should be measured to look for disseminated intravascular coagulation (see p. 91). The mortality rate for pulmonary haemorrhage is of the order of 50% even with prompt and energetic treatment; survival is often accompanied by neurodevelopmental abnormalities.

Diaphragmatic hernia

Diaphragmatic hernia is a common major malformation (Ruff *et al.*, 1980; Harrison and de Lorimier, 1981). There is a cleft in the diaphragm, usually on the left side, through which abdominal contents, stomach, spleen, liver and other viscera herniate into the left hemithorax, encouraged by fetal breathing movements. Development of the ipsilateral lung is compromised and there may also be hypoplasia of the contralateral lung. After delivery, the infant develops great difficulty with breathing because of inadequate thoracic expansion due to the diaphragmatic defect and progressive compression of the thoracic contents. There is also a progressive mediastinal shift due to gaseous distension of the hollow viscera within the thorax by swallowed air. The situation is further compounded by pulmonary hypoplasia and persistent fetal circulation (Dibbins, 1978).

Recognition

1. Prenatally, mediastinal shift and cystic structures in the left thorax may be recognized on ultrasound examination. Polyhydramnios may develop, with marked mediastinal deviation *in utero*, and is a bad prognostic sign. Infants with diaphragmatic hernia should be delivered in a regional perinatal centre because of the need for surgery and the major difficulties with respiration in the first week of life.
2. At birth the infant has: scaphoid abdomen; heart sounds loudest in the centre or on the right side of the chest; signs of respiratory distress with gasping respiration and progressive cyanosis.
3. Chest X-ray shows opacification of, or bowel gas shadows in, the left hemithorax with the heart shifted to the right and a small right lung-field. A radio-opaque nasogastric tube may be seen to go down the oesophagus into the upper abdomen and then back into the left hemithorax.
4. Differential diagnosis includes true dextrocardia, left-sided tension pneumothorax (the other major cause of apparent dextrocardia), other intrathoracic masses, left pleural effusion and eventration of the diaphragm.

Management

Respiratory support

1. Mask IPPV at delivery should **not** be given, because it will further inflate the abdominal viscera in the thorax and make the respiratory problems worse.
2. A Replogle (8 FG) tube should be inserted into the stomach and attached to continuous suction to prevent further distension of the intrathoracic abdominal viscera.
3. If facilities are available, the infant should be intubated and ventilated and an umbilical arterial catheter inserted to monitor blood gases. Management may be made easier by paralysis with pancuronium at this stage to stop further air swallowing, to limit gasping movements which suck more abdominal viscera into the thorax, and to allow controlled ventilation in a struggling dyspnoeic infant. These infants usually need high pressures and rapid rates with high inspired oxygen concentration (e.g. PIP 25–30, PEEP 3, rate 60, inspiratory time 0.5 second, FiO_2 1.00 (100%)).

Surgical treatment

The infant should be transferred to a regional perinatal centre for surgery and postoperative care. Surgical repair of the defect is usually considered an emergency although some prefer to delay repair for a few days in infants who can be stabilized from the respiratory point of view, because of the risk of severe PFC. Some prefer a selective approach to surgery because of the very poor outcome for infants requiring high concentrations of oxygen in the first few hours of life. At surgery the hernia is reduced and the defect sutured or closed with an artificial graft, using a transabdominal approach.

Postoperative care
Infants with diaphragmatic hernia are extremely prone to develop severe PFC in the postoperative period. For management of PFC, see p. 172.

Survival
The survival rate for congenital diaphragmatic hernia is around 50% for cases presenting in the first 12 hours of life. The causes of death in those who die are ventilatory failure due to pulmonary hypoplasia and PFC. The prognosis for infants who present later is much more favourable. There is some evidence that extracorporeal membrane oxygenation (ECMO) will reduce the mortality rate by around 20%.

Neonatal pleural effusion

Congenital pleural effusion is rare. The most common cause is chylothorax (see below). Haemothorax occurs occasionally in infants with bleeding disorders following trauma at delivery, or after the insertion of pleural drains, and is due to damage to the intercostal artery. A serous pleural effusion may occur in transplacental viral infections. Aspiration of fluid is usually required for diagnostic purposes.

Chylothorax

Chylothorax is an uncommon finding often associated with non-immune fetal hydrops and the neonatal Turner's (Bonneville–Ulrich) syndrome (Van Aerde *et al.*, 1984).

Recognition

1. The infant has signs of respiratory distress from birth and, if hydropic, may be extremely ill and need energetic resuscitation at delivery (p. 35).
2. A chest X-ray shows a pleural effusion on one or both sides.
3. The pleural fluid is initially serous and straw coloured and has a high lymphocyte count. The fluid becomes opalescent due to the presence of fat globules only after enteral feeding is established.
4. The infant should be carefully inspected for other signs of the Bonneville–Ulrich syndrome, e.g. webbing of the neck and lymphoedema of the hands and feet, in a girl.
5. Infants occasionally develop chylothorax as a postoperative complication of thoracic operations such as the repair of a tracheo-oesophageal fistula.

Management

1. At delivery. Emergency pleural drainage (p. 314) may be required for primary resuscitation to permit adequate lung expansion.
2. The respiratory status of the infant must be monitored by repeated blood gas measurements, and appropriate support as given above in the

general guidelines for respiratory management. A chest X-ray will confirm the diagnosis of pleural effusion.

3. If the infant develops significant respiratory difficulties in the first few hours of life, consideration should be given to pleural drainage with an underwater seal drain. Fluid production in the first few days may be extremely high (240 ml or more per day from each side of the chest) and the infant's respiratory status cannot be stabilized without effective drainage of this fluid.
4. The electrolyte and protein composition of the fluid should be analyzed to provide the necessary information for making a suitable replacement solution to be given intravenously to the infant in the same volume as the pleural losses.
5. The usual pattern of fluid production is a high rate in the first 2–3 days, falling towards the end of the first week of life. A sudden drop in fluid drainage in the first few days of life is a sign that the pleural drain is becoming blocked, leading to accumulation of fluid within the pleural space and the possibility of rapid respiratory deterioration.
6. The pleural drain or drains should be removed towards the end of the first week of life when less than 15 ml of fluid is collected per day from either hemithorax. Some infants need intermittent pleural tapping two to three times during the second or third week of life. Removal of a chest drain as early as possible is desirable to stop the continued losses of protein, fluid, electrolytes and lymphocytes.
7. A careful check needs to be kept on fluid balance and serum levels of electrolytes and protein to ensure adequate replacement.
8. Feeds should be withheld until the infant has been stable for several days without a pleural drain. Usually about 2 weeks of parenteral nutrition are required. Enteral feeds should be initiated with a formula containing medium-chain triglycerides (e.g. Pregestimil) instead of long-chain fat as this may reduce the volume of chyle produced. By 1 month after the removal of chest tube it is usually possible to change to a normal formula if repeated chest tappings have not been required.
9. Many infants are markedly lymphocytopenic for several weeks, due to drainage losses from the lymphocyte pool. When the pleural drains have been removed the immunoglobulin levels should be measured and intravenous immunoglobulin should be given if these are low. A number of infants have been found to develop repeated infections in the first year of life, associated with low immunoglobulin levels following treatment for chylothorax in the newborn period.

Congenital lobar emphysema

Congenital lobar emphysema is a condition in which there is progressive overdistension of one or several pulmonary lobes in the first week of life in an otherwise healthy infant, usually at term.

Recognition

1. A history of increasing respiratory distress in the first week of life in a term infant.

2. Clinical examination shows signs of respiratory distress and mediastinal shift.
3. Chest X-ray shows gross overdistension of one or more lobes with compression of adjacent normal lung, and mediastinal shift. There is usually no pneumothorax unless the situation is extreme.
4. This condition must be differentiated from the pre-term infant who has interstitial emphysema or cystic bronchopulmonary dysplasia.

Management

1. The respiratory condition needs to be monitored by repeated vital sign observations and blood gas measurements.
2. The usual course is of increasing overexpansion, requiring resection of the affected lung segment(s) by the end of the second week of life.
3. The ultimate prognosis is usually good.

Pulmonary hypoplasia and agenesis

Pulmonary hypoplasia or agenesis is a condition leading to severe neonatal respiratory insufficiency soon after birth, usually preceded by marked oligohydramnios from before 20 weeks' gestation. The diagnosis is often suspected before delivery because of the recognition on fetal ultrasound examination of oligohydramnios (Thiebeault *et al.*, 1985). Pulmonary agenesis most commonly occurs in association with renal agenesis. Even a small amount of amniotic fluid around the fetus appears to be sufficient to prevent significant pulmonary hypoplasia in most infants with moderate renal hypoplasia, urethral valves, or very prolonged ruptured membranes. See also p. 12 for further discussion of oligohydramnios.

Recognition

1. There is a history of oligohydramnios, and onset of respiratory difficulties at birth.
2. The infant may have deformations due to uterine compression (Potter's syndrome).
3. Severe hypoxaemia and hypercapnia develop despite energetic ventilation with 100% oxygen.
4. Chest X-ray shows small lungs which are poorly aerated despite ventilation.
5. Clinical examination and abdominal examination usually reveal major urinary tract abnormalities.
6. Infants with hydrops or pleural effusion also may present with pulmonary hypoplasia if the pleural effusion has been present for a long time and has affected growth of the lungs.

Management

1. IPPV by endotracheal tube should be started early; high pressure, rate and inspired oxygen concentration will be required.

2. Pneumothorax and other forms of displaced air are common.
3. Some infants also have PFC and may respond surprisingly well to tolazoline, dopamine, paralysis and hyperventilation (see p. 140).
4. The prognosis is uncertain and depends on the degree of pulmonary hypoplasia and coexisting PFC, RDS and renal insufficiency. Some infants survive the newborn period and die later from cor pulmonale.

Promising developments for the future in respiratory neonatal care

Treatment of RDS

There is now good evidence that the clinical course of infants with RDS can be improved by treatment with exogenous surfactant (Vidyasagar and Shimada, 1988). Clinical trials to evaluate the first pharmaceutical preparations of surfactant are currently (1991) nearing completion. Once these preparations are licensed for general use, installation of several doses of exogenous surfactant down the endotracheal tube of infants with significant RDS early in their clinical course will become an established important adjunct to management.

High-frequency oscillation for ventilatory failure

There has also been much recent interest in high-frequency oscillation as an alternative method of obtaining gas exchange in infants with ventilatory failure. Preliminary studies suggest this technique may have advantages in some infants in promoting gas exchange with less barotrauma than conventional IPPV (Hamilton *et al.*, 1983).

Extracorporeal membrane oxygenation

Extracorporeal membrane oxygenators have been used in infants, particularly those with PFC, with some success (Kirkpatrick *et al.*, 1983; French-Andrews, Roloff and Bartlett, 1984) but the efficacy and cost effectiveness of this technique requires further study in controlled trials.

Nasal and nasopharyngeal obstruction

Most newborns are obligatory nose breathers during the first 3 months of life. Minor degrees of nasal airway obstruction are common, due to the small size of the airway and the increase in airway resistance caused by even small amounts of secretions or crusts. A coryzal illness in a normal infant with a small nose may produce considerable difficulty due to airway obstruction, particularly during feeding, and the ingestion of considerable amounts of swallowed air and mucus.

Recognition

1. Complete bilateral nasal obstruction causes severe respiratory indrawing and recession with cyanosis but without stridor. The signs may be initially difficult to distinguish from other causes of respiratory distress

in the newborn (see p. 135), but they are instantly relieved when crying causes the infant to breathe through the mouth or by the insertion of an oropharyngeal airway. The most common cause is choanal atresia.

2. Incomplete or intermittent nasal obstruction, particularly if it varies with the position of the patient, is likely to be due to a nasopharyngeal tumour or nasal encephalocele. If the obstruction is incomplete, inspiration may be accompanied by a snoring or snorting noise. These tumours are often pedunculated and asymmetrically placed and usually produce variable symptoms.
3. Mild nasal obstruction developing after birth is usually due to an upper respiratory infection, or to oedema and infection from an indwelling nasal tube.
4. Nasal obstruction may occur with a nasal feeding tube *in situ* if the open nostril becomes obstructed by secretions or oedema.

Management

1. Bilateral choanal atresia is an emergency which requires experienced operative intervention. Temporary relief can be obtained by the insertion of an oropharyngeal airway provided this is adequately fixed with adhesive tape to prevent rejection by the infant. Alternatively the infant can be intubated. Suspected tumours may require similar management and should be referred to a specialist as an emergency.
2. The obstruction due to nasopharyngitis can usually be relieved by giving vasoconstrictor nose drops; crusts should be softened by cotton wool soaked in warm sterile 0.9%NaCl. Suitable nose drops are 0.5% ephedrine in 0.9% sodium chloride and should be instilled 10–20 minutes before each feed in order to relieve nasal obstruction during feeding. This treatment should not be continued for longer than 7–10 days.

Stridor

Stridor is a sign that requires urgent assessment to determine the site and severity of airway obstruction.

Diagnostic clues to the location of the obstruction include the following:

1. Inspiratory stridor suggests obstruction at or near the larynx.
2. A hoarse cry suggests involvement of the vocal cords.
3. Inspiratory and expiratory (‘to-and-fro’) stridor indicates tracheal obstruction or compression.
4. Expiratory stridor alone is likely to be due to bronchial obstruction, as in lobar emphysema, lung cyst or mediastinal displacement.
5. A honking sound accompanied by signs of airway obstruction suggests tracheal collapse due to tracheomalacia and may occur in ventilated infants with a patent endotracheal tube.
6. Stridor reduced by lying in the prone position suggests a floppy epiglottis or obstruction of the airway by the tongue.
7. Stridor accompanied by head retraction suggests tracheal compression by a goitre or vascular ring.

The following considerations relate to the severity of stridor:

1. Stridor which is intermittently present, or absent during quiet breathing, usually indicates a mild degree of obstruction.
2. Continuous stridor with tachypnoea and chest recession suggests moderate to severe airway obstruction.
3. Cyanosis, pallor and restlessness are signs of impending collapse, and urgent relief is required.

Management

1. A full history should be taken and the infant examined for external signs suggesting a cause for the stridor (e.g. history of birth trauma, signs of heart disease, abnormalities of the head and neck).
2. A chest X-ray should be performed to evaluate the lungs and to look for abnormalities in the mediastinum.
3. Blood gases should be measured and the baby observed on a transcutaneous oxygen and carbon dioxide monitor, if available, to obtain some idea of the severity of respiratory embarrassment caused by the stridor.
4. An echocardiogram should be performed to look for aberrant vessels compressing the trachea.
5. Direct laryngoscopy will be needed and should be carried out in an operating room by a competent paediatric ear, nose and throat surgeon, with an anaesthetist and facilities for intubation and tracheotomy if necessary.

Aspects of specific causes of stridor

Pierre Robin syndrome

The mandible is small, the tongue set far back in the mouth and there is a cleft in the soft palate. The airway becomes completely obstructed when the infant lies supine. Many infants can be successfully managed in a prone-lying frame for 3–4 months until the mandible and airway grow. Some require tracheotomy.

Laryngomalacia and floppy epiglottis

Airway obstruction is due to inadequate cartilaginization of the structures of the larynx. Stridor is usually intermittent and the baby is sometimes better when prone, and improves as the airway grows and the cartilage becomes firmer.

Tracheomalacia and bronchomalacia

These conditions are generally more difficult to manage than laryngomalacia and floppy epiglottis, and may produce severe respiratory difficulties. As the infant grows the situation improves but some infants require continuous positive airway pressure via an endotracheal tube or tracheotomy in order to splint the trachea and bronchi until improvement occurs.

Acute trauma to the larynx at delivery or during intubation
Acute traumatic damage to the larynx usually resolves spontaneously and may be helped by a short course of corticosteroids or by inhalation of nebulized racemic adrenaline.

Cord paralysis due to laryngeal nerve damage
Unilateral recurrent laryngeal nerve damage due to trauma at delivery or thoracic operations (e.g. ligation of a patent ductus arteriosus) rarely requires tracheotomy, but cord paralysis due to bilateral recurrent laryngeal nerve injury usually does. The latter is extremely rare.

Other aspects
Lesions in the wall of the airway (e.g. haemangiomata, granulomata, tracheal stenosis), structural abnormalities of the airway, and external structures compressing the airway (e.g. vascular ring) often require tracheotomy to permit safe corrective management of the primary lesion.

Infants who appear to have minor airway obstruction in the newborn period may develop severe airway obstruction in the first few weeks of life when they develop their first upper respiratory tract infection; parents should be advised of this potential problem and encouraged to seek medical help early.

References

Avery, M.E. and Mead, J. (1959) Surface properties in relation to atelectasis and hyaline membrane disease. *American Journal of Diseases of Children*, **97**, 517–523

Dibbins, A.W. (1978) Congenital diaphragmatic hernia, hypoplastic lung and vasoconstriction. *Clinics in Perinatology*, **5**, 93–103

French-Andrews, A., Roloff, D.W. and Bartlett, R.H. (1984) Use of extracorporeal membrane oxygenators in persistent pulmonary hypertension in the newborn. *Clinics in Perinatology*, **11**, 729–736

Goetzman, B.W., Sunshine, P., Johnson, J.D., Wennberg, R.P., Hackel, A. and Merten, D.F. (1976) Neonatal hypoxia and pulmonary vasospasm; response to tolazoline. *Journal of Pediatrics*, **89**, 617–621

Greenough, A., Morley, C. and Davis, J. (1983) Interaction of spontaneous respiration with artificial ventilation in preterm babies. *Journal of Pediatrics*, **103**, 769–773

Greenough, A., Woods, S., Morley, C.J. and Davis, J.A. (1984) Pancuronium presents pneumothoraces in ventilated premature babies who actively expire against positive pressure inflation. *Lancet*, **i**, 1–3

Hamilton, P.P., Onayemi, A., Smyth, J.A., Gillen, J.E., Cutz, E. and Froese, A.B. (1983) Comparison of conventional and high frequency ventilation: oxygenation and lung pathology. *Journal of Applied Physiology*, **55**, 131–138

Hill, A., Perlman, J.M. and Volpe, J.J. (1982) Relationship of pneumothorax to occurrence of intraventricular hemorrhage in the premature newborn. *Pediatrics*, **69**, 144–149

Harrison, M.R. and de Lorimier, A.A. (1981) Congenital diaphragmatic hernia. *Surgical Clinics of North America*, **61**, 1023–1035

Kirkpatrick, B.V., Krummel, T.M., Mueller, D.G., Ormazabal, M.A., Greenfield, L. and Salzberg, A.M. (1983) Use of extracorporeal membrane oxygenation for respiratory failure in term infants. *Pediatrics*, **72**, 872–876

Plenat, F., Vert, P., Didier, F. and Andre, M. (1978) Pulmonary interstitial emphysema. *Clinics in Perinatology*, **5**, 351–377

Primhak, R.A. (1983) Factors associated with pulmonary air leak in premature infants receiving mechanical ventilation. *Journal of Pediatrics*, **102**, 764–768

Pollitzer, M.J., Reynolds, E.O.R., Shaw, D.G. and Thomas, R.M. (1981) Pancuronium during mechanical ventilation speeds recovery of lungs of infants with hyaline membrane disease. *Lancet*, **i**, 346–348

Ruff, S.J., Campbell, J.R., Harrison, M.W. and Campbell, T.J. (1980) Pediatric diaphragmatic hernias. *American Journal of Surgery*, **139**, 641–645

Thiebeault, D.W., Beatty, E.C., Hall, R.T., Bowen, S.K. and O'Neill, D.H. (1985) Neonatal pulmonary hypoplasia with premature rupture of the membranes and oligohydramnios. *Journal of Pediatrics*, **107**, 273–277

Usher, R. (1974) Changing mortality rates with perinatal intensive care regionalisation. *Seminars in Perinatology*, **1**, 309–319

Van Aerde, J., Campbell, A.N., Smyth, J.A., Lloyd, D. and Bryan, H. (1984) Spontaneous chylothorax in newborns. *American Journal of Diseases of Children*, **138**, 961–964

Vidyasagar, D. and Shimada, S. (1987) Pulmonary surfactant replacement in respiratory distress syndrome. *Clinics in Perinatology*, **14**, 991–1016

Further reading

Reyes, H.M., Meller, T.L. and Loeff, D.C. (1989) Management of esophageal atresia and tracheoesophageal fistula. *Clinics in Perinatology*, **16**, 79–84

Stern, L. (1984) *Hyaline Membrane Disease – Pathogenesis and Pathophysiology*, Grune & Stratton, New York

Stern, L. (ed.) (1987) The respiratory system in the newborn. *Clinics in Perinatology*, **14**, 433–749

Thibeault, D.W. and Gregory, F.A. (eds) (1986) *Neonatal Pulmonary Care*, 2nd edn, Appleton Century-Crofts, Norwalk, USA

Chapter 13

Cyanosis and congenital heart disease

Cyanosis

Persistent cyanosis in the newborn requires urgent investigation.

Peripheral cyanosis

1. 'Traumatic cyanosis of the head' must be differentiated from true central cyanosis. Traumatic cyanosis of the head and face is caused by confluent petechiae, due to obstruction to external jugular blood return at the time of delivery (e.g. cord tightly around the neck or delay in delivery of the trunk, as occurs in shoulder dystocia) or by rapid uncontrolled delivery of the head. Such infants often have subconjunctival haemorrhages. Close inspection of the face reveals confluent petechiae, blue lips, but usually a pink tongue, and the scrotum or labia are always pink, confirming the local nature of the cyanosis of the head and lack of true central cyanosis. No treatment is required, apart from reassurance. Some infants are rather irritable for several days, and exaggerated jaundice is not uncommon.
2. Peripheral cyanosis in a vigorous infant with warm extremities is of no significance and disappears after 2–3 days. Blue feet are an almost universal finding in term infants during the first few hours after delivery and lead to misleading heel prick capillary blood gas results.
3. Blotchy, mottled, cold, peripheral cyanosis may be a sign of circulatory failure and shock from any cause (p. 71) or from hypothermia.

Central cyanosis

Central cyanosis is usually an indication of severe and significant underlying disease. Central cyanosis is identified as a blue plum-coloured appearance, due to more than 60 g of desaturated haemoglobin/l in the central circulation, and is apparent in the mucous membranes, tongue and nail beds.

The most important causes of central cyanosis are:

1. Polycythaemia (p. 131).
2. Cardiac causes (below).
3. Respiratory causes (p. 134).

4. Severe neonatal illness from any cause with a deterioration in circulation and respiration, e.g. hypoglycaemia, acidaemia, septicaemia.
5. Congenital or acquired methaemoglobinaemia; in this extremely rare condition, blood fails to turn red when exposed to oxygen (a simple test is to observe the persistence of the brown colour of a drop of blood on a filter paper), due to abnormalities in the oxygen-dissociation characteristics of the haemoglobin, and remains a chocolate brown colour. The congenital form is due to an autosomal recessive condition; acquired methaemoglobinaemia in the newborn may result from nitrate-contaminated water, usually from a well. The diagnosis is confirmed by haemoglobin spectroscopy and chromatography. Methaemoglobinaemia can be abolished in the more common situations (temporarily in the congenital forms) by intravenous injection of Methylene Blue (1%; 10 mg/ml); 1–2 mg/kg, followed by ascorbic acid 100 mg three to four times daily, orally.

Differential diagnosis in centrally cyanosed infants

Clinical examination

Particular attention should be paid to:

1. Heart rate.
2. Respiratory rate.
3. Grunting, chest recession, nostril flaring.
4. Presence or absence of stridor.
5. Position and quality of the apex beat.
6. Auscultation of the heart and lungs.
7. Signs of heart failure: hepatomeagly, full fontanelle, poor peripheral circulation.
8. Presence or absence of femoral pulses.
9. Urine output.

Emergency chest X-ray

This reveals cardiomegaly, lung disease, pulmonary plethora or oligaemia, pneumothorax etc.

Blood glucose

This is measured using Chemstrip (Dextrostix; see footnote to p. 59) or other strip methods, or arterial blood samples.

Cardiac investigations

Cardiac investigations and echocardiogram carried out by a competent paediatric cardiologist usually provide an accurate, or near accurate, diagnosis. An electrocardiogram may also be helpful.

Hyperoxia test

Primary respiratory causes of central cyanosis can sometimes be differentiated from those of cardiac origin by observing the rise in arterial $P\text{O}_2$ or transcutaneous Po_2 when the baby is given 100% oxygen to breathe by head box (Jones *et al.*, 1976). The procedure is as follows:

1. Insert a radial artery catheter into the right radial artery, or attach a transcutaneous oxygen monitor to the right anterior chest wall and allow to stabilize.
2. Make an arterial Po_2 or transcutaneous Po_2 measurement in air or inspired oxygen concentration 0.3 (30%).
3. Give the infant an FiO_2 of 1.00 (100%) or as near to this as can be reached by using a head box with a high oxygen flow, and allow to stabilize for 15 minutes.
4. Repeat arterial or transcutaneous Po_2 measurement.
5. Failure of the arterial Po_2 to rise above 13 kPa (>100 mmHg;torr) strongly suggests a large right-to-left shunt due to cyanotic congenital heart disease or persistent fetal circulation.

Presentation of cardiac lesions in the newborn period

Cardiac lesions may present in the neonatal period in the following ways:

1. Persistent central cyanosis due to cyanotic congenital heart disease. Central cyanosis is not usually recognized for several days because of the circulatory adaptations in the first few days of life.
2. Cardiac failure: the infant develops the following signs: pallor, tachypnoea, tachycardia, active precordium, hepatomegaly, weight gain, poor feeding, full fontanelle, poor peripheral circulation with peripheral blotchiness, hypothermia, acidosis, oliguria and apnoea.
3. Heart murmur: transient murmurs are common in the first few days of life due to circulatory adaptations, but must be carefully evaluated and followed up if accompanied by other signs, and if still present at discharge at 4–7 days.
4. Combinations of the above.

The time of appearance of signs is also an important clue to the likely diagnosis.

Cyanosis or heart failure in the first 24 hours
These signs are usually due to causes other than primary structural cardiac abnormalities.

Cyanotic congenital heart disease presenting in the first week

1. Transposition of the great vessels (this accounts for about one-third of cases).
2. Pulmonary atresia.
3. Tricuspid atresia.
4. Total anomalous pulmonary venous drainage: this can mimic respiratory causes of cyanosis.

Cardiac failure due to heart disease presenting in the first week of life

1. Hypoplastic left heart syndrome.
2. Patent ductus arteriosus in pre-term infants.

3. Coarctation of the aorta or interrupted aortic arch.
4. Complex anomalies.

Cyanosis and heart failure in the first week of life

1. Transposition of the great vessels.
2. Total anomalous pulmonary venous drainage.

Heart failure, acidosis and circulatory collapse in the second week of life

1. Missed coarctation or interrupted aortic arch following closure of the ductus arteriosus.
2. Missed transposition of the great vessels without ventriculoseptal defect, following closure of the ductus arteriosus.
3. Missed silent complex anomaly (e.g. major endocardial cushion defect).
4. Viral myocarditis, e.g. Coxsackie B virus infection.

Murmur with or without heart failure at the end of the first week or in the second week

1. Ventriculoseptal defect.
2. Fallot's tetralogy (accompanied by cyanosis).
3. Aortic or pulmonary valve lesions.
4. Patent ductus arteriosus.

Management

Infants presenting in the first week of life may deteriorate very rapidly and require urgent evaluation and discussion of management, and potential transfer to the regional paediatric cardiology centre.

The general plan is to:

1. Support the infant and prevent further deterioration by general methods.
2. Promptly reach an accurate diagnosis, if possible (see above).
3. Consider transfer to a regional paediatric cardiology centre.

Heart failure, with or without cyanosis

1. The infant should be investigated urgently, to try to establish the diagnosis.
2. Fluid intake must be conservative (60 ml/kg per day of glucose 10% parenterally). The infant's symptoms may be helped also by being nursed head up, in oxygen. Special care needs to be taken to maintain the temperature. Diuretics should be given, e.g. frusemide 0.5–2 mg i.m.
3. Digoxin should be given: a digitalizing dose over 24 hours of 40 μg/kg orally or 30 μg/kg i.m. given as three or four doses in 24 hours. Alternatively, a 24-hour maintenance dose of 10 μg/kg in two divided doses orally or intramuscularly. *Note*: digoxin levels measured by conventional radioimmunoassay methods are unreliable in pre-term and sick term infants because of cross-reactivity of the test materials with endogenously occurring substances (Seccombe *et al.*, 1984).

4. Blood gases should be monitored and metabolic acidosis treated with bicarbonate or THAM (p. 138). If there is progressive deterioration in blood gases to unacceptable levels, the infant should be ventilated.
5. Dopamine 5 μg/kg per minute should be given by continuous intravenous infusion if the blood pressure is dropping and the perfusion deteriorates.

   Drug concentration in intravenous solution = body weight (kg) ×

   $$6 \times \frac{\text{desired dose } (\mu\text{g/kg per minute})}{\text{desired intravenous fluid rate (ml/h)}}$$

6. The possibility of Coxsackie virus myocarditis and the infection risk to which adjacent patients may be exposed should be considered (see pp. 178 and 186).

Central cyanosis without heart failure

1. Investigation to establish a diagnosis (see above).
2. Watch for development of heart failure.
3. Conservative fluid intake, not more than 150 ml/kg per day orally.
4. Prostaglandin E treatment may be required if there is a ductus-dependent lesion (e.g. transposition of the great arteries, see below).
5. A palliative procedure (e.g. balloon septostomy in transposition of the great vessels) may be required soon; discuss with the regional paediatric cardiology centre.

Murmur in a well infant at the end of the first week of life

1. Chest X-ray.
2. Electrocardiogram, and echocardiogram if available.
3. Provided that the infant appears well and is free from signs of heart failure or cyanosis at the end of the first week, it can be allowed home and followed up. The baby should, however, be evaluated by a paediatric cardiologist if the murmur persists at 6 months, because of the risk of secondary pulmonary arterial changes due to pulmonary plethora with a left-to-right shunt.

Prostaglandin E_1

A continuous infusion of prostaglandin E_1 can keep open the ductus arteriosus in infants with a duct-dependent lesion long enough to permit transfer to a regional cardiology unit and the use of corrective procedures. The most common diagnoses in which this is useful are:

1. Transposition of the great vessels.
2. Coarctation of the aorta.
3. Interrupted aortic arch.
4. Hypoplastic left heart syndrome.

It may not be possible in a small unit to reach an accurate diagnosis in a rapidly deteriorating infant with heart failure, oliguria, acidosis and cyanosis: under these circumstances, in discussion with the regional paediatric cardiology centre, consideration should be given to trying prostaglandin E_1 even in the absence of a firm diagnosis, as this may be life saving.

Dosage
The dosage is 100 ng/kg per minute, reducing to 10–20 ng/kg per minute after half an hour. This must be infused at a constant rate using a syringe pump.

Infants receiving prostaglandin E_1 often develop pyrexia, leucocytosis, hypotension and apnoeic attacks, and may require ventilation. As this is only a palliative procedure, strenuous efforts must be made to transfer the infant to the regional centre for further management and investigation.

Patent ductus arteriosus in pre-term infants

Patent ductus arteriosus is a common contributory factor to the clinical course in many pre-term infants of 32 weeks gestation or less. It presents towards the end of the first week of life, and occurs to some degree in 50–70% of infants below 1.0 kg. Patent ductus arteriosus is thought to be a contributory factor in the severity of bronchopulmonary dysplasia and may adversely affect cerebral perfusion. Clinical signs appear relatively late.

Recognition

1. Systolic or continuous murmur.
2. Active precordium, visible from outside the incubator.
3. Bounding pulses, pulse pressure >20 mmHg (torr).
4. Deterioration in ventilatory status and oxygen requirement with no primary respiratory cause.
5. Signs of heart failure (see above).
6. Metabolic acidosis.
7. Cardiomegaly with or without pulmonary plethora on chest X-ray.
8. An echocardiogram may show a large left atrium/aortic ratio or large left-sided chambers, and should be carried out to exclude coincidental duct-dependent lesions or other forms of congenital heart disease.

Management

1. Reduce fluid intake to 100 ml/kg per 24 hours, as fluid overloading aggravates the symptoms.
2. Check creatinine, haemoglobin and platelet count, and measure urine output.
3. Keep the arterial PO_2 near the upper level of the acceptable range to encourage duct closure, and the haematocrit over 0.4% by transfusion if necessary; correct metabolic acidosis with bicarbonate.
4. If there are no contraindications to using indomethacin, this should be given intravenously in three doses of 0.2 mg/kg over a 24-hour period (see below). This usually closes the ductus.

5. Recheck the echocardiogram and clinical examination to confirm ductus closure.
6. If the ductus has not closed, a further course of indomethacin can be given, after 2–3 days.
7. If the ductus is still open into the second week of life, or if there are clear contraindications to the use of indomethacin, surgical closure will be required. This is an operation with a very low mortality and morbidity rate in tertiary units.

Indomethacin
Indomethacin is a prostaglandin synthetase (cyclo-oxygenase) inhibitor which favours ductal closure by influencing the ratio of E to F prostaglandins in the ductus; it is often effective in closing the ductus in pre-term infants with patent ductus arteriosus if used in the first 2 weeks of life (Gersony *et al.*, 1983).

Contraindications Active gastrointestinal bleeding is a contraindication to the use of indomethacin because of its effects on the function platelets. Signs of impaired renal function (e.g. serum creatinine >0.1 mmol/l or 1.2 mg% or urine output <1 ml/kg per hour) and thrombocytopenia (<60 × 10^9/l) are the usual contraindications. Jaundice is not a contraindication.

Side effects include oliguria and hyponatraemia for 2 or 3 days during the course of treatment, due to the drug's effects on the intrarenal prostaglandin mechanism, and tendency to bleeding, due to the effects on thromboxanes and platelet function. The risk/benefit ratio for indomethacin in the first 1.5–2 weeks of life is usually more favourable than for surgery, unless the indomethacin has proved ineffective, or has produced marked prolonged oliguria on the first administration.

Procedure for administration of indomethacin

1. Reduce the fluid intake to 100 ml/kg per 24 hours. Enteral feeds should probably be stopped. It is an advantage if the serum sodium level is a little high, because it will drop with the onset of oliguria, despite fluid restriction during the course of treatment.
2. Give three doses of indomethacin 0.2 mg i.v. 12 hours apart. All three doses should be given, even if signs of a patent ductus disappear after the first dose.
3. Monitor the electrolytes, urine output and fluid intake during the course of indomethacin and make appropriate adjustments.
4. Do not attempt to wean the infant off ventilation during the course, as this may encourage reopening of the ductus.
5. Gradually increase the fluid intake and try to wean off ventilation 24 hours after completion of the course of treatment.

Persistent fetal circulation (neonatal persistent pulmonary hypertension)

Persistent fetal circulation (PFC) is a common cause of severe central cyanosis in infants, and is an important differential diagnosis of cyanotic congenital heart disease, particularly in term infants. Severe central cyanosis is caused by delayed disappearance of the high pulmonary vascular resistance present in the fetus, which normally starts to reduce after delivery. As a result, there is right-to-left shunting to a major degree at the level of the ductus arteriosus, foramen ovale and through intrapulmonary shunts. As a result the lungs are largely bypassed. Although PFC may occur in isolation, it is most frequently associated with other, severe illnesses, such as:

1. Respiratory distress syndrome (RDS).
2. Meconium aspiration syndrome.
3. Group B streptococcal pneumonia and septicaemia.
4. Diaphragmatic hernia.
5. Severe hypoxic ischaemic encephalopathy.

The sudden dramatic deterioration seen in the above conditions, occurring 4–6 hours into their clinical course, is frequently due to the development of PFC. It does not, however, occur in all cases of these conditions, and it appears that chronic hypoxia *in utero* produces hypertrophy and distal overgrowth of the muscle layer in the pulmonary arterioles and it is infants with these muscle changes in their pulmonary arterial system who develop PFC.

Recognition

1. Presence of a predisposing factor (see above).
2. The baby requires a very high inspired oxygen concentration in order to maintain an adequate arterial $P\text{O}_2$.
3. Chest X-ray shows findings compatible with one of the predisposing causes, but no obvious change to explain the sudden deterioration in the baby's condition. The heart may be fairly large and may suggest congenital heart disease.
4. In milder cases, there may be a clinically obvious difference in colour between the part of the baby supplied by the preductal aortic arch (right arm, right chest and head) which is pink, and the rest of the body, which is blue. This difference may be confirmed using a transcutaneous oxygen monitor, a pulse oximeter, or pre- and postductal arterial blood samples using an indwelling arterial line. Severe cases are usually so desaturated they look blue all over. The $P\text{CO}_2$ may be low initially in mild cases, but rises as the condition gets worse.
5. The baby may have a murmur and signs of heart failure and is usually tachypnoeic and gasping for breath. The femoral pulses are usually easily palpable.
6. The baby may have abnormal neurological signs due to sustained severe hypoxia, due to PFC or hypoxic-ischaemic encephalopathy from perinatal causes.
7. Echocardiography is required to exclude a primary cardiac cause and Doppler flow studies to demonstrate the cardiac effects on chamber size of right-to-left shunting. Total anomalous pulmonary venous drainage is the cardiac anomaly which is most difficult to exclude; because of the difficulty in visualizing the distal aortic arch, it may be technically difficult to exclude completely a coarctation of the aorta.

8. In some cases, PFC coexists with congenital heart disease and pulmonary disease. These patients are extremely difficult to manage.

Management

1. Look for a primary cause and start appropriate treatment. The situation should be discussed with the regional paediatric cardiology centre and consideration should be given to transfer, either there, or to a tertiary neonatal unit.
2. Support the systemic blood pressure by infusions of fresh frozen plasma, blood and dopamine. The degree of shunting is influenced by the pressure differential between the pulmonary and systemic circuits, therefore the maintenance of an adequate systemic blood pressure (>70 mmHg (torr) mean blood pressure in a term infant) is important. Dopamine 5–20 μg/kg per minute by continuous intravenous infusion will assist in maintaining an adequate cardiac output.
3. Ventilation is usually required at an early stage. The infant is usually large and very distressed; paralysis with pancuronium (0.1–0.3 mg/kg per dose) is required once the patient is securely intubated.
4. Infants with PFC usually need high pressures (up to 40 cmH_2O or greater), a rapid rate (80–100 per minute), a short inspiration time (0.3 seconds) and an FiO_2 of 1.00 (100%). Optimal ventilatory characteristics can be explored by manually ventilating with a Jackson Rees anaesthetic bag system with a pressure gauge with a transcutaneous oxygen monitor attached, to find the rate and pressure which provide best oxygenation. In difficult cases very rapid rates (120 per minute) may be needed and there may be great difficulty mimicking these ventilatory characteristics on current ventilators without inadvertent positive end-expiratory pressure (PEEP). PEEP must be avoided, because overdistension and air-trapping usually develop as the disease progresses in ventilated infants. These infants may require a volume ventilator such as the Siemens servoventilator instead of the standard neonatal equipment.
5. Tolazoline, a pulmonary vasodilator and α-adrenergic blocker, may help to relieve the pulmonary arterial spasm in some cases. Tolazoline usually works well in cases with RDS, causing a dramatic rise in Po_2 but produces a much smaller response in Po_2 in PFC from other causes. Systemic arterial vasodilatation is a very important side effect and may make the situation worse (see above). Support of the systemic blood pressure is important before, during and after using tolazoline. A test dose of 2 (1–4) mg/kg i.v. is given, preferably through an intravenous line in the head. If an improvement in Po_2 occurs in the next 20 minutes, a continuous infusion of 2 mg/kg per hour is started without delay. Gastrointestinal bleeding is a frequent side effect with infants receiving tolazoline as a continuous infusion of 2 or more mg/kg per hour. If there is no response to a test dose of 4 mg/kg, it is unlikely that tolazoline treatment offers any benefit, but considerable risks.
6. Ventilator management of these infants is extremely difficult. They are exquisitely sensitive to what appear to be trivial changes in peak pressure, inspired oxygen concentration and rate, and respond with

precipitous desaturation, presenting major problems in returning them to a viable arterial $P\text{O}_2$. They usually have a critical low $P\text{CO}_2$ value, below which the pulmonary vascular bed opens up. This is usually in the range 2.5–4.0 kPa (20–30 mmHg;torr) but most severely ill infants may have to be maintained with a $P\text{CO}_2$ less than 2.5 kPa (less than 20 mmHg;torr) to keep the $P\text{O}_2$ within the viable range. Sustained low levels of $P\text{CO}_2$ are undesirable because of coincidental reduction in cerebral perfusion due to vasospasm.

7. Extracorporeal membrane oxygenation (ECMO) has been advocated for managing the most severely ill infants, and is claimed to be cost-effective and to improve survival. At the present time this technique involves tying off the right common carotid artery, with unknown effects on later neurodevelopmental outcome. The benefits or otherwise of ECMO in PFC have not been investigated in controlled clinical trials.

Arrhythmias

Congenital heart block (for prenatal diagnosis and treatment, see p. 27)

Congenital heart block is a rare condition, sometimes not associated with structural heart lesions. Some cases are genetic in origin, others occur in association with maternal collagen diseases, particularly systemic lupus erythematosus, with anti-Roh antibody. Where there is coincidental congenital heart disease, this is usually a complex anomaly.

Recognition

1. The infant usually looks quite normal, or may have mild signs of heart failure.
2. The heart rate is consistently <100 per minute (often as slow as 55–60) is regular and the pulse is of large volume. The heart rate does not increase appreciably on making the baby cry. Auscultation confirms a slow heart rate and variable intensity of the first heart sound.
3. Electrocardiography and echocardiography confirm the diagnosis and exclude major structural lesions.

Management

1. Treatment is occasionally required if there is heart failure or Stokes–Adams episodes.
2. Heart failure should be treated with diuretics, not digoxin, because digoxin will further slow the ventricular rate.
3. Dopamine 20–10 μg/kg per minute or isoprenaline 0.075 μg/kg per minute by continuous infusion can be used in patients with obvious symptoms while attempts are made to transfer the infant to a regional paediatric cardiology centre for further management and possible pacing.

Supraventricular tachycardia (for prenatal diagnosis and treatment, see p. 27)

Supraventricular tachycardia is a common arrhythmia presenting perinatally.

Recognition

1. Sustained or intermittent fetal tachycardia >200 beats per minute may be recognized prenatally. Prenatal ultrasound may pick up hydrops fetalis (with or without polyhydramnios) due to heart failure, and a detailed prenatal echocardiogram should be performed to look for cardiac anomalies. Consideration should be given to treating the mother with digoxin to control the fetal tachycardia (p. 27) and to timing of delivery if hydrops cannot be controlled by digoxin.
2. A neonate may be identified with paroxysmal episodes of regular tachycardia, tachypnoea, pallor and poor urine output, sometimes accompanied by signs of heart failure.
3. Electrocardiogram and echocardiogram confirm the diagnosis. A proportion of these infants have ventricular pre-excitation (Wolff–Parkinson–White syndrome) or a short P–R interval (Lown–Ganong–Levine syndrome).

Management

1. Commonly infants with supraventricular tachycardia *in utero* revert to sinus rhythm with delivery and have no attacks in the newborn period, but require monitoring for 24–48 hours.
2. Carotid sinus pressure and pressure on the eyeballs should not be used in the newborn to stimulate a vagal response, because of potential damage to these structures. Appropriate manoeuvres to stimulate a vagal response that may cause reversion to sinus rhythm are palpation of the abdomen, or application of a plastic bag of iced water to the upper face, including the nose, for 15–20 seconds (Bissett *et al.*, 1980).
3. If the baby vomits, the rhythm frequently reverts to sinus rhythm.
4. Digitalization (p. 169).
5. Use of a β-blocker (e.g. propranolol 0.01–0.015 mg/kg i.v. over 10 minutes followed by 0.5–1 mg/kg orally 6 hourly). The initial dose may be repeated four times if required. Verapamil, although effective, has been associated with severe hypotension and death in infants with supraventricular tachycardia (Kirk *et al.*, 1987) and is not recommended in the newborn.
6. Direct current cardioversion is rarely used in the newborn period.

External cardiac massage

For external cardiac massage, see p. 41.

Pericardial drainage

For pericardial drainage, see p. 317.

References

Bisset, G.S., Gaum, W. and Kaplan, S. (1980) The ice bag; a new technique for interruption of supraventricular tachycardia. *Journal of Pediatrics*, **97**, 593–595

Gersony, W.M., Peckham, G.J., Ellison, R.C., Miettinen, O.S. and Nadas, A.S. (1983) Effects of indomethacin in premature infants with patent ductus arteriosus: results of a national collaborative study. *Journal of Pediatrics*, **102**, 895–906

Jones, R.W.A., Bawner, J.H., Joseph, M.C. and Shinebourne, E.A. (1976) Arterial oxygenation and response to oxygen breathing in differential diagnosis of congenital heart disease in infants. *Archives of Disease in Childhood*, **51**, 667–673

Kirk, C.R., Gibbs, J.L., Thomas, R., Radley-Smith, R. and Qureshi, S.A. (1987) Cardiovascular collapse after verapamil in supraventricular tachycardia. *Archives of Disease in Childhood*, **62**, 1265–1266

Seccombe, D.W., Pudek, M.R., Whitfield, M.F., Jacobson, B.E., Wittman, B.K. and King, J.F. (1984) Perinatal changes in a digoxin-like immuno-reactive substance. *Pediatric Research*, **18**, 1097–1099

Further reading

Hastreiter, A.R. (ed.) (1988) Cardiovascular disease in the neonate. *Clinics in Perinatology*, **15(3)**, 421–719

Moller, J.H. and Neal, W.A. (1981) *Heart Disease in Infancy*, Appleton Century-Croft, New York

Rowe, R.D., Freedom, R.M., Merhizi, A. and Bloom, K.R. (1981) *The Neonate with Congenital Heart Disease*, Saunders, Philadelphia

Spitzer, A.R., Davis, J., Clarke, W.T., Bernbaum, J. and Fox, W.W. (1988) Pulmonary hypertension and persistent fetal circulation in the newborn. *Clinics in Perinatology*, **15**, 389–413

Chapter 14

Infections, including perinatal human immunodeficiency virus (HIV) infection

Administrative emergencies caused by infections in the nursery

Spreading infection in neonatal units is an ever-present risk, and requires both consistently applied preventive measures and prompt and adequate action in the face of a developing crisis. Small and sick neonates are particularly susceptible to infection and usually develop generalized infections due to their inability to localize microbiological invasion. Serious infections can easily spread from one baby to another, particularly if a number of infants are nursed together in a confined space when the unit is very busy. The prevention of spreading infection requires:

1. Microbiological surveillance of organisms obtained from nursery patients, an awareness of changing microbiological resistance patterns and a close relationship between the senior nursery medical, nursing staff and the hospital microbiologists.
2. Enforcement of routine hand washing using antiseptic soap by **all** staff members on entry to the unit and before and after handling **every** baby is the most important single measure to prevent cross-infection. Nails should be kept short.
3. Exclusion of staff and parents with active infective illnesses (e.g. gastroenteritis, respiratory infections, influenza, herpes labialis). Mothers with obstetric wound infections should be allowed into the unit, but great care must be taken with hand washing and gowning before they handle their babies.
4. Elimination of communal facilities for bathing and changing infants where cross-infection may occur.
5. Regular prophylactic cord care using drying agents with an antiseptic base (e.g. North American triple dye cord paint, hexachlorophane cord powder, regular cleaning with alcoholic chlorhexidine) to promote early drying and separation of the cord, because the cord is an important source of organisms that colonize the baby and spread from one baby to the others.
6. A well organized system for regular changing and sterilization of respiratory equipment, tubing, incubators and bedding.

Infants with early signs of infection must be recognized and isolated if there is any possibility that their infection may be a potential risk to other patients (e.g. rubella, Coxsackie virus, cytomegalovirus (CMV), herpes simplex (HSV), respiratory syncytial virus infections, diarrhoea etc.). Appropriate isolation procedures should be begun for that infant (e.g. a single room with negative air flow, gowning, and hand washing etc.); potential contacts need to be identified and kept apart as a group, and watched carefully for signs of possible infection. No new patients should be admitted into that area of the nursery until the problem is clearly contained. It is much better to overreact and then stop the isolation process later than to underreact and have spreading infection going from one baby to the next, causing major mortality among small, sick and susceptible infants.

Routes of infection

The infant may become infected *in utero*, during birth, or after delivery. Only the emergency aspects of fetal and neonatal infection are considered here.

Infections during pregnancy (congenital infections, transplacental infections)

Routine maternal screening for the TORCH (toxoplasma, rubella, CMV and herpes simplex virus) group of infections is not of much use and in any case does not include some important pathogens (see below). The more important infections acquired across the placenta, secondary to maternal infection, are CMV, rubella, herpes simplex virus, toxoplasmosis, syphilis, HIV, enterovirus infection. Infection of the fetus with the varicella-zoster virus (VZV), listeria, parvovirus B19 and tuberculosis are less common; hepatitis B virus may occasionally infect the fetus, but perinatal infection is more usual. In tropical or subtropical areas, fetal infections with malaria, brucella, African trypanosomiasis, South American trypanosomiasis (Chagas' disease), Lassa virus and Japanese encephalitis may all occur. Transplacental infection with HIV is the usual route of infection (p. 188). Intrauterine infection with *Chlamydia trachomatis* may occur with premature rupture of the membranes. Intrauterine infection with *Ascaris lumbricoides* has been reported once (Chen *et al.*, 1972).

Recognition

1. There may be a history of infectious illness during the pregnancy.
2. Clinical signs are not clearly specific for the infecting organism. Hepatosplenomegaly, thrombocytopenia and neurological symptoms are the most frequent findings. Relatively specific signs are given in Table 14.1. CMV, rubella, toxoplasmosis, enteroviruses, South American trypanosomiasis and occasionally syphilis may present a clinical appearance similar to rhesus isoimmunization, with hepatosplenomegaly, purpura, thrombocytopenia, jaundice and anaemia, with or

Table 14.1 Some relatively specific features of the commoner types of congenital and intrapartum acquired infections

Cytomegalovirus	Microcephaly with periventricular calcifications Thrombocytopenia, petechiae and hepatosplenomegaly
Toxoplasmosis	Hydrocephalus with generalized intracranial calcifications Choroidoretinitis
Rubella	'Blueberry muffin' syndrome Vertical striations of long bones ('celery stalking') Cataracts, retinal pigmentation Peripheral pulmonary arterial stenoses
Syphilis	Mucocutaneous skin lesions ('syphilitic snuffles') Periostitis, osteochondritis and bone pain
Herpes simplex	Skin vesicles CNS and hepatic involvement
Enterovirus	CNS and hepatic involvement Myocarditis

Adapted from Stagno (1981)

without hydrops ('blueberry muffin baby'). South American trypanosomiasis may also cause abortion, stillbirth, pre-term delivery, intrauterine growth retardation or a clinically normal but infected infant. Transplacental infection occurs in about 2% of infected mothers at any stage in pregnancy. African trypanosomiasis may cause congenital infection, with fever, hepatosplenomegaly, anaemia, jaundice, oedema, haemorrhage and fits, and the infant may die shortly after birth, or may appear well at delivery but show subsequent psychomotor delay (Lingam *et al.*, 1985). An expert in the appropriate form of trypanosomiasis should be consulted if the diagnosis is suspected.

3. Some infants are markedly growth retarded for gestational age, having symmetrical stunting which affects weight, length and head circumference equally. Such infants usually have other stigmata of congenital infection.
4. Congenital malaria with *Plasmodium vivax* or *Plasmodium falciparum* (or less commonly with quartan and ovale infections) occurs more often when the mother is non-immune. With *Plasmodium falciparum* infections there may be abortion, or pre-term delivery; the infant is often small for dates. The usual age of onset is 4–6 weeks, with fever, anaemia, irritability, anorexia, hypothermia, diarrhoea, vomiting, fits or respiratory distress; hepatosplenomegaly is usually present. The mother may have minimal or no signs of malaria and still transmit the infection to the fetus.

Diagnostic investigations

1. Placental histology. The placenta is a much neglected source of histological material, and of direct significance to the infant.
2. Cord blood IgM and agent-specific IgM.
3. Urine and pharyngeal secretions for virus culture, three samples should be sent (CMV and rubella).

4. Sequential maternal and neonatal serology from birth to 3 months (a falling maternal titre and rising infant titre suggests infection).
5. Neonatal examination by an ophthalmologist.
6. Skull and long bone X-rays for intracranial calcification and abnormalities of ossification of the long bones. Cranial ultrasound examination has a high sensitivity in detecting intracranial calcification.

Specific disease investigations

1. Toxoplasmosis: serial determinations of IgG, and specific IgM. Isolation of *Toxoplasma gondii* from placenta, CSF and blood.
2. Syphilis: Reagin (venereal disease reference laboratory (VDRL)), fluorescent antibody test, specific IgM and dark-field microscopy of smears from mucocutaneous lesions.
3. CMV can usually be diagnosed in the first 3 weeks of life by the detection of the virus from the urine by culture, immunofluorescence or electron microscopy. Infants with CMV excrete large quantities of virus and are highly infective, but they may have no detectable specific IgM (Best and Sutherland, 1990).
4. Neonatal herpes simplex infection can be diagnosed from the inoculation into cell cultures of lesion swabs, CSF, urine and throat and eye swabs; electron microscopy will detect virus particles most rapidly, but failure to identify virus particles does not exclude the diagnosis.
5. Malaria: placental histology, thick and thin (to distinguish the type of parasite) blood smears from mother and infant; also indirect fluorescent antibody and indirect haemagglutination tests are widely used.
6. South American trypanosomiasis (*Trypanosoma cruzi*): infant: direct blood examination with previous concentration using microhaematocrit tubes, complement fixation tests, IgM ELISA (enzyme-linked immunosorbent assay) test; placenta: histology; mother: blood culture, direct blood examination and serology (Bittencourt *et al.*, 1985).
7. African trypanosomiasis (*Trypanosoma gambiense* or *Trypanosoma rhodesiense*): can also be diagnosed serologically and by identification of the parasite in the infant's blood or CSF; specific IgM is present in blood and CSF.
8. Tuberculosis: placental histology. Maternal investigations. Look for miliary tuberculosis and tuberculous meningitis in the infant.
9. Perinatal chickenpox: history and vesicular rash, electron microscopy of vesicle fluid, serology. Rarely, intrauterine infection may cause severe cicatricial scarring with limb deformities and brain damage (p. 183).

Management

Specific management of these conditions is unsatisfactory, as considerable damage may have been sustained by several organ systems; specific cures are for the most part not available. The following considerations are of importance, however.

Infectivity
Precautions with blood and body fluid are advisable with such infants. Infants with CMV and rubella excrete virus in large quantities in the urine and other secretions and present an infective risk to pregnant staff. Infants with congenital syphilis excrete treponemes in body fluids and from mucous membranes, and should be isolated and handled with rubber gloves. (See Blood and body fluid precautions, p. 191.)

Anaemia and jaundice
This may present a major problem, due to brisk haemolytic anaemia, and rapidly increasing jaundice may require exchange transfusions. If exchange transfusion is required, care must be taken to obtain all diagnostic blood samples in the first cycle of the exchange transfusion.

Thrombocytopenia and disseminated intravascular coagulation (DIC)
Infants may require platelet transfusions and treatment for DIC, including exchange transfusion.

Specific treatments

Syphilis For this 90 mg (150 000 units) of benzylpenicillin/kg per day in three divided doses, i.m. or i.v., is given for 15 days.

Toxoplasmosis Treatment is unsatisfactory. Pyrimethamine 2 mg/kg per day orally for the first day, then 1 mg/kg per day in two divided doses for 30 days, with sulphadiazine 150 mg/kg per day in four divided doses for 30 days, and folinic acid 1 mg/kg per day orally, to reduce the marrow toxicity of pyrimethamine. Prednisolone should probably be added if there is chorioretinitis.

Trypanosomiasis For South American trypanosomiasis, nifurtimox (Lampit-Bayer 2502) has been used with some success, in a dose of 25 mg/kg per day, in three divided doses, for 90 days. Benzhidazole (Radanil, Rochagan, R07-1051) has also been used in an initial dose of 3 mg/kg per day increasing to 7.5–10 mg/kg per day for 60 days (Gutteridge, 1985). African trypanosomiasis can be treated with a combination of suramin and Melarsoprol (Mel B) (Lingam *et al.*, 1985; Gutteridge, 1985). An expert in the appropriate form of trypanosomiasis should be consulted before starting treatment.

Tuberculosis Isoniazid is the treatment of choice, with rifampicin if there is a resistant organism.

Malaria Chloroquine 10 mg/kg initially, then the same dose 6 hours later; 2 doses of 5 mg/kg are given on the second and third days. Primaquine 0.5 mg/kg daily may be given (after first excluding G-6PD deficiency in the appropriate ethnic groups) for 14 days after the chloroquine with *Pl. vivax* but is probably not necessary as relapse does not seem to occur with congenital malaria. If there is a *Pl. falciparum* infection which may be chloroquine resistant, quinine should be used instead; a specialist should be consulted on the appropriate dose and route.

Chicken pox Varicella during pregnancy may be severe or occasionally fatal, particularly if complicated by pneumonitis. Susceptible contacts should be given zoster immunoglobulin (ZIG) which prevents the infection or modifies it.

Women who develop the early signs of varicella in pregnancy should be given intravenous acyclovir; Boyd and Walker (1988) suggest a dose of 10–15 mg/kg 8-hourly for 5–6 days. If varicella develops before week 20 of pregnancy, there is a possibility that the fetus may be infected; such infants are usually small for gestational age with cutaneous scars, limb atrophy, eye defects and cortical atrophy and they develop convulsions. An infant with fetal varicella syndrome should be given acyclovir for at least 14 days, but even with treatment the likelihood of improvement is small, and death in the neonatal period sometimes occurs. About 20% of mothers with varicella in later pregnancy produce an infant with varicella. Infants born 5 or more days after the mother develops varicella may be born with a mild disease and invariably survive. Those born within 5 days of the onset of the maternal infection usually develop the rash 5–10 days after delivery, and if untreated, have a high mortality. This group should be given ZIG 250 mg/kg as soon after birth as possible, and those with clinical varicella should be treated with acyclovir 10 mg/kg i.v. 8-hourly for 10 days.

Rubella or CMV There is no proven treatment for rubella or CMV.

Recently recognized infections during pregnancy which may involve the fetus

Chlamydia psittaci of ovine origin This infection is acquired from sheep and is of importance as a cause of abortion or fetal death in the human. *Chlamydia psittaci* in sheep is responsible for ovine enzootic abortion. Infection may be fatal to the human mother and to the fetus. The diagnosis can be made by a raised titre to chlamydial group antigen in a complement fixation test. If the infection is suspected in the mother a course of tetracycline should be given. There is as yet no evidence of direct fetal infection, and death appears to be due to an acute placentitis (Johnson *et al.*, 1985). Pregnant women should avoid sheep at lambing time.

Parvovirus infection The most common manifestation of parvovirus B19 is erythema infectiosum (fifth disease) which is mainly a disease of children (Greer, 1988). Infected adults may have no rash, but may develop an arthralgia, or may have no symptoms at all. Maternal infection should be considered after contact with a case, or where a condition develops that is similar to rubella when rubella can be excluded serologically. The virus attacks mainly the erythropoietic stem cells, causing a severe anaemia resulting in a hydropic fetus; the fetus usually dies *in utero* in midtrimester or at term.

If parvovirus infection is suspected it is usually possible to detect IgM- and IgG-specific antibodies from 14 to 15 weeks of pregnancy. A raised level of maternal serum α-fetoprotein at around 16 weeks may be the first indication of fetal involvement, and shortly after this ultrasound shows evidence of fetal hydrops. It would appear that this infection may be an important cause (accounting for up to 33% of cases) of non-immune hydrops (Anand *et al.*, 1987). The fetus is affected in about one-third of infected women. There is no specific treatment but an intrauterine blood transfusion into the cord might be effective (p. 26).

Brucellosis This may, rarely, cause fetal death or the birth of an infected infant (Madkour, 1989).

Infection acquired during labour

Infection may be acquired during labour:

1. A transplacental infection resulting from maternal bacteraemia (e.g. pyelonephritis or appendicitis). Infection is usually due to a Gram-negative bacillus and the fetus may develop septicaemia with or without meningitis.
2. Chorioamnionitis, due to ascending infection, following prolonged rupture of the membranes, usually more than 48 hours, and usually indicated by maternal pyrexia and leucocytosis. Organisms implicated are most likely to be:
   (a) Streptococci: group B streptococcus, *Streptococcus pneumoniae*;
   (b) *Listeria monocytogenes*;
   (c) Gram-negative bacilli;
   (d) *Haemophilus influenzae*;
   (e) Anaerobes (e.g. Bacteroides sp. but often a mixed infection;
   (f) Herpes simplex, if there is an active lesion in the genital tract;
   (g) There is a significant risk of systemic candidiasis in babies whose mothers had a cervical suture, with candidal vaginal colonization.

Recognition

The infant may appear lethargic and respond sluggishly at delivery, with poor perfusion and developing respiratory problems, or may appear normal for 3–4 hours before developing signs of respiratory distress and a rapid downhill course with acidaemia, hypoxaemia and persistent fetal circulation, requiring energetic ventilator management.

Management

1. A full infection screen should be carried out and the infant started on an antibiotic regimen to cover the above organisms (e.g. intravenous ampicillin and gentamicin). In addition, a vaginal swab should be taken from the mother.
2. Full supportive management may be required to treat major metabolic and acid–base derangements.

Infections acquired during delivery

Gonococcal conjunctivitis (gonococcal ophthalmia)

Recognition

Gonococcal ophthalmia should be suspected with any severe purulent conjunctivitis developing within the first week (usually within 48 hours of delivery). A Gram film of the pus should be examined for Gram-negative intracellular diplococci and the pus cultured on appropriate media, usually plated out at the bedside. Gonococci will not tolerate a prolonged journey on a dry swab to the bacteriology laboratory using the hospital messenger system.

Management

1. Systemic benzylpenicillin 120 mg (200 000 units) 4-hourly i.m. or i.v., accompanied by local hygiene to the eyes and irrigation with penicillin eye drops, 12 mg/ml (20 000 units/ml).
2. Failure to improve within 24–48 hours suggests the possibility of a resistant organism, in which case erythromycin or spectinomycin should be considered.
3. The mother, her consort and other sexual contacts should be traced, investigated and treated, and the blood sent from mother and infant for VDRL and HIV investigations.

Chlamydial conjunctivitis (inclusion body conjunctivitis)

Infection is by the same route as for gonococcal ophthalmia, but *Chlamydia* sp. produces a persistent low-grade conjunctivitis, which may cause conjunctival scarring, but is particularly important because there is a significant incidence of chlamydial pneumonitis during the first 6 months of life in infants infected with *Chlamydia* sp. at birth. In some communities there is a high incidence of genital carriage of *Chlamydia* sp., and screening for both partners should be carried out at around 36 weeks of pregnancy; if either or both are positive, the infected partner or partners should be treated with erythromycin. Intrauterine infection may occur with premature rupture of the membranes.

Recognition
Low-grade conjunctivitis develops between 5 and 10 days of age. Special culture techniques are required to isolate and identify the organism. This should be arranged in conjunction with the microbiology laboratory.

Management
Erythromycin eye drops and systemic erythromycin for 2 weeks.

Herpes simplex virus

This is a potentially fatal infection acquired from active maternal genital herpes lesions. If an active lesion is recognized before delivery, the infant should be delivered by caesarean section if the membranes have not ruptured. Labial herpes presents a somewhat smaller risk.

Recognition
The disseminated form of the disease develops between 5 and 10 days after delivery. There may or may not have been an obvious active lesion in the maternal birth canal and the baby may or may not have one or more

vesicular lesions. Primary herpes infection in the genital tract is of much greater risk to the baby at the time of delivery than recurrent secondary infection. Occasionally the disease in the infant remains localized as a skin eruption, but usually the illness takes the form of a fulminating infection with respiratory, neurological and hepatic manifestations. The virus can be identified on electron microscopy of vesicle fluid and can be cultured. There is usually a CSF pleocytosis (up to 200 per mm^3) and a high CSF protein level (5–10 g/l).

Management

1. Isolation to protect other infants. Hand washing is particularly important.
2. General measures, including respiratory support, control of convulsions and management of liver failure if this develops.
3. At the present time there is no proven specific treatment. Acyclovir in a dose of 30 mg/kg per 24 hours in 8-hourly divided doses for 10–14 days appears the most promising drug but has not yet been completely evaluated; it should be infused over 60 minutes in a maximum concentration of 7 mg/ml. Side effects may be transient renal dysfunction and thrombophlebitis. If renal impairment occurs, the doses should be given at 12 or 24 hour intervals. Vidarabine (30 mg/kg daily i.v.) has been used with variable results. The prognosis in severe systemic infection with herpes simplex virus is very poor.

Enterovirus infection (e.g. Coxsackie virus)

Enterovirus infection may be acquired transplacentally following acute infection in the mother just before delivery, but presents a somewhat similar pattern to HSV infection, and therefore is considered here.

Recognition

The mother usually has symptoms of an influenza-like illness around the time of delivery, with or without a rash. Towards the end of the first week the infant develops:

1. Signs of severe systemic infection with fever, poor feeding, diarrhoea, jaundice and rash. The illness is usually a self-limiting one, but sometimes liver failure develops, due to massive hepatic necrosis, and is associated with a poor prognosis.
2. The baby develops signs of heart failure due to myocarditis sometimes with convulsions. The baby continues to deteriorate with signs of severe systemic infection and heart failure.

Management

1. There is no specific treatment.
2. Isolation of the infant, with strict barrier precautions to protect other infants is very important. It is extremely important to identify and separate as a group other potential contacts, as this infection can spread rapidly through the nursery.

3. General supportive measures.
4. The major differential diagnosis includes inborn errors of metabolism (pp. 282–287).

Infection with *Listeria monocytogenes*

Infection with *Listeria monocytogenes* is very similar clinically to group B streptococcal septicaemia.

This infection may present as:

1. A transplacentally acquired septicaemic illness with hepatosplenomegaly, respiratory features and, in a few cases, small reddish–grey skin nodules.
2. A severe generalized infection with respiratory features and septicaemia in the first week. Meningitis is common.

Management

The drug of choice for management is parenteral ampicillin 200 mg/kg i.v., accompanied by general measures for metabolic cardiac and respiratory support.

Hepatitis B

Acute hepatitis due to hepatitis B virus (HBV) may occur during pregnancy, with a high transmission rate to the infant, particularly if the disease occurs during the third trimester; alternatively the mother may be an asymptomatic carrier of the virus and the infant may come into contact with infected secretions or maternal blood during delivery. Infection of the infant is detected by the presence of hepatitis B surface antigen (HBsAg). The HBV carriage rate and transmission rate from asymptomatic carriers to their infants is particularly high in mothers of Asian origin (in the UK between 3 and 10% of Asian women are infective carriers); other high-risk groups are intravenous drug users and their partners and those who have received numerous blood transfusions for blood disorders such as β-thalassaemia or sickle-cell anaemia; individuals with the 'e' antigen (HBeAg) and no anti-e antibodies are particularly infectious, because with this combination rapid viral replication can occur; the most sensitive indicator of infectivity is by HBV DNA analysis. Infected infants become HBsAg positive after 2 and up to 5 months of age, this period presumably reflecting acquisition at delivery, followed by the incubation period; they may develop jaundice and hepatosplenomegaly, and chronic hepatitis. Only 2–5% of cases who are HBsAg positive are positive at delivery.

Recognition in the neonatal period

The mother has HBsAg; Asian and other at-risk mothers should be screened for carriage. Responses to various combinations of maternal blood results are given in Table 14.2. Health care staff should be immunized against HBV infection.

Table 14.2 Interpretation of maternal blood results for hepatitis B

Hepatitis B surface antigen	=	HBsAg
Hepatitis B core antibody	=	anti-HBc
Hepatitis B surface antibody	=	anti-HBs

Maternal results		Interpretation	Action
1. HBsAG positive or		Infectious	Give infant HBV immunoglobulin and HBV vaccine
2. HBsAg positive Anti-HBc positive Anti-HBs negative		Infectious	
3. HBsAg negative Anti-HBc positive Anti-HBs negative		May or may not be infectious, depending on clinical history	
4. HBsAg negative Anti-HBc positive Anti-HBs positive	or	negative negative positive	Past infection, now immune to HBV

Management

1. Blood and body fluid precautions should be taken (see below).
2. The infant should be handled with gloves until washed all over in the delivery room.
3. The infant should receive hepatitis B immune globulin 1.0 ml (0.5 ml in UK) (400 mg or 400 IU) i.m. within 12 hours of birth, followed by hepatitis B vaccine 0.5 ml (10 μg) i.m. at a different site. This provides the baby with both passive and active immunity. Follow-up doses of the vaccine should be given at 1 and 6 months of age.
4. There is doubt about the advisability of breast feeding because of the risk of passage of virus in the milk, but prohibition of breast feeding in less developed countries may have disastrous consequences for the infant. Non-A non-B hepatitis behaves in a similar manner clinically to HBV, but no protection is given by the immunoglobulin or HBV vaccine.

Acquired immunodeficiency syndrome

Acquired immunodeficiency syndrome (AIDS or HIV infection) was recognized in 1981. It is caused by the human immunodeficiency viruses. The virus is transmitted by sexual contact and exchange of body secretions, and parenterally by blood transfusion with infected blood, or in drug users by communal use of needles and syringes. Infection after heterosexual contact is increasing. The virus is transmitted to the fetus *in utero*, and can, less commonly, be acquired by contact with infected secretions during delivery and possibly from breast milk. It is thought that about 25% of infants of infected mothers may become infected, though Mok *et al*. (1989) found an infection rate of only 7% in HIV-positive mothers without clinical symptoms.

Recognition

Risk factors

The first step in recognition involves identification of high-risk groups of mothers:

1. Known intravenous drug users or their partners (it is uncertain whether there is the same risk for intramuscular injections, but it should be assumed that there is a risk).
2. Known prostitutes.
3. Sexual partners of men known to have AIDS or AIDS-related complex (ARC) or to have HIV antibodies.
4. Sexual partners of bisexual males.
5. Sexual contact in Africa (usually by the male partner) may be an important risk factor as AIDS is widespread throughout the general population in parts of Africa.
6. Recipients of multiple blood transfusions with potentially infected blood (before the use of universal screening of donors).

It may be extremely difficult to obtain accurate information of this kind by history, but at the present time screening for HIV antibody in infants in identified high-risk situations seems justified. Current legal opinion suggests that informed consent should be obtained in order to take the blood specimen (see below).

Clinical
Very few infants who are at risk of acquiring HIV infection have any symptoms in the newborn period. An 'AIDS embryopathy' has been described, but its existence has been questioned. Recently, screening of blood donors for HIV antibody has largely eliminated the risk of HIV acquisition by blood transfusion.

The clinical course of identified neonatal patients infected either by the mother or by blood transfusion appears to be similar.

The incubation period is shorter than in adults, with a delay of 6–24 months before symptoms appear. At the time when symptoms first appear, and the diagnosis is made, all have failure to thrive, hepatomegaly with or without lymphadenopathy and recurrent otitis media. Intractable thrush infections are common, as are repeated pyogenic bacterial infections, such as streptococcal septicaemia. There is a progressively downhill course, with repeated infections and with the acquisition of *Pneumocystis carinii* interstitial pneumonia culminating in death.

As with adults, there appears to be considerable variation in symptomatology, however, Some patients appear to have had isolated thrombocytopenia and then recovered (Saulsbury *et al.*, 1986) while other patients, although clearly infected with HIV by laboratory tests have remained clinically well for several years. Neurodevelopmental examination reveals delay, abnormalities of tone and motor dysfunction of the mouth (Harris-Copp, 1987). The clinical course appears to be more rapid in malnourished and socially deprived infants.

Laboratory diagnosis

Laboratory tests
Laboratory tests for HIV infection are of five types:

1. Screening test to detect HIV antibody (IgG). The most usual is an ELISA. This type of test is cheap, but not very specific.

2. More specific serological test for HIV antibodies (Western blot and immunofluorescence assay).
3. Identification of HIV antigen: this is most frequently used in conjunction with the virus culture.
4. Virus culture in pooled peripheral blood lymphocytes.
5. Other highly specific tests (e.g. nucleic acid probe of peripheral blood leucocytes).

Laboratory criteria for diagnosis of AIDS in infants
Laboratory diagnosis of AIDS in newborns is complicated by transferred maternal antibodies for up to 18 months after delivery (Mok *et al.*, 1989) and the delayed appearance of an IgM anti-HIV response in infected infants (Gaetano *et al.*, 1987). Current recommendations for laboratory diagnosis in infants 15 months old or less are given below.

Evidence for infection in a patient with a disease consistent with AIDS

1. If the mother is thought to have HIV infection in the child's perinatal period, the following tests should be carried out: reactive serum for HIV antibody (this should be repeated) on a screening test (ELISA) and increased serum immunoglobulin levels. In addition, at least one of the following: reduced absolute lymphocyte count; depressed helper T-cell (CD4) lymphocyte count; decreased CD4 : CD8 (suppressor T-cell) ratio, as long as subsequent antibody tests remain positive. Persistence of antibody after the age of 18 months to 2 years is strong evidence of infection in the child.
2. If the mother is not thought to have HIV infection during the child's perinatal period, the following should be carried out: Positive HIV antibody screening test (ELISA) (needs to be repeated) confirmed by one of the more specific HIV antibody tests (Western blot or immunofluorescence assay).

In either situation, infection is also shown by: a positive test result for HIV serum antigen; a positive culture result for HIV confirmed by both reverse transcriptase detection and a specific HIV antigen test; a positive result on any other highly specific test (e.g. nucleic acid probe or peripheral blood lymphocytes).

An inconclusive result is identified by:

1. A repeated reactive result on a screening test followed by a negative or inconclusive result of a supplementary test without culture or antigen confirmation.
2. A serum specimen from a child of less than 15–18 months, whose mother is thought to have HIV infection in the child's perinatal period, which is repeatedly reactive on a screening test for HIV antibody, even if a supplementary test gives a positive result without additional evidence of immune deficiency and without positive culture or serum antigen for HIV.

Current medicolegal recommendations are that blood samples drawn for AIDS testing must only be taken after obtaining fully informed consent from the patient or, in this instance, the parent or guardian, in view of the potential consequences medically and socially of a positive result. It must be stressed at that time that repeated positive results are required in order to confirm the diagnosis, not just one positive test.

Management

There is no proven specific treatment for AIDS. The role of azidothymidine (AZT), a retrovirus reverse transcriptase inhibitor, has not yet been established in children or infants.

Treatment of repeated bacterial and fungal infections is difficult, with early recurrence despite adequate treatment.

Pneumocystis carinii pneumonia may respond to co-trimoxazole and pentamidine but there appears to be a high incidence of hypersensitivity to these drugs in AIDS patients. Alternative combinations are dapsone with trimethoprim and pyrimethamine with sulphadiazine.

Prevention of AIDS

There is no available immunization against AIDS. Preventive methods include testing of donor blood for AIDS antibody, and public education and recommendations to prevent spread by the venereal route or by exchange of body fluids by other means.

Protection and isolation procedures

AIDS is not highly infective and is a fragile virus, easily killed by oxidizing agents, such as household bleach. The risk to health care workers of being infected with the virus, other than by sexual contact with an infected person, is extremely small. In one study of health care workers exposed to HIV-infected blood or body fluids, none of the 74 workers with mucous membrane exposure seroconverted, while only 3 (0.9%) of 351 cases of percutaneous exposure seroconverted. Seroconversion following percutaneous exposure is usually associated with direct accidental injection of several millilitres of infected blood.

Blood and body fluid: general precautions

Because of the inability to recognize the patients who present a risk to health care workers, blood and body fluid precautions should be used in **all** situations where a significant risk may occur.

1. Gloves should be used where contact with blood and body fluids, mucous membranes and non-intact skin is likely. Eyeshields and masks should be used for procedures that might produce droplets of secretions or blood.
2. Hands should be washed immediately if contaminated with blood or body fluids.
3. Precautions should be taken against needle injuries.
4. Although saliva has not been implicated in AIDS transmission, resuscitation equipment should be used, rather than mouth-to-mouth

resuscitation, and gloves should be worn for endotracheal tube suctioning.

5. Health care workers with open skin lesions, such as eczema, should avoid direct patient care while the lesion is present.
6. Potentially infected waste should be collected separately in labelled containers and incinerated.

Maternal contact

The mother must have access to her baby, but must be aware of the potential risks of infection to the baby from body fluids, such as saliva. Breast feeding should probably be discouraged because of the risk of further infection of the infant through the milk (but see p. 000 and Further reading).

Termination

A request for a termination by an infected or clinically affected mother should be accepted, although counselling should be given before a definite decision is reached.

Acute postnatal infections

Newborns, particularly pre-term infants, are more susceptible to generalized infections than older children and may be considered relatively immunocompromised. An attempt to define an anatomical site of infection in the newborn must recognize that infections become disseminated very quickly, although localized infections may develop from seeding during a period of bacteraemia (e.g. osteomyelitis). Occasionally, also, term infants appear to develop localized pyelonephritis.

Acute septicaemia

Recognition

Symptoms requiring immediate investigation include:

1. A sudden change in behaviour or appearance, such as grey pallor, lethargy, deterioration in feeding performance. These are more likely to be noticed by the mother or nurse.
2. A rise or fall in temperature.
3. Apnoeic attacks, tachypnoea, dyspnoea or cyanosis.
4. Abdominal distension.
5. Exacerbation of jaundice, with or without hepatosplenomegaly.
6. Sudden diarrhoea or vomiting.
7. Sudden shock.
8. Bleeding or oozing from puncture sites (possibility of DIC).

It should be remembered, however, that similar symptoms, including jaundice, may also be due to various inborn errors of metabolism.

Investigation

Full infection screen A standard plan of investigation should be used in all cases and should be completed even after one of the investigations is found to be abnormal.

1. Blood culture taken with full aseptic precautions from a vein or artery, but not from a catheter. Any baby with a positive blood culture should have a lumbar puncture.
2. Lumbar puncture with examination of the fluid for glucose, protein, cell count and Gram film. Coagglutination tests for group B streptococcus may be available, with protein, cell count and Gram film.
3. Because of the difficulty in obtaining a clean specimen, suprapubic bladder tap should be carried out, any growth being indicative of infection.
4. Chest X-ray.
5. Swabs from throat, umbilicus and rectum are the most fruitful, in addition to any clearly infected lesions.

Management of infections in general

1. Shock: this usually occurs in any septicaemic illness and is treated with colloids such as fresh frozen plasma, albumin or whole blood (20 ml/kg, the first 10 ml/kg given over 30 minutes) with monitoring of blood pressure. Dopamine 5 μg/kg per minute may also be required.
2. Antibiotics (Table 14.3): the initial choice depends on the antibiotic policy of the nursery and on the patterns of infection and microbiological sensitivity of the organism in that particular nursery. The combination should cover Gram-positive organisms including streptococci and staphylococci and Gram-negative bacilli and *Haemophilus influenzae*. The choice depends on the local bacterial flora, but penicillin or

Table 14.3 Neonatal antibiotic dosage (dose/kg per 24 hours)

Antibiotic	*Dose for*	
	<7 days	*7–28 days*
Benzylpenicillin (penicillin G)	30–60 mg (50 000–100 000 units) in 2 doses	60–150 mg (100 000–250 000 units) in 3 doses
Cloxacillin	50–100 mg in 2 doses	100–200 mg in 3 doses
Ampicillin	100 mg in 2 doses	200–300 mg in 3 doses
Gentamicin	5 mg in 2 doses	7.5 mg in 3 doses
Kanamycin	15 mg in 2 doses	15 mg in 2 doses
Tobramycin	4 mg in 2 doses	6 mg in 3 doses
Chloramphenicol	25 mg pre-term 25 mg term in 2 doses	25 mg pre-term 50 mg term in 2 doses
Vancomycin	30 mg in 2 doses	45 mg in 2 doses
Cefotaxime	100 mg in 3 doses	150 mg in 3 doses
Levels	Gentamicin and tobramycin	Peak 5–10; trough <2 mg/l
	Kanamycin	Peak 15–25; trough <2 mg/l
	Chloramphenicol	Peak 15–25 mg/l
	Vancomycin	Peak 25–30; trough 5–10 mg/l

ampicillin combined with gentamicin usually provide adequate cover. Cloxacillin should be added if there is a chance of deep-seated staphylococcal infection with a penicillinase producer. In meningitis the initial choice could be chloramphenicol and gentamicin or ampicillin, gentamicin and cefotaxime (one of the third-generation cephalosporins, which has good CSF penetration). Choice should be modified according to the results of culture and sensitivity.

3. Ventilatory support where blood gases are significantly deranged.
4. Careful fluid and electrolyte balance and maintenance of the haemoglobin level.
5. Where these measures appear to be unsuccessful, exchange transfusion, transfusion with fresh frozen plasma or granulocyte transfusions have been tried with some success.

Infections requiring special attention

Neonatal meningitis

Recognition
Neonatal meningitis is a serious infection with a significant mortality and long-term morbidity rate. Clinical signs are non-specific and occur late, and a high index of suspicion of meningitis has to be maintained in any infant with a general deterioration in condition.

Predisposing factors for neonatal meningitis include a history of chorioamnionitis and prolonged ruptured membranes in the mother, and illness accompanied by invasive investigations in the newborn.

Clinical signs
Clinical signs of meningitis in the newborn are vague and non-specific. Poor feeding, lethargy, irritability, apnoeic episodes or respiratory irregularity, feeding intolerance or abdominal distension, temperature instability and increasing or persistent jaundice are frequent findings. Late signs include seizures, circulatory failure and shock. The diagnosis may or may not be suspected at the time when a full infection screen is carried out which reveals CSF pleocytosis and organisms on Gram film. Blood staining of the CSF is a not infrequent finding in neonatal meningitis.

Organisms
Common organisms causing neonatal meningitis are: *Escherichia coli*, group B streptococcus, *Listeria monocytogenes*, *Staphylococcus aureus* and *Staphylococcus epidermidis* (albus).

Management
Antibiotic choice is discussed above. Infants with meningitis may be severely ill and require vigorous cardiorespiratory management with ventilation and treatment for shock (p. 72) or may have much less severe symptoms. Antibiotic treatment should be continued for 10–14 days; the lumbar puncture should be repeated 2–3 days after stopping antibiotics. There is no evidence that the injection of antibiotics into the ventricles has any effect on the ultimate outcome (McCracken *et al.*, 1980).

Complications of neonatal meningitis include: persistent ventriculitis, postmeningitis hydrocephalus, cranial nerve damage including sensorineural deafness and cognitive deficits detected at follow up.

Group B haemolytic streptococcal infection

This may present as:

1. A fulminating septicaemic illness with pneumonia and respiratory symptoms in the first 12 hours of life, following acquisition of the organism in the birth canal.
2. Isolated meningitis between 1 and 12 weeks of age. Infants with group B streptococcal infection may also develop arthritis, osteitis and empyema. Colonization at delivery is a common finding and it is only between 1 in 500 and 1 in 1000 of such infants who develop fulminating disease. At the present time there are no generally available tests that can identify the infants who are particularly at risk.

Management

1. Prophylaxis: group B streptococcal disease occurs so soon after delivery and can be so devastating and is so difficult to differentiate from other, more benign, forms of respiratory distress that prophylactic ampicillin 100 mg/kg per day i.v. should be given to any infant with respiratory symptoms, after an initial blood culture, gastric aspirate and white count have been sent. Urine from a suprapubic tap should also be sent for the group B streptococcal coagglutination test. In the majority of infants, ampicillin prophylaxis will prevent or modify the development of fulminating disease and can be stopped if the cultures are negative.
2. Infants who have strongly suspected or proven streptococcal septicaemia, should be treated with intravenous ampicillin 200 mg/kg per day and an aminoglycoside for between 10 days and 3 weeks.
3. Supportive treatment is extremely important, particularly in attempting to treat shock. Fresh frozen plasma should be given for shock (p. 72) and dopamine (p. 170) may also be required.
4. The infant is likely to develop persistent fetal circulation and require energetic ventilator management (p. 138).

Osteitis (osteomyelitis)

Osteitis in the newborn differs from osteitis in other age groups in four ways:

1. Infection of the upper metaphysis of the humerus or femur may involve the shoulder and hip joints respectively, causing a septic arthritis.
2. More than one bone may be involved.
3. Unusual sites may be infected (e.g. the maxilla or premaxilla).
4. Numerous organisms may cause osteitis, the most common being *Staphylococcus aureus*. Less commonly, osteitis may be due to Gram-negative bacilli, streptococci, pneumococci, gonococci and meningococci.

Recognition

1. The initial symptoms may be those of a septicaemia and evidence of bone involvement may only become apparent later. The risk of osteomyelitis emphasizes the importance of treating neonatal staphylococcal pustular disease seriously.
2. Localizing symptoms are those of swelling and loss of movement, or crying when the affected area is touched or moved.
3. Infection of the shaft of the long bones is usually obvious because of the swelling, but involvement of the upper end of the humerus or femur is less obvious, because the swelling is not easy to recognize around the joint. The main differential diagnosis is fracture of a long bone.
4. Confirmation of the diagnosis may be provided by aspiration and culture of pus from an obvious swelling, or from blood culture. Aspiration of the shoulder or hip joint should be done by an orthopaedic surgeon.

Osteitis at special sites

Sites that are difficult to detect

1. The vertebrae: osteitis of a vertebra is particularly difficult to detect clinically. Infection of cervical vertebrae may cause torticollis with little apparent swelling or abscess.
2. Sacrum, or sacroiliac joint: infection may only become obvious at a very late stage, unless it is included in a skeletal survey as part of a search for osteitis.

Osteitis of the maxilla

This infection is rarely seen outside the neonatal period. It may present with swelling of the cheek, periorbital oedema, proptosis or chemosis of the conjunctiva. Pus may be discharged at the inner or outer canthus of the eye, the midpoint of the lower lid, the outer surface of the alveolar margin near the site of the first molar, through the hard palate or through the nose on the affected side. The condition may be mistaken for orbital cellulitis. Radiography is rarely helpful but culture of the blood or pus usually yields a growth of *Staphylococcus aureus*. Early diagnosis and treatment will avoid damage to the primary dentition and facial asymmetry.

Osteitis of the premaxilla

This causes similar symptoms but the first sign is swelling of the upper alveolar margin near the midline. Infection is usually confined to the premaxilla, but may spread to the maxillary sinus. Investigation is as for maxillary osteomyelitis.

Management

1. In the absence of contrary evidence, it should be assumed that the infection is a staphylococcal one. An orthopaedic surgeon should be asked to see infections involving the long bones or joints and a dental surgeon should be involved in managing infections in the maxilla and premaxilla.

2. Antibiotics: treatment should be started with cloxacillin and with gentamicin in addition if the organism is not known. Staphylococcal infections which do not respond to cloxacillin may respond to erythromycin, fusidic acid (Fucidin), lincomycin or clindamycin.
3. Duration of treatment: antibiotic treatment should be continued for a minimum of 2 weeks after all signs of infection have disappeared and in any case for not less than 4 weeks. The X-ray appearance takes much longer to return to normal. The prognosis for growth and joint function in neonatal osteomyelitis in general is surprisingly good.

Pyelonephritis

Acute pyelonephritis in the newborn may develop in one of two ways:

1. As part of a septicaemic illness in which infection of the renal tissue occurs as part of the septicaemia. Subsequent investigation of the renal tract usually shows no abnormality.
2. As a primary infection in an abnormal urinary tract, often with secondary septicaemia. In either case jaundice may be a presenting feature.

Recognition

The infant may present with jaundice and a septicaemic illness, or with poor feeding, slow weight gain and non-specific symptoms. The diagnosis is usually made after a full infection screen. It is important not to omit a suprapubic urine specimen as part of a full infection screen in infants in the second week of life, who are more likely to have infection in the urinary tract.

Management

1. Antibiotics: gentamicin (reduced dose with poor renal function) and ampicillin should be used in the initial septicaemic illness. When sensitivities are available, treatment may continue with ampicillin alone, if the organism is sensitive. Treatment should be continued for 2 weeks.
2. Blood urea, creatinine and electrolytes should be measured.
3. All infants should have ultrasound examination of the renal tract and those found to have abnormalities may require further radiological investigation.
4. Infants with a significant abnormality of the renal tract should receive a maintenance dose of an appropriate antibiotic (e.g. co-trimoxazole) and the opinion of a urologist should be sought.

Acute gastrointestinal infections

Diarrhoea is an important symptom in newborns, and may occur for a variety of reasons, only some of which are infective; but the possibility of infective diarrhoea requires that serious consideration be given to the isolating and segregating of patients (see above). Infective diarrhoea may be due to enteropathogenic *E.coli*, *Campylobacter* sp. rotavirus, *Shigella* or *Salmonella* spp. and occasionally to staphylococcal or candida enterocolitis. Blood-stained diarrhoea may also be a symptom of necrotizing enterocolitis.

Recognition

The sudden onset of frequent loose stools, with vomiting or deterioration in feeding, raises the possibility of acute gastroenteritis. Blood and mucus in the stool may occur with *Campylobacter*, *Shigella* or *Salmonella* spp., but are rare with *E.coli*. Other conditions which must be considered are:

1. Mismanagement of feeds with underfeeding.
2. Profuse diarrhoea within a few hours of starting milk, due to lactase deficiency (lactose intolerance).
3. Necrotizing enterocolitis or intussusception.
4. Diarrhoea with abdominal distension preceded by delayed passage of meconium, due to Hirschsprung's disease.
5. Cow's milk allergy.
6. Acute adrenal failure, due to congenital adrenal hyperplasia.
7. Orally administered drugs, which might cause frequent stools (e.g. ampicillin, ferrous sulphate, calcium gluconate).
8. Incarceration of an inguinal hernia.
9. A septicaemic illness presenting with abdominal distension and diarrhoea.
10. Infants showing signs of withdrawal from opiates (narcotic abstinence syndrome) frequently have diarrhoea as a presenting feature (see also Chapter 28).
11. Breast milk from a mother taking laxatives or an excessive amount of fruit (orange juice, plums etc.).

Infants maintained on a low fluid intake and hyperosmolar feeds, and diuretics, such as those with bronchopulmonary dysplasia, are particularly sensitive to the circulatory effects of sudden fluid depletion caused by diarrhoea. Such infants readily develop circulatory collapse and it is particularly important to recognize gastrointestinal symptoms in these patients early and to provide an adequate fluid intake.

Management

1. Isolation and sending of stools for bacteriological analysis. A full 'infection screen' should be carried out if the infant appears systemically unwell.
2. If there is moderately severe dehydration or the infant is not tolerating feeds adequately, intravenous fluids should be started.
3. In term infants with mild dehydration who can tolerate feeds, oral replacement with a standard clear fluid and electrolyte mixture can be attempted. An alternative solution is sodium chloride 0.45% in glucose 2.5% with potassium added, depending on electrolyte results.
4. Antibiotics are not generally indicated and are not of proven value in gastroenteritis due to pathogenic *E.coli*. Oral amoxycillin or systemic ampicillin should be given in salmonella or shigella infections.

Administrative aspects of infective gastroenteritis in a maternity unit

Single cases An infant developing sudden diarrhoea should be regarded as potentially infective and should be transferred to an isolation room and investigated. When the infection is confirmed, the baby should be kept in effective isolation with appropriate hand washing precautions and if necessary transferred to suitable facilities in another unit.

Stool specimens should be sent from infants nursed in the same room as the index case, and no further patients admitted to that room until the test results are known to be negative.

In presumed viral infections, a period of 10 days without symptoms in a contact should be regarded as evidence of non-infectivity.

More than one case occurring simultaneously This raises the possibility of infection from a common source, such as contamination of the milk supply. Serious consideration should be given under these circumstances to closing the unit to further admissions, if possible.

Antibiotic policy in the newborn

1. Local applications should not contain any antibiotic which could be used systemically, because of the risk of inducing resistant organisms.
2. In general the following antibiotics are contraindicated in the newborn: bacitracin, neomycin, novobiocin, polymyxin, tetracyclines and sulphonamides in the presence of jaundice. Co-trimoxazole can be used for urinary infections in low doses in the absence of jaundice. Chloramphenicol may be used for the treatment of meningitis due to Gram-negative bacilli.
3. Antibiotic policy is based on continuous surveillance of the resistance characteristics of the local organisms.

Antimicrobial drug dosage

For antimicrobial drug dosages, see Table 14.3.

References

Anand, A., Gray, E.S., Brown, T., Clewly, P. and Cohen, B. (1987) Human parvovirus infection in pregnancy and hydrops fetalis. *New England Journal of Medicine*, **316**, 183–186

Best, J.M. and Sutherland, S. (1990) Diagnosis and prevention of congenital and perinatal infections. *British Medical Journal*, **301**, 888–889

Bittencourt, A.L., Mota, E., Ribeiro Filho, R., Fernandes, L.G., de Almeida, P.R. and Sherlock, I. (1985) Incidence of congenital Chagas' disease in Bahia (Brazil). *Journal of Tropical Paediatrics*, **31**, 242–248

Boyd, K. and Walker, E. (1988) Use of acyclovir to treat chickenpox in pregnancy. *British Medical Journal*, **296**, 393–394

Chen, W.G., Chen, P.M. and Huang, C.C. (1972) Neonatal ascariasis. *Journal of Pediatrics*, **81**, 783–785

Gaetano, C., Scano, G., Carbonari, M., Giannini, G., Mezzaroma, I., Aiuti, F., Marolla, L., Casadei, A.M. and Carapella, E. (1987) Delayed and defective anti-HIV IgM response in infants. *Lancet*, **i**, 631

Greer, I.A. (1988) Complications of erythema infectiosum in pregnancy. *British Medical Journal*, **296**, 862–863

Gutteridge, W.E. (1985) Trypanosomiasis: existing chemotherapy and its limitations. *British Medical Bulletin*, **41**, 162–168

Harris-Copp, M. (1987) Neurodevelopmental findings in infants and children with HIV infection (Abstract). *Developmental Medicine and Child Neurology*, **29** (Suppl. 55), 43–44

Johnson, F.W.A., Matheson, B.A., Williams, H., Laing, A.G., Jandial, V., Davidson-Lamb, R., Halliday, G.J., Hobson, D., Wong, S.Y., Hadley, K.M., Moffat, M.A.J. and Postlethwaite, R. (1985) Abortion due to infection with *Chlamydia psittaci* in a sheep farmer's wife. *British Medical Journal*, **290**, 592–594

Lingam, S., Marshall, W.C., Wilson, J., Gould, J.M., Reinhardt, M.C. and Evans, D.A. (1985) Congenital trypanosomiasis in a child born in London. *Developmental Medicine and Neurology*, **27**, 670–674

McCracken, G.H., Mize, S.G. and Threlkeld, N. (1980) Intraventricular gentamicin therapy in Gram-negative bacillary meningitis in infancy. *Lancet*, **i**, 787–791

Madkour, M.M. (1989) *Brucellosis*, Butterworths, London, p. 203

Mok, J.Y.Q., Hague, R.A., Yap, P.L., Hargreaves, F.D., Inglis, J.M., Whitelaw, J.M., Steel, C.M., Eden, O.B., Rebens, S., Peutherer, J.P., Ludlam, C., Taylor, R., MacCallum, L.R. and Brettle, R.P. (1989) Vertical transmission of HIV: a prospective study. *Archives of Disease in Childhood*, **64**, 1140–1145

Saulsbury, F.T., Boyle, R.J., Wykoff, R.F. and Howard, T.H. (1986) Thrombocytopenia as the presenting manifestation of human T-lymphotropic virus type III infection in infants. *Journal of Pediatrics*, **109**, 30–34

Stagno, S. (1981) Diagnosis of viral infections of the newborn infant. *Clinics in Perinatology*, **8**, 579–589

Further reading

Freij, B.J. and Sever, J.L. (eds) (1988) Infectious complications of pregnancy. *Clinics in Perinatology*, **15**, 163–419

McCracken, G.H. and Nelson, J.C. (1983) *Antimicrobial Therapy for Newborns*, 2nd edn, Grune and Stratton, New York

MacLeod, C. (ed.) (1988) *Parasitic Infections in Pregnancy and the Newborn*, Oxford Medical, Oxford

Plotkin, S.A. and Star, S.E. (1981) Symposium on Perinatal Infections. *Clinics in Perinatology*, **8**, 395–637

Remington, J.S. and Klein, J.O. (1983) *Infectious Diseases of the Fetus and Newborn Infant*, 2nd edn, Saunders, Philadelphia

Task Force on Pediatric AIDS (1988) Pediatric guidelines for infection control of HIV in hospitals, medical offices, schools and other settings. *Pediatrics*, **82**, 801–807

Chapter 15

Convulsions

Causes

Fits in the newborn are usually due to hypoxic-ischaemic encephalopathy, cerebral injury associated with intraventricular haemorrhage, hypoglycaemia, hypocalcaemia or hypomagnesaemia, and the probable causes can be inferred from the perinatal history. In the severely ill infant more than one of these causes may be present. The categories of fits have been subdivided into the common (Table 15.1) and less common (Table 15.2)

Table 15.1 Common causes of convulsions in the newborn

Aetiology	*Cause*	*Clinical condition before fit*	*Type of fit*
Onset in the first 72 hours after delivery			
Perinatal hypoxia	Hypoxic-ischaemic encephalopathy	Ill	Generalized clonic or tonic
Mechanically difficult delivery	Acute subdural haemorrhage (anterior or posterior fossa)	Ill	As above, occasionally focal
Infant of diabetic mother	Hypoglycaemia Hypocalcaemia†	Well	Focal, multicentric focal or generalized clonic
Small-for-dates infant	Hypoglycaemia	Well	As above
Smaller of twins	Hypoglycaemia	Well	As above
Small pre-term infant	Intraventricular haemorrhage*, periventricular leucomalacia	Ill	Tonic
4 hours up to 7 days			
Infant of diabetic mother	Hypocalcaemia†	Well	Focal, multicentric focal or generalized clonic
Onset from 5 days onwards			
Infection	Meningitis*: occasionally earlier than 5 days	Ill	Focal, generalized clonal or tonic
High phosphorus cow's milk feeds	Hypocalcaemia†	Well	Focal, multicentric focal or generalized clonic

*Hypoglycaemia and/or hypocalcaemia may also be present.
†Hypocalcaemia and hypomagnesaemia often occur together and therefore it should be routine for both ions to be estimated by the laboratory even if only calcium is requested.

Table 15.2 Less common causes of convulsions in the newborn

Cause of fit	*Aetiology*	
Metabolic		
Hypoglycaemia	Galactosaemia Fructose intolerance Nesidioblastosis Islet cell tumour or hyperplasia Wiedemann–Beckwith syndrome Glycogen storage disease (Type I)	Chapter 27
Hypocalcaemia	Maternal vitamin D deficiency Maternal hyperparathyroidism Idiopathic hypoparathyroidism Taitz–DiGeorge syndrome (third and fourth arch syndrome with hypoparathyroidism and deficiency of thymus	Chapter 16
Hypocalcaemia–hypomagnesaemia	Maternal magnesium malabsorption Specific magnesium malabsorption	
Hyponatraemia (water intoxication)	Excess low electrolyte fluids Inappropriate antidiuretic hormone secretion with intracranial haemorrhage or IPPV Accidental injection of oxytocic drug into infant	Chapter 20
Hypernatraemia	Accidental addition of salt to feeds and other causes	
Hyperbilirubinaemia with kernicterus		
Pyridoxine dependency	Probably autosomal recessive	
Drug related		
Toxic effects of local anaesthetic	Accidental injection into fetus High fetal blood levels	p. 48
Maternal drug abuse, neonatal withdrawal symptoms	Narcotics Barbiturates Alcohol	Chapter 28
Infective		
Congenital	Toxoplasmosis, rubella, cytomegalovirus, herpes, Coxsackie B virus	Chapter 14
Late transplacental	Coliform meningitis present at birth (pp. 194–195)	
Malformations		
Sturge–Weber syndrome	Unknown	
Incontinentia pigmenti	X-linked dominant, lethal in male	
Microcephaly, other cerebral malformations without microcephaly	Various: occasionally autosomal recessive	

causes. Meningitis must be excluded in any infant with fits even if it appears well.

One of the less common causes of neonatal convulsions should be suspected when there is no clue in the perinatal history and the commoner causes have been excluded, and also when the fits are resistant to the usual anticonvulsant drugs.

Recognition

The recognition that an infant is having a fit is not always easy, partly because other conditions may be mistaken for a fit and partly because the clinical manifestations may be easily missed or misinterpreted.

The following conditions must be distinguished from fits:

1. Jitteriness: a hyperexcitable state in which any stimulus, even a sound, produces a symmetrical rhythmical tremor of the limbs, predominantly the arms. This occurs in cerebral oedema, hypoglycaemia, hypocalcaemia, hypomagnesaemia or, quite frequently, from no apparent cause.
2. Apnoeic attacks: these may, if prolonged, result in an hypoxic tonic–clonic fit. Careful observation will show that apnoea is the first event, whereas in tonic fits the apnoea results from the tonic spasm of the respiratory muscles.
3. The random uncoordinated movements of a single limb which occur in infants of 30 weeks' gestation or less.

The type of fit can be as follows:

1. Minor or atypical fits: transient nystagmus, deviation of the eyes, repetitive chewing movements or smacking of the lips, apnoea, bradycardia, cyanosis.
2. Focal or multicentric focal: these may affect either side alternately or different parts of the body sequentially; their focal nature does not imply a localized lesion and they are commonly associated with hypoglycaemia, hypocalcaemia or hypomagnesaemia. The frequency is usually 1–3 per second, and between fits the child looks well and alert.
3. Generalized tonic–clonic fits: This is the most common type of fit, and may be due to any of the causes already mentioned (p. 202), but is most likely to occur in an ill infant (Table 15.1).
4. Tonic fits: These have the worst prognosis as they commonly occur in infants with severe hypoxic brain damage or in pre-term infants with intraventricular haemorrhage.

Accompanying physical signs

These may give an indication of the probable cause of the fits. Fits and other neurological abnormalities in the jaundiced infant may indicate kernicterus. Head retraction or a tense or bulging fontanelle occurs in meningitis or intracranial haemorrhage, hepatosplenomegaly and a papular purpuric rash occur in congenital infections, and hepatomegaly alone occurs in galactosaemia, fructose intolerance and glycogen storage disease. A port wine stain on the upper face with or without buphthalmos occurs in the Sturge–Weber syndrome.

Management

Initial diagnosis

1. Dextrostix (or Chemstrip, see footnote to p. 59) estimation: since this can be done immediately and with minimal trauma this is a most useful

investigation, although the finding of hypoglycaemia should not be taken to indicate that this is the sole cause of the fits, unless the perinatal history makes this very probable (Table 15.1). If the glucose strip reads <1.4 mmol/l (<25 mg%), this is proof of significant hypoglycaemia, although before starting treatment blood should be taken for laboratory confirmation of the blood glucose which should be <1.7 mmol/l (<30 mg%) (pp. 209–210). It has been shown (Lucas, Morley and Cole, 1989) that may be important to maintain the blood glucose above 2.5 mmol/l (47 mg%) in order to avoid brain damage (p.000). A lumbar puncture should be carried out in all cases except in a very ill infant where there is a risk that it might produce apnoeic attacks and serious deterioration. In these circumstances it should be delayed until the infant's condition has improved even if this means starting treatment for meningitis without adequate proof. Although there may be circumstances when the evidence is strong enough to treat hypoglycaemia without doing a lumbar puncture, confirmation of this diagnosis requires clear evidence of improvement or loss of symptoms within 10–20 minutes of correcting the hypoglycaemia. If hypocalcaemia or hypomagnesaemia is suspected there is inevitably a longer delay in obtaining a result, and it is best to exclude hypoglycaemia and perform a lumbar puncture while waiting to see whether hypocalcaemia or hypomagnesaemia has been confirmed. Intravenous treatment for hypocalcaemia or hypomagnesaemia should never be given until there is proof of the diagnosis.

2. If meningitis is suspected, a full infection screen should be done, not merely a lumbar puncture (pp. 194–195).
3. Hyponatraemia should be considered where hypoglycaemia, hypocalcaemia, hypomagnesaemia, meningitis and intraventricular haemorrhage have been excluded and where the serum sodium is <120 mmol/l (see pp. 230–231) for list of causes and for management).
4. Hypernatraemia (pp. 235–236).
5. A metabolic disorder should be suspected when all the more common causes of fits have been excluded, but particularly in the presence of fits which are resistant to the treatment, and are accompanied by a persistent metabolic acidosis, or in which ketone bodies are present in the urine.

Treatment

1. Any biochemical cause which has been discovered should be treated: hypoglycaemia (p. 211), hypocalcaemia (p. 220), hypomagnesaemia (p. 223), hyponatraemia (p. 234), hypernatraemia (p. 238).
2. For the routine treatment of recurrent fits phenobarbitone should be used as it can be continued on a maintenance basis whereas diazepam cannot. The initial dose should be 10 mg/kg i.v. as a single dose, followed by a further 10 mg/kg dose if the convulsion cannot be controlled within 10 minutes. Further doses of 5 mg/kg boluses at 20–30 min. intervals, if fits continue, up to a loading dose of 40 mg/kg. A trough level of 60–70 μmol/l is required for a therapeutic effect.
3. If phenobarbitone is unsuccessful in controlling fits, or does so only

with an unacceptably large dose, phenytoin should be added in a dose of 10 mg/kg i.v. and repeated if necessary after 10 minutes. Phenytoin can also be given intramuscularly or orally in divided doses 12-hourly; maintenance dose 4–6 mg/kg/24 hours; trough level 40–80 μmol/l.

4. For status epilepticus or very frequently recurring fits which cannot be controlled by phenobarbitone or phenytoin, diazepam should be given intravenously or intramuscularly according to the degree of urgency. Facilities for immediate intubation should be available when using intravenous diazepam because of the danger of apnoea. Diazepam in its usually available parenteral form contains sodium benzoate which competes with bilirubin for binding sites and may therefore lower the threshold for the development of kernicterus in jaundiced infants, particularly the pre-term infant. Recently an emulsion of diazepam without sodium benzoate has become available (Diazemuls, KabiVitrum, London; ampoules of 10 mg in 2 ml) for intravenous use only; this should **not** be mixed with saline solution but can be given as a slow drip in glucose 5% or 10%; this preparation can be given safely to jaundiced infants. With the usual preparation of parenteral diazepam the dose is 0.25–1.0 mg/kg by slow intravenous injection over 2–3 minutes.
5. In status epilepticus resistant to phenobarbitone, phenytoin and diazepam, paraldehyde i.v. should be tried: loading dose 3 ml/kg/hr of a 5% solution for 3 hours, then 0.4 mg/kg/hr. Tubing must be protected from light, and the solution changed every 4 hours. Alternatively, it may be necessary to curarize the infant and use intermittent positive pressure ventilation (IPPV). Avoid theophyllines in apnoea due to fits.
6. In treatment of fits for presumed cerebral oedema in the posthypoxic state, intravenous mannitol may be given as a 20% solution in a dose of 1–2 g/kg (4–8 ml/kg) over a period of 45–90 minutes, preceded by a test dose of 0.2 g/kg (1.0 ml/kg) over 5 minutes (Swyer, 1975). However, if there is oliguria due to renal failure, mannitol should not be given. In addition dexamethasone may be given in a dose of 0.2–0.4 mg/kg i.v. initially, followed by 0.1–0.2 mg/kg every 6 hours i.v. or i.m. There is no evidence that the use of mannitol and dexamethasone affects neurodevelopmental outcome. IPPV and hyperventilation ($P\text{CO}_2$ reduced to 4 kPa (30 mmHg; torr)) can be used in infants who are known to have suffered from severe hypoxia. At present, however, a definite diagnosis of cerebral oedema is difficult to make, though obliteration or narrowing of the lateral ventricles shown by sector scanner or computerized tomography would be good evidence in favour of cerebral oedema.
7. In fits thought to be due to pyridoxine dependency (AR) on clinical grounds or because of a previously affected child, pyridoxine 50 mg should be injected intravenously preferably with EEG control. Intramuscular injection can also be used but is likely to produce a less clear cut result. An injection of pyridoxine should be given empirically to all infants with intractable fits.

Prognosis

In hypoxic-ischaemic encephalopathy in term infants cerebral parenchymal hypodensity on a CT scan at 4 days of age is a good indicator of later prognosis; generalized hypodensity has a very poor prognosis (Fitzhardinge, Floodmak, Fitz and Ashby, 1981); interpretation of CT scans in asphyxiated preterm infants is less helpful (Fitzhardinge, Floodmak, Fitz and Ashby, 1982).

References

Fitzhardinge, P.M., Floodmak, O., Fitz, C.R. and Ashby, S. (1981) The prognostic value of computed tomography as an adjunct to assessment of the preterm infant with post-asphyxial encephalopathy. *Journal of Pediatrics*, **99**, 777–785.

Fitzhardinge, P.M., Floodmak, O., Fitz, C.R. and Ashby, S. (1982) The prognostic value of computed tomography of the brain in asphyxiated premature infants. *Journal of Pediatrics*, **100**, 476–481.

Lucas, A., Morley, R. and Cole, T.J. (1989) Adverse neurodevelopmental outcome of moderate neonatal hypoglycaemia. *British Medical Journal*, **297**, 1304–1308.

Swyer, P.R. (1975) The intensive care of the newly born infant. *Monographis in Paediatrics*, **6**, 152, Karger, Basel.

Further reading

Tarby, T.C. and Volpe, J.J. (1986) Neonatal seizures. In *Textbook of Neonatology* (ed. N.R.C. Robertson). Churchill Livingstone, Edinburgh, Chapter 21 (Part II), pp. 533–542.

Chapter 16

Hypoglycaemia and hyperglycaemia

Hypoglycaemia

Since glucose and dextrose are identical, in the interests of clarity the term 'glucose' is used throughout. There is no justification for retaining 'dextrose' in descriptions of intravenous glucose solutions.

Estimations of 'blood sugar' give results of 0.5–0.8 mmol/l (10–15 mg%) higher than those which estimate true glucose only.

Plasma glucose estimations give, for practical purposes, the same results as with whole blood.

Definition

In the light of the findings in a large survey of hypoglycaemia in the newborn (Lucas, Morley and Cole, 1989), levels of blood glucose previously regarded as unlikely to cause brain damage must be revised upwards. Lucas, Morley and Cole showed a clear correlation between neurodevelopmental impairment (as shown by cerebral palsy or developmental delay at 18 months) and recurrent hypoglycaemia at levels of below 2.5 mmol/l (47 mg%). These results were obtained in both term and preterm infants. The developmental delay was correlated with the number of days on which levels of <2.5 mmol/l (<47 mg%) were found, and was very significant for hypoglycaemia occurring on 3 or more days. Recurring moderate hypoglycaemia was more significant than severe but less frequent hypoglycaemia episodes.

Normal range

This is the range within which blood glucose should be maintained: 2.5–5.0 mmol/l (47–90 mg%). The various causes of hypoglycaemia in the newborn are shown in Fig. 16.1.

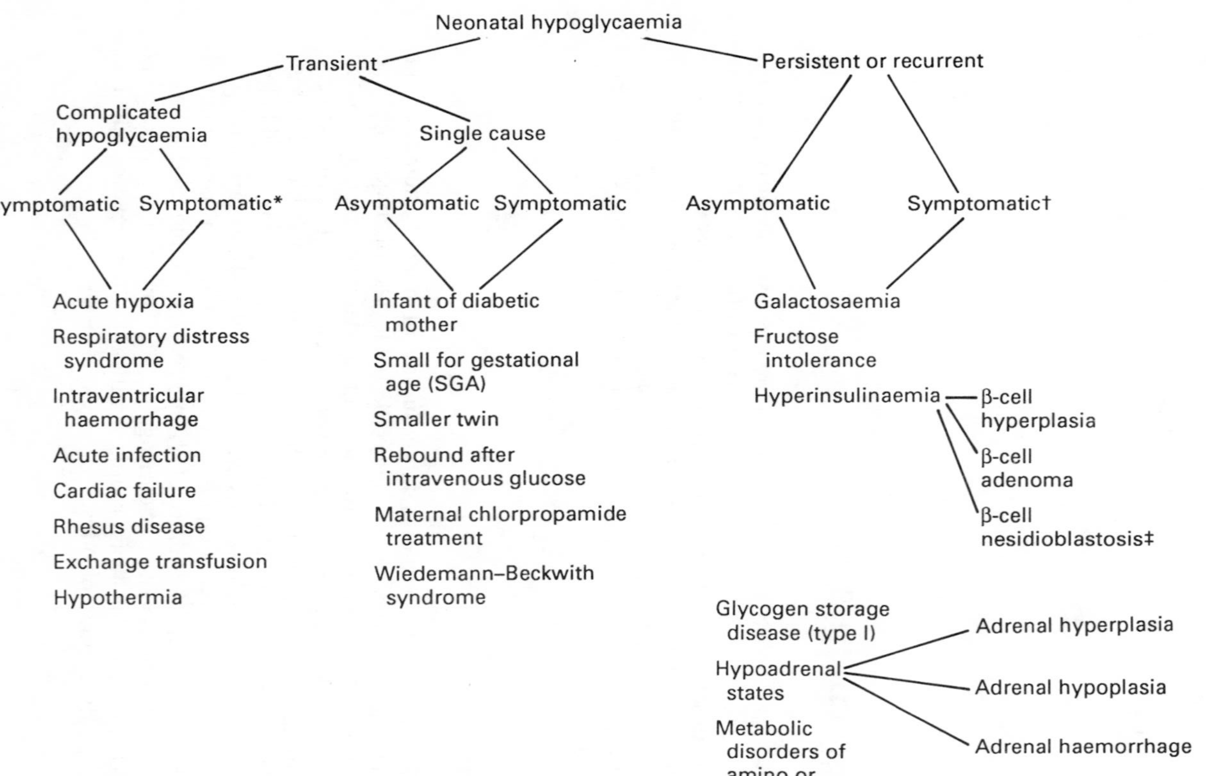

Figure 16.1 Neonatal hypoglycaemia. *In this group it is usually impossible to attribute symptoms to hypoglycaemia with any certainty, but it is nevertheless important to treat it when detected chemically. †In these conditions hypoglycaemia is usually symptomatic at some stage but infants may be severely hypoglycaemic for long periods without symptoms. ‡From Aynsley-Green *et al*. (1981)

Transient hypoglycaemia

1. Hypoglycaemia with other complicating conditions occurs in very sick infants, often in association with a metabolic acidosis and hypocalcaemia. Even in the absence of symptoms related to hypoglycaemia, the blood glucose should be maintained within the normal range. Usually the blood glucose returns to normal when the primary condition has been corrected. Blood glucose levels in the sick infant should be measured regularly, by Chemstrip or Dextrostix (see footnote to p. 59), and confirmed when necessary by glood glucose estimations.
2. Transient hypoglycaemia from a single cause can often be prevented by early milk feeds, particularly in the infant of the diabetic mother (IDM) and the small-for-gestational-age (SGA) infant, and in the smaller twin. Rebound hypoglycaemia after stopping an intravenous glucose drip can be prevented by slowing the rate of delivery of glucose and overlapping this with gradually increasing milk feeds. The hypoglycaemia from maternal chlorpropamide treatment for diabetes is avoidable in the sense that chlorpropamide should not be used in diabetes in pregnancy, but where this has been given the hypoglycaemic effect may be expected to last for as long as 3–4 days (Zucker and Simon, 1968). The Wiedemann–Beckwith syndrome of exomphalos, macroglossia and visceromegaly may be obvious clinically.

Hypoglycaemia from a persistent cause

With the exception of adrenal haemorrhage and masculinized females with adrenal hyperplasia, there are no characteristic physical signs in this group, though infants with nesidioblastosis may resemble those of the diabetic mother (Aynsley-Green *et al.*, 1981). The clinical pictures in galactosaemia and fructose intolerance are described elsewhere (pp. 288–291), and glycogen storage disease (usually type I) may present with hepatomegaly. In the inherited disorders of amino and organic acid metabolism, hypoglycaemia is often associated with a metabolic acidosis and the blood glucose returns to normal as soon as the metabolic disorder is appropriately treated.

Recognition of hypoglycaemia

1. Asymptomatic hypoglycaemia obviously cannot be detected on clinical grounds, but should be looked for in all acutely ill infants, whatever the cause.
2. Symptomatic hypoglycaemia should be considered in any infant with the following symptoms (however, it should be recognized that these symptoms are in no way specific to hypoglycaemia and may be due to other associated diseases).
   (a) Jitteriness, irritability (p. 203);
   (b) Fits: focal, multicentric focal or generalized;

(c) Unexplained persistent cyanosis, apnoeic attacks, shallow respiration, tachypnoea or bradycardia;
(d) Lethargy, unresponsiveness or coma;
(e) Vomiting.

In contrast with other age groups, newborn infants with hypoglycaemia rarely become pale and sweaty when hypoglycaemic. The only exception to the definition of hypoglycaemia given on p. 207 is when the blood glucose level falls very rapidly, as in an infant of a diabetic mother (p. 217) when symptoms may occur at levels between 2.2 and 2.8 mmol/l (40–50 mg%).

Management

Asymptomatic hypoglycaemia or hypoglycaemia associated with non-specific symptoms

In view of the findings of Lucas, Morley and Cole (1989), previously discussed, the policy in neonatal units should be to maintain a blood glucose level at >2.5 mmol/l (>47 mg%) at all times. Clearly there is a limit to the number of estimations which should be performed in any 24 hour period, and the frequency of estimation will vary with the degree of clinical illness in the infant. Small pre-term infants will require frequent estimations; although symptoms (p. 59) may not be specific to hypoglycaemia, their occurrence, or indeed any sudden clinical deterioration, should be an indication for a glucose strip or blood glucose estimation. In sick infants, repeated estimations should be continued until it is clear that a safe level of blood glucose can be maintained without the aid of intravenous glucose; in very small sick infants blood glucose estimations may have to be continued for several weeks. Where it is clear that a single self-limiting factor is operating, as in the IDM, the duration of blood glucose monitoring can be quite short.

The majority of infants, requiring frequent blood glucose estimations will be receiving intravenous fluids, and the correction of hypoglycaemia will usually only require an adjustment to the rate of administration of intravenous glucose or its concentration. Severe hypoglycaemia (levels <1.7 mmol/l or <30 mg%) without obvious symptoms will require the same treatment as for symptomatic hypoglycaemia.

Symptomatic hypoglycaemia

Fits appear to be the only symptom that can be clearly associated with hypoglycaemia in the newborn, and even here a fit in an already ill infant may be due to some other cause or causes, such as intraventricular haemorrhage or meningitis. It is only when there is known to be either a well-recognized predisposing cause, as in the IDM, or in recurring hypoglycaemia in an otherwise well infant (e.g. in nesidioblastosis, Weidemann–Beckwith syndrome, maternal treatment with chlorpropamide or a metabolic disorder such as galactosaemia) that a fit can be assumed to be due to hypoglycaemia alone. In these circumstances the fit will be terminated by intravenous glucose (see below).

Treatment of symptomatic hypoglycaemia

1. In an acute emergency, as in severe fits, coma or shock, in which the symptoms can with reasonable certainty be attributed to hypoglycaemia, a test dose of 2–4 ml/kg (0.5–1.0 g/kg) of glucose 25% (glucose 10% in a dose of 6 ml/kg will be adequate if the 25% solution is not immediately available) should be given at the rate of 1 ml/minute without waiting for confirmation by glucose strip or biochemical estimation. Nevertheless, blood **must** be taken before injection of the glucose for subsequent confirmation that hypoglycaemia did in fact exist. Normally, if the symptoms are solely due to hypoglycaemia, the infant will return to normal within 10–20 minutes and at this stage a further glucose strip or blood glucose estimation should be carried out to confirm that a normal level has been achieved, and further estimations at hourly intervals for 4–6 hours to detect a rebound or recurrence hypoglycaemia. There are two possible difficulties in the use of the test dose of glucose; first, an infant who has been severely hypoglycaemic for some hours may recover more slowly than expected even when the blood glucose has been corrected; secondly, a spurious and usually transient improvement may result in infants with cerebral oedema (generally in the posthypoxic state), due to the osmotic effect of the hypertonic glucose.
2. If symptomatic hypoglycaemia is confirmed by a test dose, as described above (or for maintenance treatment of asymptomatic hypoglycaemia), an intravenous infusion of glucose 10% should be started at the rate of 2–3 ml/kg per hour (50–75 ml/kg per 24 hours), increasing the rate according to the age of the child up to a maximum of 100 ml/kg per day by the second day, with 0.18% sodium chloride in 4.3% glucose to make up the total volume of 150 ml/kg per 24 hours if the plasma sodium is low or starts to fall. The aim is to keep the blood glucose level between 2.5 and 5.0 mmol/l (47–90 mg%) or blood glucose strip estimation between 2.5 mmol/l (47 mg%) and 5.9 mmol/l (108 mg%). The normal maintenance requirement for glucose in this age group is 6–8 mg/kg per minute, but higher rates may be needed.

   If these rates of delivery of glucose are inadequate to maintain normal blood glucose the strength of glucose should be increased to 15 or 20% at the same rate as before. Failure to control hypoglycaemia at the rates of delivery of glucose given above should suggest the possibility of hyperinsulinaemia.
3. Failure to maintain adequate blood glucose levels with intravenous glucose alone requires the addition of one of the following:
   (a) Hydrocortisone 15 mg/kg orally or i.v. for 24 hours given at 6-hourly intervals, or more frequently as indicated by blood glucose levels; maintenance glucocorticoids can be used orally in the form of prednisolone in a dose of 1–3 mg/kg per 24 hours divided into 4 doses, 6-hourly; or

(b) Glucagon should be used as a continuous infusion of 0.5–2.0 mg over 24 hours where infants need an infusion rate of glucose of >14 mg/kg/minute. A single dose should not exceed 1.0 mg (1000 μg).

Notes

1. Glucagon is less effective in infants with depleted liver glycogen (posthypoxic states, SGA infants, the smaller twin) and is ineffective where glycogen is not available for release, as in glycogen storage disease, galactosaemia or fructose intolerance. Glucagon stimulates gluconeogenesis and acts as a stimulant to the production of insulin and should not be given repeatedly in hyperinsulinaemic states.
2. Fructose (laevulose, invert sugar) should **never** be used in neonatal hypoglycaemia because it will produce severe, possibly fatal, hypoglycaemia in unrecognized fructose intolerance and may cause a metabolic acidosis in the normal neonate.

Subsequent management

In transient hypoglycaemia, intravenous glucose should be slowly reduced as described above. Oral glucose by itself should not be used for the maintenance or treatment of hypoglycaemia because it is a potent stimulus for insulin production. Hypertonic glucose solution given orally may produce a dumping syndrome.

In persistent hyperinsulinaemic states feeds may have to be given round the clock at 2-hourly intervals and in resistant cases with proved high plasma insulin levels diazoxide may be required in a dose of 10–25 mg/kg per 24 hours divided into three doses; or oral prednisolone (dose as above) may be tried. In nesidioblastosis prevention of hypoglycaemia with drugs and frequent oral feeds is usually unsuccessful and partial pancreatectomy is required (Aynsley-Green *et al.*, 1981).

Hyperglycaemia

Definition

This has been defined, for the neonatal period, as a blood glucose level greater than 6.9 mmol/l (>125 mg%) (Cornblath and Schwartz, 1976), although glycosuria is unlikely unless the blood glucose exceeds 10.0 mmol/l (>180 mg%), and clinical syndromes rarely present unless the blood glucose is >14.0 mmol/l (>250 mg%).

The causes of neonatal hyperglycaemia are:

1. Ill low-birth-weight infants on intravenous glucose infusions or total parenteral nutrition (TPN).
2. As a complication of intraventricular haemorrhage (IVH) in low-birth-weight infants.
3. Transient neonatal diabetes, which may be inherited as an autosomal recessive.
4. Congenital absence of the islet cells (Dodge and Laurence, 1977)
5. Septicaemia is the commonest cause of a sudden deterioration of glucose tolerance.

Recognition

1. All ill low-birth-weight infants should have regular (twice daily or more frequently) blood glucose checks carried out when on glucose infusion or TPN and the urine should be tested with Clinitest when blood levels exceed 10.0mmol/l (180mg%).
2. When an IVH is suspected the diagnosis should be confirmed by a computerized tomography (CT) scan or sector scanner.
3. The diagnosis of transient neonatal diabetes should be suspected on the following evidence:
   (a) An infant which is exceptionally small for gestational age;
   (b) Rapidly developing skin pallor, loss of weight and dehydration in spite of conventionally adequate intake of calories and fluid;
   (c) Polyuria in the presence of indications in (b);
   (d) Glycosuria without ketonuria;
   (e) Hyperglycaemia without ketoacidosis: the blood glucose levels are much higher than in the other form of neonatal hyperglycaemia, usually greater than 33mmol/l (500mg%). Plasma sodium is low due to sodium depletion due to polyuria. Plasma levels of urea and potassium are often moderately raised, and there is a metabolic acidosis. The condition is easily distinguished from adrenal failure and renal hypoplasia once the presence of glycosuria and hyperglycaemia has been discovered.
4. Congenital absence of the islets (? AR or XR); this very rare condition presents in a manner similar to that described in transient diabetes, but histology of the pancreas shows a complete absence of islet cells (Dodge and Laurence, 1977).

Management

Hyperglycaemia in the ill low-birth-weight infant

This should be managed by reducing the glucose load until blood levels return to normal (the usual requirement for glucose is 6–8mg/kg per hour). Insulin should not be used unless the hyperglycaemia cannot be controlled by manipulating the glucose intake; the usual dose, given as an infusion, is 0.05 units/kg/hr (10 units to 100ml fluid: 1ml/kg/hr = 0.1 unit/kg/hr).

Transient diabetes

1. Rehydration with 0.9% sodium chloride initially, changing to 0.9% sodium chloride with glucose 5% as soon as the blood glucose starts to fall.
2. Short-acting insulin (soluble, Actrapid or other similar insulins) should be given in a daily dose of 1–3 units/kg per 24 hours given preferably by infusion pump, or in divided dose twice or three times in the 24 hours. The dose of insulin is regulated according to 4-hourly blood glucose strip or biochemical glucose estimations.

3. Potassium supplements are often required as soon as the blood glucose falls, and should be given only when the plasma potassium is normal or low and when the ECG shows evidence of depletion.
4. The duration of treatment is unpredictable; insulin may be required for days, weeks or months, and hypoglycaemia may occur when the insulin requirement falls.

References

Aynsley-Green, A., Polak, J.M., Bloom, S.R., Gouch, M.H., Keeling, J., Ashcroft, S.J.H., Turner, R.C. and Baum, J.D. (1981) Nesidioblastosis of the pancreas. *Archives of Disease in Childhood*, **56**, 496–508

Cornblath, M. and Schwartz, R. (1976) *Disorders of Carbohydrate Metabolism in Infants*, 2nd edn, Saunders, London

Dodge, J.A. and Laurence, K.M. (1977) Congenital absence of islets of Langerhans. *Archives of Disease in childhood*, **52**, 411–419

Lucas, A., Morley, R. and Cole, T.J. (1989) Adverse neurodevelopmental outcome of moderate neonatal hypoglycaemia. *British Medical Journal*, **297**, 1304–1308

Zucker, P. and Simon, G. (1968) Prolonged symptomatic neonatal hypoglycaemia associated with maternal chlorpropamide therapy. *Pediatrics*, **42**, 824–825

Further reading

Gentz, J.C.H. and Cornblath, M. (1969) Transient diabetes of the newborn. *Advances in Pediatrics*, **16**, 345–363

Milner, R.D.G. (1979) Neonatal hypoglycaemia. *Journal of Perinatal Medicine*, **7**, 185–194

Chapter 17

The infant of the diabetic mother

Pregnancy in a mother with diabetes constitutes a high-risk pregnancy and the infant of the diabetic mother (IDM) is an infant at high risk requiring special observation in the immediate neonatal period. The IDM is classically macrosomic and the birth of a macrosomic infant of more than 4.5 kg at term suggests that the mother is prediabetic even though abnormal glucose tolerance may not have been documented before or during pregnancy. With diligent prepregnant and prenatal management by a combined team of obstetric and diabetic specialists, a normally grown infant can be produced without any significant increase in neonatal problems over normal term infants.

Recognition

1. A history of diabetes before the pregnancy, or abnormal glucose tolerance requiring treatment by diet or insulin during the pregnancy may be available from the mother's records. Particular attention should be paid to the use of oral hypoglycaemic agents during pregnancy, as IDMs born to mothers receiving oral hypoglycaemics may develop severe prolonged hypoglycaemia lasting 4 or 5 days in the newborn. For this reason, oral hypoglycaemics are not now used during pregnancy. At delivery, the infant may be obviously macrosomic, may be of normal appearance with birth parameters appropriate for gestational age, or, particularly where there have been pregnancy complications or the mother has vascular complications of diabetes, the baby may be small for gestational age and the placenta is unexpectedly small. Such infants are probably at greater risk of hypoglycaemia and neurological injury.
2. Macrosomia (greater than 4.5 kg at term). There may or may not be any indications that the mother has diabetes but a macrosomic infant above the 90th percentile in weight for gestational age should be managed as an infant of a diabetic mother. IDMs are truly macrosomic, with all organ weights at the top end of normal, due to the growth factor effect of insulin *in utero*.

Possible problems in the IDM include:

1. Increased prematurity rate due to obstetric complications such as polyhydramnios, pre-eclampsia and placental abruption, all of which are more common in diabetic pregnancies.

2. Macrosomia: this increases the risk of delivery problems such as shoulder dystocia (pp. 43 and 44) and hypoxia.
3. Hypoglycaemia, hyperinsulinaemia coupled with low glucagon and catecholamine levels induces reduced glucose production from the liver in the face of a high glucose utilization rate. Maintenance of blood glucose is dependent on gluconeogenesis which is diminished.
4. Respiratory distress:

   (a) There is an increase in the incidence of transient tachypnoea of the newborn;
   (b) Respiratory distress syndrome is more frequent and more severe due to a delay in the appearance of phosphatidylglycerol, one of the components of surfactant, even though the lecithin production may be adequate as reflected by a mature amniotic fluid lecithin/sphingomyelin (L/S) ratio. Respiratory distress syndrome may occur in a term infant who is an IDM.
5. Malformations: There is about a four times increase in major malformations, including rib and vertebral abnormalities, seen in its most severe form as the caudal deletion syndrome (sacral agenesis) which has a 600 times increase in incidence over non-IDMs and is present in 1% of IDMs. Sacral agenesis is easily missed; however, the following features are usually present. The infant appears to have a waist because the iliac bones are closer together than normal, there is clawing of the toes, and evidence of a weak or paralysed bladder, as shown by passive dribbling of urine on crying, or with suprapubic pressure; there is a lax anal sphincter. There is an increased incidence of the small left colon syndrome (Davis and Campbell, 1975), neural tube defects and of congenital heart disease, transposition of the great vessels, ventricular septal defect and coarctation of the aorta being the most common. Transient interventricular septal hypertrophy with ventricular outflow obstruction is a transient echocardiogram finding in some IDMs.
6. Polycythemia and hyperviscosity syndrome: 34% of all IDMs have a packed cell volume (PCV) greater than 0.7 in the first 8 hours, and this is frequently associated with thrombocytopenia and hypoglycaemia. In severe cases this may warrant haemodilution by a partial exchange transfusion (p. 132).
7. Hypocalcaemia (p. 219 and hypomagnesaemia p. 223).
8. Jaundice (p. 103).
9. Renal vein thrombosis (p. 79): renal vein thrombosis is common in IDMs and presents with fever, vomiting, hypertension, haematuria, proteinuria and deterioration in renal function. Venous thrombosis may occur in other sites, e.g. adrenal and lung. It is not clear whether this problem is related to polycythemia or has other causes.

Management

A preliminary explanation should be given to the parents of the reasons why the baby is having its blood glucose monitored, otherwise they may jump to the conclusion that their baby is a diabetic. There is no reason why the diabetic mother should not breast feed; a glass of milk or 2–3 10g portions of carbohydrate should be taken before starting to breast feed, to avoid hypoglycaemia. A watchful approach should be adopted in looking for the problems outlined above. In the absence of hypoxia and respiratory problems maintenance of the blood glucose is the most important problem in the first few hours after delivery.

1. Early initiation of milk feeds within the first 2–3 hours. Use of a normal baby formula will prevent hypoglycaemia in the majority of infants, tends to damp down insulin–glucose oscillations and favours a switchover to fat metabolism and gluconeogenesis. Feeds should be started at 60ml/kg per day and increased to 150ml/kg per day by the 4th day. There is little place for glucose 10% orally as it is slowly absorbed and delays gastric emptying.
2. The blood glucose should be monitored by formal blood glucose measurements or a quick method such as Chemstrip (see footnote on p. 59) or equivalent during the first 48 hours and should be monitored 1 to 2 hourly until feeding is well established. The aim is to maintain the blood glucose greater than 2.6mmol per litre (47mg%) (p. 210).
3. If (a) the infant develops signs of clinical hypoglycaemia or (b) the blood glucose level is recorded at less than 2.6mmol/l with or without symptoms, the blood glucose measurement should be repeated and the infant started on glucose 10% 60ml/kg per day (glucose 4mg per kg per minute*) as a continuous infusion in addition to continuation of oral milk feeds. Large intravenous boluses of glucose should be avoided. In a severely symptomatic hypoglycaemic infant, symptoms may be abolished by delivering around 3ml/kg glucose 10% extra in addition to the calculated infusion rate during the first half hour of the infusion.
4. If the blood glucose remains low 1–1½ hours after commencement of the infusion, the rate should be increased to 6mg/kg per minute (90ml/kg per day).
5. If the blood glucose continues to remain low, glucagon 1mg daily should be given as a continuous infusion in addition to the current glucose infusion rate. The purpose of adding glucagon is not to stimulate glycogenolysis but to normalize the insulin/glucagon ratio to favour gluconeogenesis from glycerol, alanine and acetyl-CoA. After starting glucagon, it is usually possible to reduce gradually the glucose infusion rate towards 4mg/kg per minute. Further reductions in the glucose infusion rate should not be made until the infant is tolerating 150ml of milk/kg per day orally (see also note, p. 212).
6. Other anticipated problems that occur should be managed as outlined in the appropriate chapters.

References

Davis, W.S. and Campbell, J.B. (1975) Neonatal small colon syndrome. *American Journal of Diseases of Children*, **129**, 1024–1027

*1mg of glucose is contained in 0.01ml of glucose 10%.

Further reading

Cummins, M. and Norrish, M. (1980) Follow up of children of diabetic mothers. *Archives of Disease in Childhood*, **55**, 259–264

Day, R.E. and Insley, J. (1976) Maternal diabetes mellitus and congenital malformations: survey of 205 cases. *Archives of Disease in Childhood*, **51**, 935–938

Dignan, P.S. (1981) Teratogenic risk and counselling in diabetes. *Clinical Obstetrics and Gynecology*, **24**, 149–159

Farquhar, J.W. (1976) The infant of the diabetic mother. *Clinics in Endocrinology and Metabolism*, **5**, 237–264

Tsang, R.C., Ballard, J. and Brown, C. (1981) The infant of the diabetic mother: today and tomorrow. *Clinical Obstetrics and Gynecology*, **24**, 125–147

Chapter 18

Hypocalcaemia and hypercalcaemia

Hypocalcaemia

This can be defined as a serum level of <1.75mmol/l (<3.5mequiv./l or <7.0mg%). Symptoms occasionally develop at levels up to 1.9mmol/l (3.8 mequiv./l ≡ 7.5mg%). ECG tracings may be helpful in the diagnosis of hypocalcaemia in the newborn, but are difficult to interpret.

Normal range: 1.75–2.4mmol/l (3.5–4.8mequiv./l = 7.0–9.5mg%)

In the neonate in particular hypomagnesaemia may accompany hypocalcaemia, and in these circumstances the hypocalcaemia is resistant to the usual treatment, but corrects itself or becomes responsive to treatment when the hypomagnesaemia is treated. It should therefore be a routine in all laboratories dealing with the newborn to estimate both calcium and magnesium even if a request is made for calcium or magnesium only; the additional laboratory work is very small.

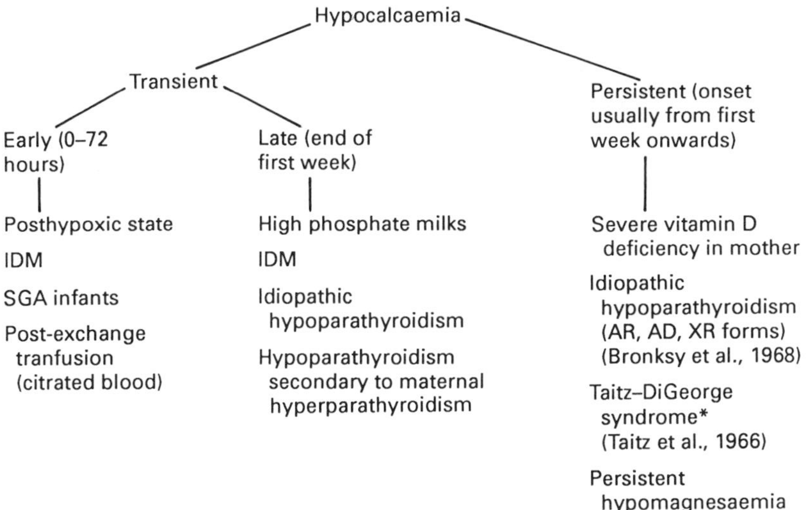

Figure 18.1 Causes of neonatal hypocalcaemia. *Mode of inheritance uncertain, possibly autosomal recessive

There is no evidence that transient hypocalcaemia is damaging to the brain and asymptomatic hypocalcaemia often corrects itself when the infant recovers from the acute illness. However, it is important to ensure that hypocalcaemia is not persistent, by repeating the serum calcium estimate after treatment has stopped to make certain that a normal level can be maintained without treatment. Long-continued hypocalcaemia is clearly associated with mental retardation. The causes of neonatal hypocalcaemia are given in Figure 18.1.

Recognition

In posthypoxic states and in the very-low-birth-weight infant who is severely ill, hypocalcaemia is usually an incidental finding; if asymptomatic, it requires no treatment and the serum calcium returns to normal when the infant has recovered.

Symptomatic hypocalcaemia may have the following symptoms or signs:

1. Hyperirritability or jitteriness.
2. Increased muscle tone, in the absence of other demonstrable cause.
3. Fits which are focal or multifocal with rhythmical jerking at 1–3 per second but with the infant remaining alert between fits. Either side of the body may be affected or the sides may alternate.
4. Rare symptoms of hypocalcaemia are:
   (a) Oedema (Benson and Parsons, 1964);
   (b) Cardiac failure.

All these signs and symptoms may have causes other than hypocalcaemia, and intravenous calcium gluconate should not be used as a therapeutic test because of the danger of sloughing of the subcutaneous tissues if there is extravasation out of the vein and also because of the possibility of cardiac arrest. When symptomatic hypocalcaemia is suspected, other causes of the symptoms should be excluded before treatment of hypocalcaemia is started.

Management

1. Where a high phosphate milk is the cause, change to a low phosphate milk.
2. For minor symptoms such as jitteriness, **oral** calcium supplements should be given, using the parenteral preparation of 10% calcium gluconate in an initial dose of 5–10 ml three or four times daily (1 ml of 10% calcium gluconate contains 9 mg of elemental calcium in 100 mg of calcium gluconate).
3. Only if fits are severe or recurrent should intravenous 10% calcium gluconate be used. It should be given at not more than 1 ml/minute (monitored by ECG and stethoscope at the apex) in a total dose of 1–2 ml/kg; the injection should be stopped immediately there is slowing of the heart rate. The maximum dose for a pre-term infant is 5 ml (500 mg calcium gluconate) and for a term infant 10 ml. Alternatively,

calcium gluconate can be given by slow infusion; it cannot be mixed with sodium bicarbonate or other alkaline solution and should only be given into a peripheral vein, with glucose saline.

Treatment of persistent hypocalcaemia

Calciferol can be used orally in an initial dose of 1000 units daily. The serum calcium should be checked at weekly intervals initially.

Resistant hypocalcaemia

When hypocalcaemia is unaltered by adequate treatment with the preparations described above, the possibility of coexistent hypomagnesaemia should be considered (see also p. 223).

Hypercalcaemia

This is an uncommon condition in the newborn; it can be defined as a serum level of >2.8 mmol/l (>5.6 mequiv./l ≡ 11.0 mg%).

Normal range see p. 219.

Causes of neonatal hypercalcaemia

1. Maternal hypoparathyroidism (Bronsky *et al.*, 1972); the hypercalcaemia rarely lasts more than a few days.
2. Maternal treatment with large doses of vitamin D as in the treatment of maternal hypoparathyroidism. Again, the hypercalcaemia is transient and not severe enough to cause symptoms.
3. Idiopathic hyperparathyroidism (Goldbloom *et al.*, 1972).
4. Subcutaneous fat necrosis (Veldhuis *et al.*, 1979).
5. Idiopathic hypercalcaemia may be detected in the neonatal period because of failure to thrive, 'elfin face' and systolic murmur.

Recognition

Minor symptoms of hypercalcaemia are hypotonia and constipation. In idiopathic hyperparathyroidism there are, in addition, poor feeding, failure to thrive, polyuria and polydipsia; radiological changes of hyperparathyroidism may be present and bone resorbtion may cause fractures.

Management

1. Minor symptoms can be treated with an increased fluid intake up to 200–250 ml/kg per 24 hours. Intravenous 0.9% sodium chloride may be used with the addition of frusemide (1.0 mg/kg every 6 hours). Thiazide

diuretics may increase hypercalcaemia and should not be used. If these measures fail to reduce the serum calcium level oral cortisone or prednisolone can be given when the hypercalcaemia is due to a vitamin D effect, idiopathic hypercalcaemia, or is associated with subcutaneous fat necrosis. However, corticosteroids have no effect in hyperparathyroidism.

2. Severe symptoms in idiopathic hyperparathyroidism usually require subtotal or total parathyroidectomy (Tsang *et al.*, 1979).
3. Idiopathic hypercalcaemia usually requires treatment with a low calcium milk and the temporarily omission of vitamin D from the diet.

References

Benson, P.F. and Parsons, V. (1964) Hereditary hypoparathyroidism presenting with oedema in the neonatal period. *Quarterly Journal of Medicine*, **33**, 197–208

Bronsky, D., Kiamko, R.T. and Waldstein, S.S. (1968) Familial idiopathic hypoparathyroidism. *Journal of Clinical Endocrinology*, **28**, 61–65

Bronsky, D., Kiamko, R.T., Moncada, R. and Rosenthal, I.M. (1972) Intrauterine hyperparathyroidism secondary to maternal hypoparathyroidism. *Pediatrics*, **42**, 606–613

Goldbloom, R.B., Gillis, D.A. and Prasad, M. (1972) Hereditary hyperparathyroidism; a surgical emergency of early infancy. *Pediatrics*, **49**, 514–523

Taitz, L.S., Zarate-Salvador, C. and Schwartz, E. (1966) Congenital absence of parathyroid and thymus glands in an infant. *Pediatrics*, **35**, 412–415

Tsang, R.C., Noguchi, A. and Steichen, J.J. (1979) Pediatric parathyroid disorders. *Pediatric Clinics of North America*, **26**, 223–249

Veldhuis, J.D., Kulin, H.E., Demers, L.M. and Lambert, P.W. (1979) Infantile hypercalcemia with subcutaneous fat necrosis: endocrine studies. *Journal of Pediatrics*, **95**, 460–462

Further reading

De Luca, H. and Anast, C.S. (1980) *Pediatric Diseases Related to Calcium*, Blackwell Scientific, Oxford

Forfar, J.O. (ed.) (1976) Normal and abnormal calcium, phosphorus and magnesium metabolism in the perinatal period. *Clinics in Endocrinology and Metabolism*, **5**, 123–148

Hughes, I.A. and Davies, P.A. (1980) Neonatal endocrine and metabolic emergencies. *Clinics in Endocrinology and Metabolism*, **9**, 583–604

Tsang, R.C., Noguchi, A. and Steichen, J.J. (1979) Pediatric parathyroid disorders. *Pediatric Clinics of North America*, **26**, 223–249

Chapter 19

Hypomagnesaemia and hypermagnesaemia

Hypomagnesaemia

Definition

This can be defined as a level of <0.5 mmol/l (<1.0 mequiv./l ≡ 1.2 mg%). ECG changes are rarely specific and are difficult to interpret in the newborn. The normal range is 0.75–1.25 mmol/l (1.5–2.5 mequiv./l ≡ 1.8–3.8 mg%).

Causes

1. Any of the usual causes of neonatal hypocalcaemia may be associated with hypomagnesaemia.
2. Maternal magnesium depletion can cause symptomatic hypocalcaemia and hypomagnesaemia in the newborn (Davis *et al.*, 1965).
3. A specific form of magnesium malabsorption may cause neonatal hypocalcaemia–hypomagnesaemia, but more commonly symptoms do not develop until the age of a few months (Tsang, 1972).
4. Other causes of neonatal hypomagnesaemia are: the SGA infant (for 3–4 days after birth), in the infant of the diabetic mother (IDM) with hypocalcaemia, after exchange transfusion with citrated blood, and neonatal 'hepatitis'.

Recognition

1. It is impossible to distinguish in the newborn between the symptoms due to hypomagnesaemia and those due to hypocalcaemia, particularly as both conditions often occur together.
2. Hypomagnesaemia should be considered when hypocalcaemia is resistant to the usual forms of treatment.

Management

Non-urgent symptoms

Non-urgent symptoms (irritability, jitteriness, occasional or brief fits), magnesium sulphate can usually be tolerated orally if the usual 50%

solution is diluted to 25% or 12.5%. The initial dose should be 0.125–0.5 ml of the 50% solution/kg (0.25–1.0 mmol/kg or 0.5–2.0 mequiv./kg) which is then diluted to 25% or 12.5%; this is given in divided doses. An alternative preparation which may be better tolerated is the standard (8%) magnesium hydroxide solution which is 6.8 mmol (13.6 mequiv.) in 5 ml; the dose is 1–2 ml three times daily. Turner *et al.* (1977) have successfully used intramuscular magnesium sulphate in the treatment of high phosphate load hypocalcaemic tetany even in the absence of low serum magnesium levels; two or three injections at 12-hourly intervals are usually adequate.

Resistant hypocalcaemia

Resistant hypocalcaemia accompanied by hypomagnesaemia may require calcium supplements (p. 220) in addition to magnesium salts, as above.

Severe or repeated fits

These should be treated with magnesium sulphate intramuscularly or, in an emergency, intravenously.

Intramuscular route

This is the method normally used for the relief of acute symptoms. The 50% magnesium sulphate solution should be used in a dose of 0.1–0.25 ml/kg at 12-hourly intervals. Transient hypomagnesaemia is usually relieved by 2–3 doses. In very small infants the solution should be diluted to 25% or 12.5%; it is very irritant and should be injected deep into the muscle of the mid-thigh.

Intravenous route

A 1% solution of magnesium sulphate should be used (containing 0.04 mmol or 0.08 mequiv. of magnesium sulphate per ml) in a dose of 6–10 ml at a rate of not more than 1 ml/minute using ECG control and listening at the apex with the stethoscope because magnesium has similar effects on the heart to calcium. If there is slowing of the heart rate, the injection must be stopped. Since intravenous magnesium sulphate also lowers the blood pressure, this should be checked, if practicable, before, during and after the injection.

Hypermagnesaemia

Definition

This can be defined as a level of >1.25 mmol/l (2.5 mequiv./l ≡ 3.0 mg%). For the normal range, p. 223.

Causes

1. Asymptomatic hypermagnesaemia occurs in the posthypoxic state, but requires no treatment.

2. Neonatal hypermagnesaemia has resulted from the treatment of the mother with intramuscular magnesium sulphate just before delivery (Brady and Williams, 1967; Lipsitz and English, 1967).

Recognition

The possibility of hypermagnesaemia should be considered when, associated with maternal treatment with magnesium sulphate, the infant is drowsy and hypotonic; in severe cases respiratory paralysis develops. An emergency serum magnesium level should be requested if hypermagnesaemia is suspected; ECG changes are not helpful.

Management

In the newborn it is difficult to relate the severity of symptoms to specific serum magnesium levels, but in the older child or adult drowsiness develops at a level of 2.5–3.5 mmol/l (5.0–7.0 mequiv./l ≡ 6.0–8.5 mg%) and respiratory depression at 5.0 mmol/l (10.0 mequiv./l ≡ 12.0 mg%).

1. In the absence of respiratory weakness there is usually no need for specific treatment apart from increasing the fluid intake.
2. Respiratory paralysis may require intermittent positive pressure ventilation (IPPV) (Brady and Williams, 1967). The serum magnesium can be rapidly lowered by an exchange transfusion.

References

Brady, J.P. and Williams, H.C. (1967) Magnesium intoxication in a premature infant. *Pediatrics*, **40**, 100–103

Davis, J.A., Harvey, D.R. and Yu, J.S. (1965) Neonatal fits associated with hypomagnesaemia. *Archives of Disease in Childhood*, **40**, 286–290

Lipsitz, P.J. and English, I.C. (1967) Hypermagnesaemia in the newborn infant. *Pediatrics*, **40**, 856–862

Tsang, R.C. (1973) Neonatal magnesium disturbances. *American Journal of Diseases in Children*, **124**, 282–293

Turner, T.L., Cockburn, F. and Forfar, J.O. (1977) Magnesium therapy in neonatal tetany. *Lancet* **i**, 283–285

Further reading

Goldberger, E. (1980). *A Primer of Water, Electrolyte and Acid–Base Syndromes*, 6th edn, Lea and Febiger, Philadelphia, pp. 358–364

Tsang, R.C. (1972) Neonatal magnesium disturbances. *American Journal of Diseases of Children*, **124**, 282–293

Chapter 20

Hyponatraemia and hypernatraemia

Hyponatraemia

Definition

In the first 12 hours of life <124mmol/l and after 12 hours of age <128mmol/l. Significant hyponatraemia is likely to be associated with symptoms at <120mmol/l. The normal ranges (Cockburn and Drillien, 1974) are:

Serum sodium: 136–148mmol/l.
Osmolality: serum 280–300mosmol/kg.

Causes

The more common causes of hyponatraemia are given in Figure 20.1.

Recognition

It is important to work out the cause of hyponatraemia, as without this a logical plan of treatment cannot be made.

Asymptomatic hyponatraemia (Table 20.1)

The serum sodium level in this condition is usually between 120 and 128mmol/l (120–124mmol/l in the first 12 hours of life). At levels of 120 mmol/l or less there may be no symptoms but they are likely to develop if corrective action is not taken, particularly if there is a small increase in water intake or a sudden change in the clinical condition.

Dilutional hyponatraemia with oedema (hypervolaemia)
The appearance of oedema is usually preceded by weight gain. There may be both sodium and water retention or sodium depletion due to excessive use of diuretics.

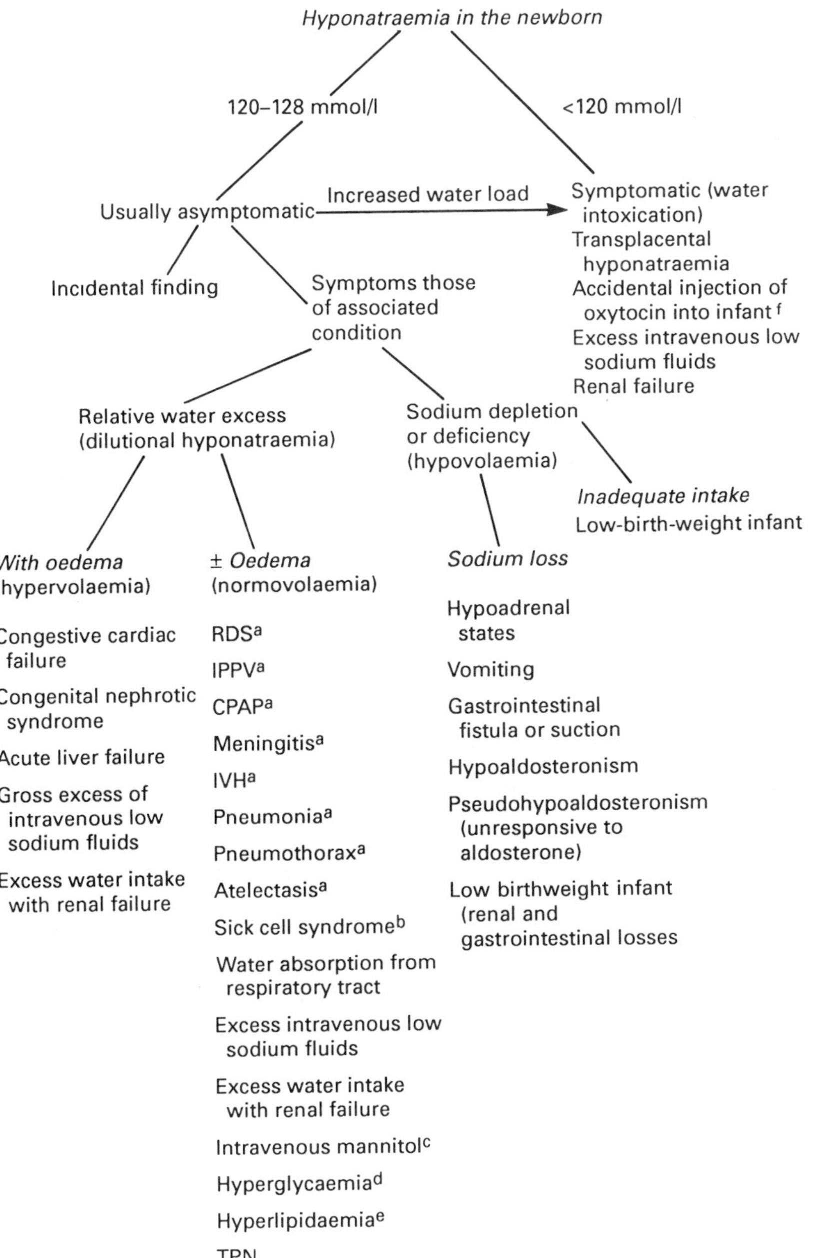

Figure 20.1 Hyponatraemia in the newborn. [a]Thought to be due to syndrome of inappropriate antidiuretic hormone secretion (SIADH). [b]Any severe illness, with tissue hypoxia. [c]Hyponatraemia due to withdrawal of intracellular fluid. [d]Hyperglycaemia from intravenous glucose causes negligible hyponatraemia in the newborn (Uttley and Habel, 1976i). [e]Spurious hyponatraemia due to displacement of plasma by chylomicrons; centrifuge and estimate sodium in true plasma. [f]Oxytocin with ergometrine (Syntometrine) (see pp. 230–233)

Table 20.1 Asymptomatic hyponatraemia in the newborn

*Causes**	*Body weight*	*Serum sodium*	*Serum osmolality*	*Urine volume*	*Urine sodium*	*Urine osmolality*
Hypervolaemia						
Cardiac failure Nephrotic syndrome Liver failure	↑↑ (oedema)	↓ (120–128 mmol/l)	↓	↓	Variable often <20 mmol/l	↑
Normovolaemia						
SIADH ± Sick cell syndrome	Slight ↑ or no change; ± oedema	As above	↓	↓	Variable	↑ or normal
Hypovolaemia						
Sodium depletion from sodium-losing states	↓	↓ (often <120 mmol/l) (K↑)	↑	↓	↑ (>50 mmol/l)	↑
Sodium depletion						
From extrarenal loss or inadequate intake	↓	↓	↑	↓	↓ (<10 mmol/l)	↑

*See Figure 20.1 for full list of causes.

Dilutional hyponatraemia without oedema (normovolaemia)

This occurs in a large number of conditions with varying combinations of syndromes of inappropriate antidiuretic hormone secretion (SIADH) and sick cell syndrome. There may be slight weight gain if the antidiuretic hormone (ADH) effect is predominant. (See Figure 20.1 for causes.)

Sodium deficiency

In sodium deficiency due to inadequate intake (as in very low birthweight infants) with reduced extracellular fluid (ECF) there is failure to gain weight which is corrected by sodium supplements. Such infants may also have excessively high gastrointestinal losses of sodium. It is important to collect a single (not 24-hour) specimen or urine as soon as hyponatraemia has been recognized and before corrective treatment has started, because a simultaneous estimate of the sodium content will distinguish between a renal sodium-losing state (as in hypoadrenalism, hypoaldosteronism and pseudo-hypoaldosteronism) and extrarenal losses or inadequate intake (Table 20.1).

Acute sodium (salt)-losing states

In any condition associated with acute sodium loss there is rapid loss in weight, with reduction in tissue turgor, progressing to shock, hypotension and oliguria. Other symptoms are vomiting, occasionally mistaken for pyloric stenosis, and less commonly watery stools and hypoglycaemia. (For causes, see Figure 20.1.)

Table 20.2 Sodium (salt)-losing states in infancy*

Condition	*Mode of inheritance*	*Male genotype*	*Female genotype*	*Response to mineralo-corticoids*
21-Hydroxylase deficiency (commonest type of CAH)	AR	N	Masculinization, variable degree	+
20,22-Desmolase deficiency (lipoid hyperplasia) (rare form of CAH)	AR	Incomplete masculinization	N	+
3β-Hydroxysteroid dehydrogenase deficiency (rare form of CAH)	AR	As above	N or slight masculinization	+
18-Hydroxylase or 18-dehydrogenase deficiency (hypoaldosteronism)	AR	N	N	+
Pseudohypoaldosteronism (renal insensitivity to aldosterone)	?AR	N	N	0
Adrenal hypoplasia	?AR	N	N	+
Adrenal hypoplasia (cytomegalic type)	XR	Males only	0	+
Acute adrenal haemorrhage	0	N	N	+
Adrenal suppression due to corticosteroid treatment during pregnancy	0	N	N	+
Danazol given during pregnancy (p. 000)	0	N	Masculinization, variable degree	Transient sodium losing effect
Renal sodium-losing states	?	N	N	0
Neonatal diabetes†	?AR	N	N	0

CAH = congenital adrenal hyperplasia. N = normal.
*For further details of investigation of steroid metabolism as an aid to diagnosis, see Table 24.2 (p. 229) and pp. 270–271.
†Polyuria with glycosuria: may show hyponatraemia with hyperkalaemia initially (see also p. 213).

Acute sodium-losing states may occur as part of a total adrenal insufficiency with failure of cortisol production as well as aldosterone, or it may be due to isolated aldosterone deficiency, or renal insensitivity to aldosterone (pseudohypoaldosteronism). Other acute sodium-losing states include renal salt loss and neonatal diabetes (p. 213). Where the diagnosis of adrenal hyperplasia of a sodium-losing variety is obvious it can be assumed that there is a lack of cortisol production which is contributing to the state of shock; similarly with adrenal hypoplasia and acute adrenal haemorrhage. Confirmation of a sodium-losing state is shown by:

1. Hyponatraemia: serum sodium <128 mmol/l and often <120 mmol/l, accompanied by a urine sodium level of >50 mmol/l (often as high as 100 mmol/l) at a time when there is unequivocal hyponatraemia.
2. Hyperkalaemia: this may precede the development of obvious hyponatraemia and may occur transiently in neonatal diabetes (p. 213) as well as in hypoadrenal states.

Symptomatic hyponatraemia

There are no symptoms due to hyponatraemia itself; they are due to water intoxication with cerebral oedema. Symptoms are usual at serum sodium levels below 120 mmol/l but may occur above this figure if the level has fallen very rapidly. In spite of the reduced ECF in sodium depletion it is possible to induce symptoms of water intoxication by giving water, glucose or low-electrolyte solutions particularly in hypoadrenal states where water is excreted slowly.

Pure water intoxication without sodium retention or depletion is seen in the following situations (Table 20.3).

Table 20.3 Water overload in the newborn

Cause	*Weight*	*Serum*		*Urine volume*	*Urine sodium*	*Urine osmolality*
		Sodium	*Osmolality*			
Maternal hyponatraemia with excess water load	↓ Post-natally	↓	↓	↑	↓	↓
Accidental injection of oxytocin	↑ After injection	↓	↓	↓	↑	↑
Excess water intake with normal renal function	↑ ± Oedema	↓	↓	↑	↓	↓
Excess water intake with renal insufficiency	↑ ± Oedema	↓	↓	Small or none	Variable	Fixed

1. Transplacental hyponatraemia with excess water load due to maternal water retention or intoxication during labour (Tarnow-Mordi *et al.*, 1981); this is due to a combination of excessive water intake (usually intravenous glucose 5%) and may be accentuated by endogenous ADH production and intravenous oxytocic drugs (Schwartz and Jones, 1978; Singhi *et al.*, 1985). The infant is overloaded with water at birth and rapidly loses weight postnatally. Symptoms of water intoxication (see below) are not uncommon.
2. Accidental injection of oxytocic drugs into the infant (Whitfield and Salfield, 1980). The preparation involved is usually a combination of oxytocin and ergometrine (Syntometrine) producing water intoxication and direct cerebral effects of the ergometrine. Within a quarter to half an hour of the injection grunting respiration develops followed by respiratory depression requiring intermittent positive pressure ventilation (IPPV). Fits usually occur within 3–4 hours. The serum sodium is normal just after the injection but falls rapidly, with the development of oliguria.
3. An intake of low-electrolyte fluid in excess of the ability of the kidney to excrete the water load. This may occur with a very high intake and normal renal function, or in the presence of an endogenous ADH effect in the postoperative state or possibly after a traumatic delivery.
4. In unrecognized renal insufficiency (as in agenesis or hypoplasia of the kidneys, bilateral obstruction of the renal tract, bilateral renal vein

thrombosis or cortical necrosis) even a normal intake of low-sodium fluid or feed may cause water intoxication.

In complex situations it may be difficult to decide whether symptoms are due to the primary condition, as in meningitis, intraventricular haemorrhage or severe hypoxic brain damage, or to the accompanying hyponatraemia. On occasion, the diagnosis of water intoxication may have to be one of exclusion.

The symptoms which are usually attributable to water intoxication are: hypotonia; respiratory distress; lethargy; apnoeic or cyanotic attacks; poor feeding; fits.

There are no specific physical signs of water intoxication in the newborn. Clinical evidence of raised intracranial pressure is rare. Serial measurements of the size of the lateral ventricles (flattening or obliteration) by sector scanning may help.

Management

In all cases where there is clinical or biochemical evidence of excessive water retention or hyponatraemia the fluid intake and, where possible, the urine output must be carefully measured and the effect checked by twice daily weighing. Similarly, serum sodium and the other electrolytes should be estimated daily with minor degrees of hyponatraemia and twice daily when levels are <120 mmol/l and where corrective treatment has been given.

Asymptomatic hyponatraemia

Dilutional hyponatraemia with oedema (hypervolaemia)
The primary condition (Figure 20.1) should be treated. Oedema can be reduced by decreasing the fluid intake by 10–25%, with if necessary frusemide intramuscularly or intravenously. The loss of oedema may reveal a true hyponatraemia and sodium depletion which should be corrected slowly (see below).

Dilutional hyponatraemia without oedema (normovolaemia)
With serum sodium levels of 120–124 mmol/l the hyponatraemia usually corrects itself with recovery from the primary condition. However, if the sodium level continues to fall the fluid intake should be decreased as described above. At levels of 120 mmol/l or less additional sodium should be given by changing the maintenance fluid to 0.9% sodium chloride with glucose 5% or adding supplements of sodium chloride (in divided doses) in an initial dose of 1–2 mmol of sodium chloride per kg per 24 hours. Diuretics should not be used.

Sodium deficiency
In the very low birthweight infants sodium supplements should be given routinely in a dose of 2 mmol/kg per 24 hours after the first 24 hours of life, or from the age of 48 hours while on an intravenous infusion. Sodium

may need to be added if the baby is growing fast on a low sodium milk (Al-Dahhan *et al.*, 1983). Regular attempts should be made to reduce the sodium supplements once the serum sodium is normal and weight gain is satisfactory.

Acute sodium (salt)-losing crisis
This may occur spontaneously or as a result of stress of any kind, but in adrenal hyperplasia and hypoplasia symptoms usually develop within the first 2–3 weeks of life.

If a diagnosis of adrenal disease has not been made a complete 24-hour collection of urine should be made for steroid estimations (p. 270) but treatment should be witheld during the collection.

Intravenous fluid
Initial treatment should consist of 0.9% sodium chloride in glucose 5% at an initial rate of 20ml/kg per hour for the first 1 or 2 hours, or until shock has been relieved. In very severely shocked infants plasma or equivalent at 20ml/kg per hour should be substituted for the saline for the first hour. Subsequently, the saline solution should be continued up to a total of 120ml/kg per 24 hours.

Salt-retaining preparations
Where deoxycortone (in USA desoxycorticosterone) acetate (DOCA) is available, it should be given in a dose of 2mg i.m. twice daily on the first day, then 1mg twice daily until vomiting has ceased and oral treatment can be started (see below). Alternatively, deoxycortone glucoside (available in the UK from Ciba (Horsham, West Sussex) on a named patient basis supported by a consultant's request) can be used. This is supplied as 50mg in 5ml; it is a water-soluble preparation which can be given intravenously but is usually given intramuscularly in a dose of 5mg twice daily initially, reducing the dose as described above for DOCA. With both these preparations the adequacy of the dosage should be checked by frequent comparisons of sodium concentration in the serum and in random specimens of urine. If neither DOCA nor the glucoside is available, treatment should be continued with 0.9% sodium chloride in glucose 5% until oral treatment can be started.

Fludrocortisone is started as soon as vomiting has ceased, in a dose of 0.1–0.2mg/day; this is continued as a maintenance treatment.

Glucocorticoids
Hydrocortisone sodium succinate should be given as soon as the diagnosis of adrenal failure is suspected: an initial dose of 100mg is given intravenously followed by 25mg at 6-hourly intervals, reducing gradually to 25mg twice daily, followed by cortisone 12.5mg orally twice daily then 5mg/24 hours in three divided doses (2.5, 1.25, 1.25mg) as maintenance treatment. After the acute state, hydrocortisone–sodium phosphate i.m. can be substituted for the intravenous preparation.

Sodium supplements
As soon as oral treatment is practicable, additional sodium chloride should be given in a dose of 15–30mmol/day in divided doses; this should be

continued until the serum sodium is maintained within normal limits and fludrocortisone has been given for at least 2 days. Oral sodium chloride and fludrocortisone should not be given together for longer than a few days, otherwise hypertension may develop.

Symptomatic hyponatraemia (water intoxication)

Transplacental water intoxication

In this condition the infant can usually be left to excrete the additional load of water and to correct the hyponatraemia in this way. Once the condition is recognized the fluid intake should be reduced by 50% until there is a demonstrable weight loss and the serum sodium is above 125 mmol/litre.

Accidental injection of oxytocin

In accidental injection of oxytocin (usually combined with ergometrine, as Syntometrine, p. 230) a reduction in total fluid intake to 25–50% of the normal should be used in an attempt to maintain the body weight constant (twice daily weighing); continued weight gain indicates an excessive intake. The antidiuretic effect of the very large dose (for an infant) of oxytocin may continue for 48 hours (Whitfield and Salfield, 1980). Respiratory failure may necessitate IPPV. Fits should be treated with diazepam or phenobarbitone (p. 204).

Hyponatraemia from excessive intravenous water

If the hyponatraemia is due to an excessive intravenous water or low sodium fluid intake, the quickest and safest way to raise the sodium level is to change the maintenance intravenous fluid to 0.9% sodium chloride with glucose 5% and to reduce the total fluid intake per 24 hours by 25% or, if this is insufficient, by 50%, particularly if an ADH effect is suspected. Sodium-retaining steroids such as fludrocortisone should not be given.

Water intoxication with renal insufficiency

The management of this condition is difficult because the kidney cannot be used to excrete the excess water and there is often a considerable water load and hypervolaemia by the time the condition is recognized. With mild symptoms (i.e. without fits) the serum sodium can be brought down slowly by giving the minimal daily requirement of fluid (33 ml/kg per 24 hours) (Uttley and Habel, 1976ii) plus the previous day's urine output; if there is considerable fluid overload, the fluid intake can be stopped completely for 24 hours or until a clear loss in weight with serum sodium above 120 mmol/l can be achieved. For management of fits, see below. Nursing under a radiant heater may decrease the water load by increasing transepidermal water loss.

Water intoxication with sodium depletion

In the rare cases of water intoxication with the presence of sodium depletion, as in hypoadrenal states, the sodium deficit should be replaced by the use of 0.9% sodium chloride in glucose 5% at a rate of 150 ml/kg per 24 hours, with additional plasma if there is a state of hypovolaemic shock.

Fits

The fits in water intoxication are notoriously resistant to anticonvulsants but there is nothing to be lost by attempting to control them with standard doses of diazepam i.m. or i.v. or phenobarbitone i.m., but these drugs should not be used in the presence of respiratory distress or apnoeic attacks. Anticonvulsant treatment should of course be accompanied by correction of the hyponatraemia as described above.

Evidence of tentorial herniation or foramen magnum coning

Emergency treatment is required if there is evidence of midbrain or brainstem compression. The symptoms which suggest the onset of these complications are:

1. Tonic fits or decerebrate spasms.
2. Constant hypertonia.
3. Hemiplegia.
4. Unequal pupils or rapidly changing pupil size.

Methods of treatment

Hyperventilation with IPPV Hyperventilation, which has a rather transient effect, should achieve a $P\text{CO}_2$ of 2.6–3.3 kPa (20–25 mmHg:Torr). To avoid cerebral ischaemia (from vasoconstriction the $P\text{CO}_2$ should be lowered gradually.

Mannitol In the presence of these signs it is a matter of extreme urgency to reduce the intracranial pressure. In the presence of normal renal function this can be most rapidly achieved by intravenous 20% mannitol in a dose of 1–2 g/kg given over 30–60 minutes (for a 3 kg infant this would be a total infusion of 15–20 ml per dose). This can be repeated after 1–2 hours. It should be remembered that this form of treatment will produce a dangerous degree of hypervolaemia unless each dose is followed by a diuresis, and that the serum sodium level may be temporarily reduced during the phase when the mannitol has withdrawn water from the cells and before the diuresis has started. Mannitol will cause excretion of sodium as well as water, with relatively more water than sodium. However, it may be necessary to replace sodium slowly after the mannitol. Mannitol will overcome an ADH effect, whether endogenous or exogenous (e.g. accidental oxytocin injection).

Hypertonic saline An alternative form of treatment is the use of hypertonic saline, which can be given with impaired renal function. The aim should be to raise the serum sodium by 10 mmol/l by infusing a hypertonic solution of sodium chloride over 1 hour, or in a less urgent situation over 4 hours. Calculations are based on the fact that 6 mmol/kg will raise the serum sodium by 10 mmol/l. Therefore to raise the serum sodium of a 3 kg infant from 115 to 125 mmol/l 18 mmol sodium will be required. This is based upon the following:

Body weight in kg × 0.6 × desired rise in serum sodium in mmol/l (10 mmol/l).
Therefore for a 3 kg infant: 3.0 × 0.6 × 10 = 18 mmol of sodium chloride. A 3% solution of sodium chloride contains 0.5 mmol of sodium per ml (1 mmol per 2 ml).
Therefore volume to be infused will be 36 ml (12 ml/kg).
A 5% solution contains 0.85 mmol of sodium chloride per 1 ml (1 mmol per 1 ml).
Therefore volume to be infused will be 21 ml (7 ml/kg).

Exchange transfusion
In anuric and oliguric renal failure an alternative method of treatment particularly in the presence of a dangerous amount of fluid overload and hypervolaemia would be an exchange transfusion (p. 119–130).

Hypernatraemia

Definition

Serum sodium of 150 mmol/l per litre or above. For the normal range of serum sodium, see p. 226.

Causes of hypernatraemia (Figure 20.2)

Hypernatraemia may be due to a deficit of water or an excess of sodium in the ECF or occasionally to a combination of both factors. Asymptomatic hypernatraemia with moderately raised serum sodium levels (150–155 mmol/l) is not uncommon in the newborn, particularly in the small preterm infant. More severe hypernatraemia is due to a variety of causes, some being iatrogenic, and is associated with cerebral symptoms and occasionally with disseminated intravascular coagulation (DIC) or cerebral venous thrombosis.

Recognition

Asymptomatic

This is usually discovered on routine estimation of the serum electrolytes in very low birthweight infants, especially in the first week of life in those with an oedematous gelatinous skin. In infants who are already ill from other causes it is often impossible to know which symptoms, if any, can be attributed to the hypernatraemia. Nevertheless hypernatraemia indicates a serious imbalance between water and sodium which should be corrected.

Symptomatic (general symptoms)

General symptoms are alternating periods of irritability and drowsiness, with high pitched cry and increased muscle tone. In hypernatraemic

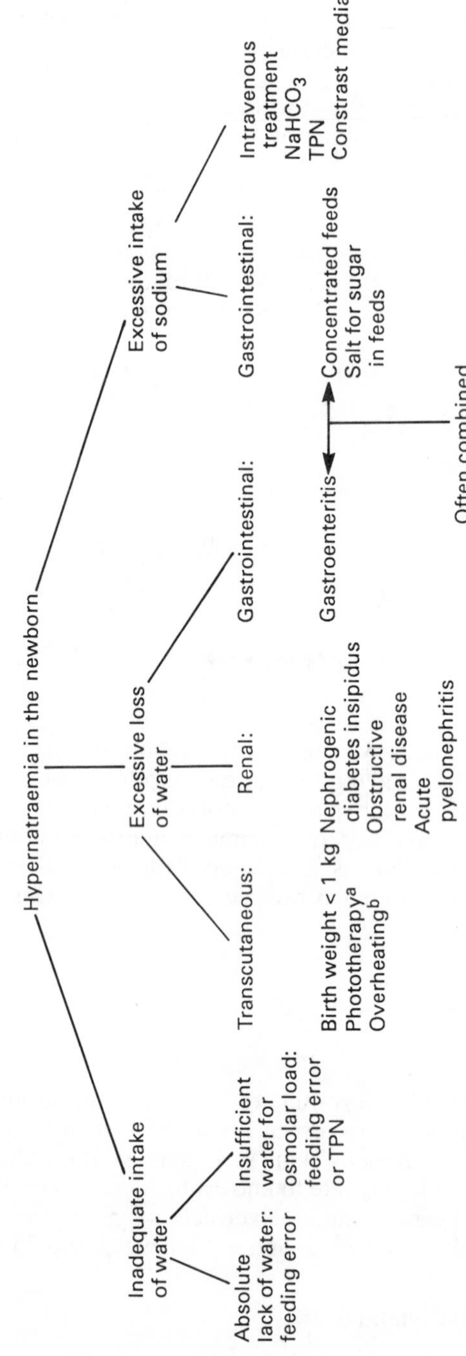

Figure 20.2 Hypernatraemia in the newborn. [a]Oh and Karecki (1972); [b]Williams and Oh (1974); [c]Ansell (1970)

dehydration due to gastroenteritis with continued high sodium intake, the skin feels firm and rubbery which makes the clinical assessment of the degree of fluid deficit difficult to judge. A tense and bulging fontanelle or fits before the start of treatment usually indicates venous thrombosis, acute subdural haematoma from shrinkage of the brain or diffuse intracerebral haemorrhage. The persistence of polyuria may indicate transient diabetes insipidus, or renal tubular necrosis, as one manifestation of DIC.

Nephrogenic diabetes insipidus (XR)

This is not easily recognized unless there is a clear family history of the condition which is rare since affected survivors have usually been labelled non-specifically as mentally retarded. Characteristic symptoms are refusal or vomiting of feeds and failure to thrive; glucose, water or diluted fruit juice is taken eagerly in preference to milk feeds. Clinical dehydration develops quickly, with a serum sodium of 170 mmol/l or more with a moderately raised blood urea. The urine is usually of low osmolality (50–100 mosmol/kg) except in states of extreme dehydration when the urine osmolality may paradoxically exceed that of the plasma. Failure to recognize and treat nephrogenic diabetes insipidus causes severe mental retardation.

Congenital obstructive disease of the renal tract

This may present with symptoms similar to NDI with polyuria and hypernatraemia. The distinction from NDI is important as surgical correction may be required.

Iatrogenic salt poisoning

This may be recognized because a number of infants are affected by an error in making up the feeds in a hospital nursery (Finberg *et al.*, 1963) or by the mother who notices that she has substituted salt for sugar in the feeds. The symptoms are usually persistent vomiting and dehydration. Serum sodium levels may be as high as 200 mmol/l (Saunders *et al.*, 1976).

Management

Asymptomatic

A critical revew of the water and sodium intake and possible causes of excessive water loss or inadequate intake will usually indicate the necessary adjustments to be made. Even in moderate hypernatraemia (serum sodium 150–155 mmol/l), a rapid increase in water intake should be avoided. The daily intake should be increased by 10% initially on the first 24 hours, with further similar increases every 24 hours as required. The additional fluid should be given orally if this is practicable, by diluting the feeds, or by the addition of glucose 5% to the calculated amount of the 24 hour total.

Symptomatic

Gastroenteritis

The most important consideration is to avoid fits from cerebral oedema which result from lowering the serum sodium too quickly, aiming at a reduction of 15 mmol/l per day (Potter, 1973). Owing to the difficulty in assessing the fluid deficit (see above), an initial deficit of 50 ml/kg should be assumed and half of this should be replaced in the first 4 hours, together with the usual maintenance requirement of 150 ml/kg per 24 hours. If shock is present, plasma should be used initially in a volume of 20–30 ml/kg otherwise 0.9% sodium chloride without glucose should be used until the serum sodium has fallen below 150 mmol/l. Insulin should not be given for hyperglycaemia. If fits due to cerebral oedema develop, intravenous mannitol and intravenous or intramuscular dexamethasone should be given, with intravenous diazepam if necessary, to control the fits (see also p. 204): IPPV with hyperventilation may be necessary (p. 234).

Nephrogenic diabetes insipidus

If the infant is breast fed, an additional 50% of solute-free water should be given in addition to the normal intake. Even larger amounts of additional water will be required if a high-solute artificial milk is used; however, such milks should not be used because the difficulty of maintaining a very large fluid intake makes it difficult for the infant to take the normal feeds and to maintain an adequate calorie intake. If artificial feeds are used they should be of a composition similar to that of breast milk.

Congenital obstruction of the renal tract

This requires urgent investigation in a neonatal surgical unit.

Iatrogenic salt poisoning

This may require peritoneal dialysis using a dialysate fluid containing a sodium concentration of 140 mmol/l (Saunders *et al.*, 1976). An exchange transfusion would be a practical alternative.

References

Al-Dahhan, J., Haycock, G.B., Chantler, C. and Stimmler, L. (1983) Sodium homeostasis in term and preterm neonates. *Archives of Disease in Childhood*, **58**, 335–345

Ansell, G. (1970) Fatal dose of contrast medium in infants. *British Journal of Radiology*, **43**, 395–396

Cockburn, F. and Drillien, C.M. (1974) *Neonatal Medicine*, Blackwell Scientific, Oxford, pp. 799–801.

Finberg, L., Kiley, J. and Luttrell, C.N. (1963) Mass accidental poisoning in infancy. A study of a hospital disaster. *Journal of American Medical Association*, **184**, 187–190

Oh, W. and Karecki, H. (1972) Phototherapy and insensible water loss in the newborn infant. *American Journal of Diseases of Children*, **124**, 230–232

Potter, D. (1973) *Pediatric Emergencies* (eds D.J. Pascoe and M. Grossman), Lippincott, Philadelphia, p. 193

Saunders, J., Balfe, J.W. and Laski, B. (1976) Severe salt poisoning in an infant. *Journal of Pediatrics*, **88**, 258–261

Schwartz, R.H. and Jones, R.W. (1978) Transplacental hyponatraemia due to oxytocin. *British Medical Journal*, **i**, 152–153

Singhi, S., Chookang, E., Hall, J.St.E. and Kalghatgi, S. (1985) Iatrogenic neonatal and maternal hyponatraemia following oxytocin and aqueous glucose infusion during labour. *British Journal of Obstetrics and Gynaecology*, **92**, 356–363

Tarnow-Mordi, W.O., Shaw, J.C.L., Liu, D., Gardner, D.A. and Flynn, F.V. (1981) Iatrogenic hyponatraemia in the newborn due to maternal fluid overload; a prospective study. *British Medical Journal*, **283**, 639–642

Uttley, W.S. and Habel, A.H. (1976) Fluid and electrolyte metabolism in the newborn infant. *Clinics in Endocrinology and Metabolism*, **5**, (i) 29; (ii) 10

Whitfield, M.F. and Salfield, S.A.W. (1980) Accidental administration of syntometrine in adult dosage to the newborn. *Archives of Disease in Childhood*, **55**, 68–70

Williams, P.R. and Oh, W. (1974) Effect of radiant heat warmer on insensible water loss in newborn infants. *American Journal of Diseases of Children*, **128**, 511–514

Further reading

Finberg, L. (1969) Hypernatraemic dehydration. *Advances in Pediatrics*, Yearbook Medical Publishers, Chicago, vol. 16

Flear, C.J.G. and Gill, G.V. (1981) Hyponatraemia: mechanisms and management. *Lancet*, **ii**, 26–31

Rivers, R.P.A., Forsling, M.L. and Olver, R.P. (1981) Inappropriate secretion of antidiuretic hormone in infants with respiratory infections. *Archives of Disease in Childhood*, **56**, 358–363

Uttley, W.S. and Habel, A.H. (1976) Fluid and electrolyte metabolism in the newborn infant. *Clinics in Endocrinology and Metabolism*, **5**, 3–30

Chapter 21

Hypothermia and hyperthermia

Hypothermia

Low-reading thermometers should be available in all maternity units and special care baby units, and should be used whenever hypothermia is suspected. Hypothermia, particularly in the pre-term infant, may predispose to a metabolic acidosis and impair the production of surfactant causing respiratory distress syndrome (RDS). The avoidance of hypothermia is therefore an important part of the management of the pre-term infant.

Transient or primary hypothermia after delivery

Even the normal term infant delivered into a warm (i.e. comfortable for an adult) environment may drop its rectal temperature by 1–2°C shortly after birth and may not achieve a normal stable body temperature until the age of 4–8 hours. In low birthweight infants the fall in body temperature may be much greater and more rapid unless special precautions are taken immediately after birth. Situations which may contribute to transient hypothermia after delivery are:

1. Low birth weight.
2. Intra- and post-partum hypoxia.
3. Prolonged resuscitation without protection against heat loss (e.g. a radiant heater or silver swaddler).
4. Delivery into a cold environment.
5. Failure to dry the infant at delivery and/or delay in wrapping after drying.
6. Bathing the term infant too soon after delivery; this should not be done until the baby is at least 8–12 hours old. Pre-term infants should not be bathed at all.
7. Drugs given to the mother during labour or delivery; the most important are the morphia group, diazepam and any general anaesthetic.
8. Hypoglycaemia from any cause.

Recognition

In mild hypothermia the extremities are blue and cold but the face and trunk are pink and warm. In more severe cases, particularly after a hypoxic delivery, the trunk is cold.

Management

If the rectal temperature is <35°C, the infant should be warmed up quickly by wrapping in a warm towel, and should be kept in a room temperature of not less than 26.5°C. However, the use of a double-walled incubator is preferable; this should be set at 33–34°C for a term infant, 34–35°C for a low-birth-weight infant of <1.5 kg, or 35–36°C for an infant of <1.2 kg body weight. If an incubator is used, the infant should be placed under a Perspex shield. A 'silver swaddler' will stop the infant from gaining heat from its environment and should only be used to prevent heat loss during transport. Particularly in very-low-birth-weight infants (<1.5 kg) who do not warm up with maximum incubator settings, plastic cooking material (Clingfilm) can be used to reduce heat losses by convection.

Secondary hypothermia*

This occurs when the body temperature falls, due to factors other than those immediately associated with delivery. Hypothermia is frequently an important sign of severe and worsening illness in a sick newborn.

Important contributory factors are:

1. Low birthweight.
2. Acute infections, especially septicaemia.
3. Severe respiratory distress syndrome.
4. Hypoglycaemia from any cause.
5. Acute blood loss.
6. Intracranial haemorrhage, particularly intraventricular haemorrhage in RDS.
7. Exchange transfusion if inadequate precautions are not taken to prevent heat loss (p. 124).
8. Withdrawal states following maternal drug dependence during pregnancy (p. 298); also a direct effect of diazepam if taken by the mother up till delivery.
9. Severe cardiac failure.
10. Hypothyroidism.

Management

The management is that of the primary condition; the hypothermia is treated as described above.

*The use of a servo-controlled incubator with a skin or rectal temperature sensor may mask the temperature fall due to an infection, thus removing an important piece of evidence.

Acute hypothermia

If a term infant is exposed to a cold environment for up to 6 hours, or for a proportionately shorter time for a low-birth-weight infant, the body temperature will fall, but can safely be raised by rapid rewarming, as described above.

Situations which may cause acute hypothermia are:

1. Unattended delivery at home, or delivery in an ambulance. In cold weather the risk of hypothermia is obviously greater.
2. Delivery into a lavatory; this is nearly always associated with an unattended and often pre-term delivery; the infant is usually severely hypoxic.
3. Transport from one place to another without a portable incubator.
4. Undetected failure of incubator heating (all incubators should have an alarm).

Management

This is as described above.

Cold injury

This is the most serious form of hypothermia and is now rare in the UK, but may be seen in undeveloped countries where the nights are cold. It occurs almost exclusively in the home and rarely involves pre-term infants because they are invariably delivered in or admitted to hospital. There is a strong association with poor socioeconomic circumstances. Conditions which may cause cold injury are:

1. Inadequate heating of the infant's room, especially at night.
2. Unexpected cold spells.
3. Contributory factors such as infection, underfeeding.

Recognition

The frog-like coldness of the infant should be instantly recognizable to the touch, and a thermometer should not be necessary to make the diagnosis. However a rectal thermometer is likely to indicate a temperature of <30°C.

Management

Apart from the lack of facial expression, these infants look misleadingly normal with bright red extremities and tip of the nose. There may be pitting oedema and hardening of subcutaneous tissues. Both heart and respiration rates are slow.

1. Infection: all infants with cold injury should be assumed to be infected and should have a full infection screen as soon as their clinical condition

permits. The aminoglycoside group of antibiotics should be used w care (monitoring of blood levels) because of poor renal excretion, a should be combined with penicillin.

2. Rewarming: rapid rewarming is dangerous because it may precipita severe hypoglycaemia. The infant should therefore be warmed u slowly, using a rectal temperature probe and maintaining the enviroı mental temperature at 1°C above the rectal temperature. Th recommended rate of rewarming is 1°C every 4 hours.
3. Circulatory support, with fresh frozen plasma, is often required.
4. If ventilation is needed, the inspired gases should be warmed to 37.5°C to warm the baby.
5. Hypoglycaemia: even with slow rewarming there is a danger of hypoglycaemia and an intravenous infusion of glucose 10% should be given at 3 ml/kg per hour (half the normal rate), with Dextrostix or Chemstrip (see footnote, p. 59) readings every hour. If hypoglycaemia occurs in spite of the intravenous glucose, 20% should be given at the same rate as before.
6. Feeding: only when a normal body temperature has been achieved should tube feeding with milk be started. Bottle feeding should be started when the baby appears to be eager to suck.
7. After recovery, hypothyroidism should be excluded (serum thyroid-stimulating hormone and thyroxine) and careful follow up, both medical and social, is required. Permanent brain damage is an occasional sequel.

Hyperthermia (fever)

This indicates a rise of the body temperature above normal, and is best detected by routine or continuous temperature recording. Hyperthermia may be due to:

1. Infection: particularly in the pre-term infant, a fall in body temperature is a more common response to an infection. The infected infant looks unwell and has cool hands and feet and the abdominal skin temperature exceeds the hand skin temperature by more than 3°C (Rutter, 1986).
2. Overheating from excessive external heating; warm pink hands and feet; abdominal skin temperature exceeds skin temperature by less than 2°C (Rutter, 1986).
3. Incubator temperature set too high.
4. Exposure to a radiant heater, phototherapy or placing an incubator or cot too near a hot wall radiator.
5. Incubator in direct sunlight.
6. Failure of a warning device; detachment of servo-probe of heating device.
7. Withdrawal states following maternal drug dependence during pregnancy (Table 28.3, p. 298).
8. Mother pyrexial at delivery.

Table 21.1 Incubator and room temperatures necessary to provide adequate warmth for infants of different birth weight at different ages

Birth weight (kg)	*Effective* incubator temperature*			*Room temperature*		
	35°C	34°C	33°C	32°C	26.5°C	24°C
1.0	for 10 days→	after 10 days→	after 3 weeks→	after 5 weeks	—	—
1.5	—	for 10 days →	after 10 days →	after 4 weeks	—	—
2.0	—	for 2 days →	after 2 days →	after 3 weeks	for 1 week→	after 1 week
3.0	—	—	for 2 days →	after 2 days	for 1 day →	after 1 day

*To obtain an estimate of the effective environmental temperature within a single-walled incubator, subtract 1°C from incubator air temperature for every 7°C by which this temperature exceeds room temperature.
Reproduced from Simpson (1974) with permission of author and publishers.

Management

The best treatment is to place the infant, unclothed, in an incubator set at the neutral thermal environmental temperature for the infant's body weight. Table 21.1 lists the incubator and room temperatures necessary.

References

Rutter, N. (1986) Temperature control and its disorders. In *Textbook of Neonatology* (ed. N.R.C. Roberton), Churchill Livingstone, Edinburgh, p. 159

Simpson, H. (1974) Disorders of respiration. In *Neonatal Medicine* (eds F. Cockburn and C.M. Drillien), Blackwell Scientific, Oxford, p. 189

Further reading

Hey, E.N. (1972) Thermal regulation in the newborn. *British Journal of Hospital Medicine*, **8**, 51–64

Hey, E.N. (1975) Thermal neutrality. *British Medical Bulletin*, **31**, 69–74

Hull, D. (1976) Temperature regulation and disturbance in the newborn infant. *Clinics in Endocrinology and Metabolism*, **5**, 39–54

Chapter 22

Gastrointestinal symptoms and emergencies

Vomiting

Vomiting in the newborn infant should always be regarded as being of potential significance particularly when it occurs repeatedly and in the first week of life. However, it must be recognized that most newborn infants vomit occasionally for no obvious reason. Vomited material should be kept for inspection if it is yellow, green, brown or contains fresh blood.

Vomiting in relation to delivery

Many infants vomit after a difficult or hypoxic delivery, and especially after a caesarean section. The vomit may consist of clear mucus, milk, blood or swallowed meconium (see below). After a concealed accidental haemorrhage (abruptio placentae), the infant may continue to vomit maternal blood during the first 24 hours after birth (p. 99).

Feeding difficulties and errors

Breast-fed infants
Vomiting may be due to a too rapid flow of milk; there is choking and gulping during feeds. Unrecognized underfeeding may also cause vomiting, probably due to air-swallowing, accompanied by small watery greenish–yellow stools; this must be distinguished from gastroenteritis in which there is reluctance to feed and the stools are large and watery.

Bottle-fed infants
Vomiting may result from similar causes to those described above, but is due to a too large or too small hole in the teat.

Maternal emotional and psychiatric disorders
Vomiting with or without underfeeding may result from a disorganized or erratic feeding schedule or frequently interrupted feeds. Possible causes are maternal depression, obsessional or anxiety states, thyrotoxicosis or withdrawal symptoms with maternal drug abuse (p. 298).

Forcible or projectile vomiting

This may occur in the following conditions:

1. Pyloric stenosis, rarely before the age of 2–3 weeks.
2. 'Mucous gastritis' (see below).
3. Gross underfeeding (see below).
4. Hiatus hernia; vomiting usually begins in the first week of life and the vomit may contain fresh or altered blood (p. 99). Weight gain is usually slow.
5. Duodenal atresia or stenosis (see under Down's syndrome).
6. Malrotation with duodenal obstruction.
7. Acute sodium-losing crisis due to adrenal insufficiency (p. 229).

Other causes of repeated vomiting are summarized in Figure 22.1.

Green vomiting

This may be due to:

1. Swallowed meconium; there is a history of meconium-stained amniotic fluid. Vomited meconium can be distinguished from bile-stained vomiting because it appears as flecks or lumps of dark-green material whereas in bile-stained vomiting the material is uniformly green (or yellow).
2. Bile-stained vomiting occurs in intestinal obstruction from any cause, initially as clear yellow material and rapidly becomes clear green and finally of a murky green or brown appearance. Transient bile-stained vomiting may occur in small pre-term infants but actual intestinal obstruction should be carefully excluded clinically and radiologically. Bile-stained material may also drain spontaneously from a nasojejunal feeding tube, or from a gastric tube whose tip has passed through the pylorus; however, a true obstruction may be masked by this drainage. In intestinal obstruction which is present before delivery, green bile in the amniotic fluid may be mistaken for meconium.

'Mucous gastritis'

In this ill-understood condition there is forcible vomiting in the first 12–24 hours after birth, without evidence of obstruction. The vomited material consists of bright-yellow curds which are negative to chemical tests for bilirubin. It is usually treated by one or two stomach wash-outs with glucose 5%, but is a self-limited condition.

Vomiting with salivation, choking and cyanosis

This may be due to:

1. Oesophageal atresia with or without tracheo-oesophageal fistula (p. 148).
2. Incoordinated swallowing which occurs transiently in apparently normal infants, or in infants which have suffered severe perinatal hypoxia.

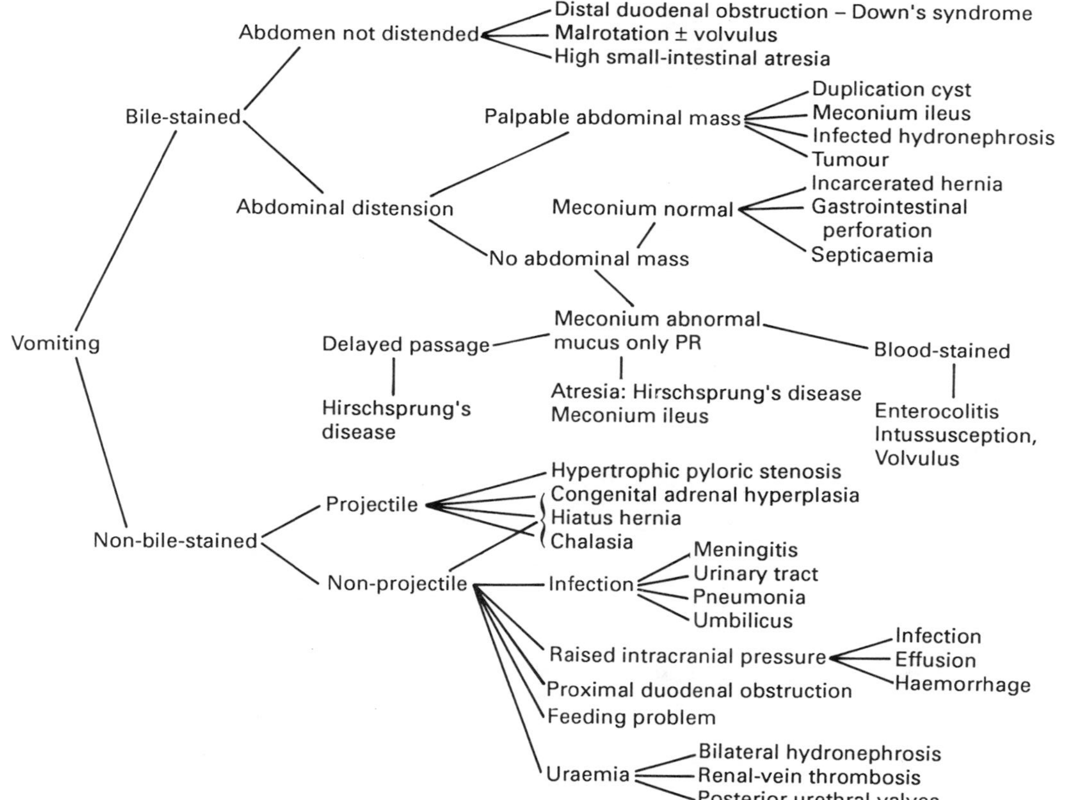

Figure 22.1 Diagnostic approach to vomiting in the newborn. PR, per rectum. Reproduced from Spitz (1987) with permission of the author and publishers

Vomiting with a tense or bulging fontanelle

This may be due to hydrocephalus, meningitis (p. 194) or intracranial haemorrhage (p. 96).

Vomiting with diarrhoea

Infective gastroenteritis (p. 197) is the most common cause, but, where symptoms develop within the first 24 hours of life, lactose intolerance (lactase deficiency) should be considered. Lactose intolerance may also cause acute intestinal distension similar to an ileus. Where the stool contains blood and mucus, necrotizing enterocolitis (p. 256) and salmonella and shigella infections should be considered.

Vomiting in Down's syndrome

Vomiting in the first 24–72 hours of life is usually due to duodenal atresia or stenosis which may be above or below the entrance of the common bile duct. Delay in the onset of vomit may be due to dilatation of the stomach and duodenum. The vomiting may be forcible or projectile and may contain fresh blood. The presence or absence of bile in the vomit depends upon the site of the obstruction. Atresias of the intestinal tract at lower levels may also be present.

Other causes of vomiting which must be considered are:

1. Acute septicaemic illness (p. 192).
2. Oral drugs, especially iron or calcium preparations.
3. Metabolic disorders such as galactosaemia or fructose intolerance (pp. 288–291).

Diarrhoea

See under diarrhoea and vomiting above. Occasionally Hirschsprung's disease may present with severe diarrhoea instead of lower intestinal obstruction.

Delay in the passage of meconium

In a term infant, failure to pass meconium within 48 hours of delivery requires a full examination of the infant. In the pre-term infant delay of up to 48 hours is common in an otherwise normal infant. The commonest cause of apparent delay is the unrecorded passage of meconium in the delivery room.

The causes of delayed passage of meconium are:

1. Mucus plug syndrome: there is usually a moderate degree of gaseous abdominal distension and coils of bowel filled with meconium may be visible through the abdominal wall. A whitish plug of mucus can often be seen just above the anal margin, and after introducing a finger into the anal canal and then withdrawing it a large amount of meconium

and flatus is passed, preceded by the plug of mucus. This condition is not necessarily associated with any abnormality of the meconium, but the possibility of abnormally sticky meconium due to cystic fibrosis or Hirschsprung's disease must be considered.

2. Immature function of the bowel in a small pre-term infant (see under intestinal obstruction).
3. Meconium ileus: in most cases this is due to cystic fibrosis and the meconium when obtained should be tested for a high protein content by making a suspension of meconium in a test-tube and using an 'albustix' or Boehringer-Mannheim (BM) test paper; this test can, however, give both false negative and false positive results in cystic fibrosis, and the results should never be regarded as conclusive. Meconium ileus may produce delayed passage of meconium with minimal signs of obstruction, or meconium peritonitis in which perforation has already occurred *in utero*.
4. Hirschsprung's disease: this condition may cause delay in passage of meconium with evidence of large or small intestinal obstruction, according to the site and length of bowel affected. In the common form, with a narrow aganglionic segment at the lower end of the rectum the obstruction can often be temporarily relieved by passing a finger or a catheter above the narrow segment, with the passage of a large amount of flatus or meconium and partial diminution of the abdominal distension.
5. Imperforate anus: this may be due to a simple skin-covered anal opening through which the dark meconium can be seen or to a more complete atresia of the anal canal. In the skin-covered type, there may be a minute hole through which a 'fly-speck' of meconium is forced.
6. Anal stenosis and ectopic anus: where the anus is anteriorly placed there may be stenosis accompanied by a rectovaginal or rectourethral fistula, with the passage of meconium through vagina or urethra.

Abdominal distension

Present at delivery

This may be due to enlarged renal masses (p. 264), hepatosplenomegaly from severe rhesus isoimmunization (p. 117), chronic fetomaternal (p. 81) or twin-to-twin haemorrhage (p. 81), meconium peritonitis or ascites (see below), or less commonly teratoma, neuroblastoma, hepatoblastoma or megacystis.

Developing after delivery

This may be due to renal-vein thrombosis or adrenal haemorrhage (p. 78), excess air in the bowel in tracheo-oesophageal fistula or as a result of resuscitation, intestinal obstruction from any cause, necrotizing enterocolitis, haemoperitoneum or peritonitis.

Meconium peritonitis
This is invariably due to meconium ileus developing *in utero* and causing a sterile perforation. Cystic fibrosis is the primary condition in nearly every case.

Recognition The gross abdominal distension will be detected prenatally either clinically or by ultrasound. In long-standing meconium peritonitis, flecks of calcification can often be seen on X-ray, outlining the peritoneal cavity: this calcification may be detectable before delivery. A characteristic finding in a postnatal X-ray is the granular or foamy appearance of the distended loops of bowel, in contrast with the fluid levels seen in other types of obstruction.

Management This is a surgical emergency; the infant should be transferred to a neonatal surgical unit as soon as possible. A tube (see p. 69) should be passed into the stomach to reduce the risk of vomiting and inhalation.

Ascites
For a list of causes of ascites with generalized oedema (hydrops fetalis), see p. 274. Ascites without oedema may be due to:

1. Hepatitis or other liver disease.
2. Biliary ascites due to a perforation in the biliary tract (p. 114).
3. Chylous ascites due to lymphatic obstruction within the abdomen or to the thoracic duct.
4. Urinary ascites due to congenital obstruction of the lower renal tract (p. 264).
5. Peritonitis from any cause, including necrotizing enterocolitis (p. 256).
6. Haemoperitoneum from rupture of the liver or spleen (p. 75), torsion of an ovarian cyst (p. 265) or traumatic perforation by a catheter of the aorta (p. 310) or umbilical vein (p. 127).

Intestinal obstruction

Recognition

Apart from meconium peritonitis, other types of intestinal obstruction only become apparent after delivery. The main difficulty is in distinguishing between a functional ileus and an organic obstruction since an ileus may be transient or can be treated medically according to its cause, while an organic obstruction requires immediate surgery.

The signs and symptoms of intestinal obstruction in the newborn are: vomiting, abdominal distension with delay in the passage of meconium if the obstruction is a lower intestinal one and the cause was present at delivery.

1. Vomiting is one of the earliest signs of intestinal obstruction and apart from conditions where the obstruction is above the opening of the common bile duct (e.g. pyloric stenosis, high duodenal obstruction, oesophageal atresia), the vomited material rapidly becomes bile-stained (p. 246).

2. Abdominal distension: the degree of distension is greatest with large bowel obstruction and least in duodenal or pyloric obstruction in which gastric peristalsis may be obvious. In general, the lower the site of the obstruction, the later the distension appears and the more gradual its onset.
3. Delay in the passage of meconium for more than 24 hours in a term infant or more than 48 hours in a pre-term infant requires investigation (p. 252). It is important to recognize that meconium may be passed normally for a few hours after delivery when an intestinal atresia is present.

Causes of intestinal obstruction

These can be subdivided according to the presence or absence of the obstruction at birth.

Obstruction present at birth:

1. Oesophageal atresia (considered separately on p. 148).
2. Duodenal stenosis or atresia.
3. Intestinal atresia.
4. Meconium ileus.
5. Mucus plug syndrome.
6. Rectal stenosis or atresia.
7. Imperforate anus.

Obstruction developing after birth
Mechanical cause

1. Malrotation with or without volvulus.
2. Duplication of stomach or bowel.
3. Meconium disease of very low birthweight infants, usually a few days after birth (Vinograd *et al.*, 1983).
4. Inspissated milk syndrome.
5. Incarcerated inguinal hernia (p. 266)
6. Necrotizing enterocolitis (p. 258).
7. Hydrocolpos (p. 265).
8. Hirschsprung's disease.
9. Postoperative adhesions.

Non-mechanical cause, i.e. functional ileus

1. Immature bowel syndrome (very-low-birth-weight infants).
2. Ileus in severe respiratory distress syndrome (RDS).
3. Septicaemia with or without pneumonia, meningitis, pyelonephritis (pp. 192–194).
4. Gastrointestinal perforation (p. 253).
5. Hypothyroidism.
6. Lactose intolerance (lactase deficiency).

Management

Unless it is obvious that the symptoms are due to a functional ileus the combination of bile-stained vomiting and abdominal distension should be assumed to be due to a mechanical cause and investigated appropriately.

Investigation

If there is delay in the passage of meconium, a rectal examination should be performed; if a mucus plug is present the stimulus of the examination will cause the plug, followed by meconium, to be passed and the obstruction will be relieved. In Hirschsprung's disease, the anal canal and lower rectum are usually empty and if a finger can be passed above a short aganglionic segment, its withdrawal will be followed by the passage of a large amount of flatus and meconium, with temporary relief of the obstruction. If the upper end of the narrow segment cannot be reached by a finger, a soft rubber catheter should be passed in an attempt to get above the narrow segment; the open end should be kept in a receptacle containing sterile water or saline to detect the passage of flatus. The temporary relief of obstruction in this way is virtually diagnostic of Hirschsprung's disease, but the diagnosis must be confirmed by contrast medium enema and suction biopsy of the mucosa if the narrow segment is accessible to this approach.

Radiological investigation is essential in all cases except where the diagnosis is obvious and simple, as in skin-covered anus. Initially a plain film of the abdomen should be taken in the erect and supine position; a chest X-ray should also be requested to exclude pneumonia or other intrathoracic disease. A contrast medium enema may be useful in Hirschsprung's disease, using initially a small amount of medium to outline the duodenum in suspected malrotation. Aspiration of the stomach contents followed by radiography after the injection of 20 ml of air is a simple method of using air as a contrast medium. Gastrografin should **never** be used for a swallow or meal as its inhalation into the lungs causes severe pneumonitis.

Preoperative care

Ideally an infant with intestinal obstruction should be seen by a paediatric surgeon in the special care baby unit (SCBU), when the diagnosis can be discussed. In hospitals where the SCBU and neonatal surgical unit are in the same building this should present no difficulty and the infant can be returned to the SCBU postoperatively. Where transfer by ambulance is necessary, it may not be possible to obtain a paediatric surgical opinion in the maternity unit and the infant may have to be transferred even if the diagnosis is still uncertain. Before transfer the following points should receive attention (see also Transport of the sick neonate, Chapter 5).

1. Exclusion of septicaemia or other infection (pp. 192–195).
2. Passage of a tube (8–10 FG) into the stomach with frequent aspiration of the stomach contents; the top end of the tube should be left open to allow free drainage of fluid and gas.

3. Satisfactory acid–base status and electrolyte balance should be maintained with an intravenous drip of 10% glucose with 2.5 mmol/kg of NaCl, supplying the infant's basic requirements, to which is added the amount of fluid aspirated or drained from the gastric tube in the previous 12 hour period.
4. The infant should be accompanied by 5–10 ml of the mother's blood and an operation consent form signed by one parent.
5. For care during transfer, see Chapter 5.

Important conditions presenting as gastrointestinal emergencies

Tracheo-oesophageal fistula with oesophageal atresia (p. 148)

Diaphragmatic hernia (p. 156)

Exomphalos (or gastroschisis)

Recognition
The diagnosis is obvious; the association with the Beckwith–Wiedemann syndrome (exomphalos, gigantism, hypoglycaemia, with a later tendency to neoplasia) should be remembered. In all cases malrotation of the intestine is common.

Management
Surgical repair should be done as soon as possible, and until the operation, the whole of the infant's lower half should be enclosed in 'clingfilm' or a sterile plastic bag tied just above the abdominal defect. Hypothermia is common and therefore the infant should be kept in an incubator.

Perforation of the stomach

Recognition
Perforation usually occurs spontaneously, though it may be due to an indwelling nylon or polythene gastric tube which has become rigid or to overdistension during resuscitation, particularly if an endotracheal tube is mistakenly passed into the oesophagus; there is also an association with distal obstruction. Clinically, there is sudden shock, with vomiting which may be blood-stained. The abdomen rapidly becomes distended and hyperresonant and there may be respiratory embarrassment if the distension is extreme. X-ray of the abdomen in the upright position shows free air below one or both diaphragms. The diagnosis can be confirmed and the distension reduced by aspiration of as much air as possible from a hyperresonant area.

Management
Shock should be treated preoperatively (p. 72) and repair of the defect in the stomach should be done as an emergency. Antibiotics should be given on the assumption that peritonitis may develop.

Perforation of the oesophagus (Wiseman et al., 1959; Chunn and Geppert, 1962)

Recognition
This condition is more common in the pre-term than in the term infant. Rupture is usually spontaneous but may also be associated with oesophagitis and repeated vomiting or the passage of a feeding tube. Shock develops rapidly, and pneumothorax occasionally under tension develops on either the right or left side. Mediastinal or subcutaneous emphysema are rare complications. Confirmation is by an erect chest X-ray. The possibility of ruptured oesophagus should always be considered when an X-ray shows a combination of pneumothorax and fluid in the pleural cavity. Confirmation of the origin of the fluid is by the aspiration of fluid containing milk of a high acidity from regurgitated gastric contents.

Management
Management is as for perforation of the stomach except that thoracotomy will of course be required and the pneumothorax should be aspirated or drained continuously before operation.

Sacrococcygeal tumour

Recognition
This rare tumour may be detected prenatally by ultrasound, or a large mass attached to the sacrum is found at or after delivery. Small tumours may displace the anus or cause bulging of the perineum, and are easily missed.

Complications
1. Perinatal hypoxia due to difficult delivery.
2. Shock from fluid loss or bleeding into the tumour.
3. Obstruction to the lower gastrointestinal or renal tracts.
4. Early malignant change, irrespective of size of the tumour.

Management
Referral in the first week of life for immediate removal by an experienced neonatal surgeon.

References

Chunn, V.C. and Geppert, L.J. (1962) Spontaneous rupture of the esophagus in the newborn. *Journal of Pediatrics*, **60**, 404–407

Spitz, L. (1987) Acute abdominal emergencies. In *Paediatric Emergencies*, 2nd edn (ed. J.A. Black), Butterworths, London, p. 364

Vinograd, I., Mogle, P., Peleg, O. and Lernau, O.Z. (1983) Meconium disease in premature infants with very low birth weight. *Journal of Pediatrics*, **103**, 963–966

Wiseman, H.J., Celano, E.R. and Hester, F.C. (1959) Spontaneous rupture of esophagus in a newborn infant. *Journal of Pediatrics*, **55**, 207–210

Further reading

Lister, J. and Irving, I.M. (eds) (1990) *Neonatal Surgery*, 3rd edn, Butterworths, London

Chapter 23

Necrotizing enterocolitis

Aetiology

Necrotizing enterocolitis (NEC) is the most common cause of sudden general deterioration with abdominal distension and shock in the newborn period, and is a relatively recent disease (Touloukian *et al.*, 1973; Santulli *et al.*, 1975). In the British Columbia Provincial Neonatal Intensive Care Unit the incidence of necrotizing enterocolitis is 5.6% in infants of 1.5 kg or less at birth. The exact aetiology of NEC is not fully understood but superinfection of the bowel with overgrowth of a single strain of organism, with the production of endotoxin and hypoxic damage to the intestinal mucosal barrier appear to be important factors. Pentration of the bowel wall by organisms usually restricted to the colonic lumen produces bubbles of gas within the bowel ('intramural air') and a gas-gangrene-like pathology in the bowel. These bubbles may enter the portal circulation and sometimes enter the systemic circulation if there are portosystemic anastomoses. There are extensive third space fluid losses, the infant develops circulatory collapse with great rapidity and may be septicaemic and in severe cases may need ventilation. NEC usually occurs within the first 4 weeks of life but occasionally occurs later in infants, and sometimes affects older children with immune defects. It is mainly a disease of infants who have the following risk factors:

1. Prematurity.
2. Severe perinatal hypoxia and intrauterine growth retardation.
3. Respiratory distress syndrome.
4. Cyanotic congenital heart disease or patent ductus arteriosus.
5. Umbilical catheterization and exchange transfusion.
6. Polycythaemia.
7. Extensive intraventricular haemorrhage.
8. Bronchopulmonary dysplasia.

NEC tends to occur in clusters or epidemics with one or two organisms being grown from the blood cultures. It does not, however, seem to be a simple infectious disease of the bowel. Ill infants who have a number of the problems listed above tend to be at a higher risk of also developing NEC. Prenatal corticosteroid administration seems to be moderately protective (Bauer *et al.*, 1984). Enteral feeding appears to be a prerequisite for the development of full-blown NEC, because feeds provide a substrate for intraluminal bacterial multiplication. Some infants who have never been fed enterally do, however, develop NEC and these do not have radiologically evident intramural air. One third of infants have a positive blood culture. The organism obtained in the blood culture depends on the predominant organism in the bowel of infants in the nursery: *Escherichia coli, Klebsiella* and anaerobes including *Clostridium* and *Staphylococcus epidermidis* are common organisms. Cerebrospinal fluid culture is positive in about 8% of those with a positive blood culture.

Complications

1. During the acute phase, intestinal perforation, peritonitis, massive intestinal infarction.
2. During the convalescent phase, strictures, adhesions, intestinal malabsorptions.

Recognition

1. The infant has usually one of the risk factors described above.
2. Within a few days or weeks of starting feeds, the infant develops in sequence:
   (a) Increasing gastric aspirates.
   (b) Green bile-stained gastric aspirates.
   (c) Frank blood and mucus in the stool indicating colitis.
   (d) Abdominal distension and ileus.
   (e) Circulatory collapse, apnoea and a need for ventilation. In severe cases all these symptoms may suddenly appear together.
3. Abdominal X-ray shows intramural air (except in early cases where the infant has not been fed), usually in the colon but sometimes throughout the bowel, and in about 20% of cases, there is gas in the portal system and in the liver. There may also be bowel-wall thickening and free fluid or gas in the peritoneal cavity if perforation has occurred.
4. In busy neonatal units there is a tendency to assume that any acutely sick infant with apparent abdominal pathology has necrotizing enterocolitis. It is most important that the differential diagnosis is carefully considered if an accurate diagnosis is to be made and inappropriate management avoided.

Differential diagnosis of necrotizing enterocolitis

Causes of blood in the stools

1. Gastroenteritis (*Shigella, Salmonella, Campylobacter*, rotavirus).
2. Anal fissure.
3. Bleeding disorders.
4. Swallowed maternal blood in the first week of life.

5. Milk intolerance.
6. Ingested maternal blood during breast feeding.

Causes of abdominal distension and ileus

1. Septicaemia and/or meningitis.
2. Intestinal obstruction (e.g. malrotation, Hirschsprung's disease, volvulus, intussusception, strangulated inguinal, umbilical or internal hernia).
3. Neonatal appendicitis (rare) (p. 254).
4. Severe electrolyte or other metabolic disturbances.

Causes of intolerance to feeds

1. Delayed gastric emptying, intestinal hypoperistalsis or delayed maturation of enterohormonal responses to enteral feeding.
2. Constipation.
3. Milk intolerance.
4. Disaccharidase deficiency.

Causes of free air in the peritoneal cavity

1. Pneumoperitoneum associated with pneumothorax with a patent pleuroperitoneal canal.
2. Acute gastric perforation.
3. Meconium peritonitis with perforation.

The diagnosis of NEC should be considered:

1. 'Suspect' when there is no intramural gas on several abdominal X-rays but the infant has the symptoms given above, usually in the mild form; or
2. 'Proven' if there is intramural gas and/or typical findings at operation or pathological examination.

Management

1. The infant requires urgent transfer to an area where full intensive support can be provided.
2. The feeds should be stopped, and the infant started on 'drip and suck'; total parenteral nutrition (TPN) should be introduced after 48 hours.
3. Ventilation and bicarbonate for acid–base correction are nearly always needed in severe NEC.
4. A full infection screen should be performed including lumbar puncture, and the infant should be started on appropriate antibiotics. The choice of antibiotic depends on the local blood culture results and evidence of bowel superinfection in infants developing NEC in each neonatal unit. Gram-negative organisms, anaerobes and *Clostridium*

should be covered by the antibiotics chosen. Ampicillin and gentamicin may be appropriate. In a unit with a high incidence of toxin-producing *Staphylococcus epidermidis*, cephotaxime and vancomycin appear to be most appropriate and effective.

5. Circulatory support should be given with fresh frozen plasma (FFP) and blood if necessary. Because of rapid third space losses, 10–20 ml of FFP per kg may be required two or three times a day in the first few days of the illness and in severe cases dopamine (2–5 μg/kg per minute) may be required for severe hypotension.
6. Adequate analgesia with morphine (0.1–0.2 mg/kg per dose or as an infusion of 0.015 mg/kg/hr) should be given to reduce shock, recognizing that this may precipitate a need for ventilation in a previously unventilated infant.
7. Blood gases, electrolytes, plasma proteins, haemoglobin, white cell count, platelets and vital signs should be followed carefully for the first 72 hours, by which time usually there has been considerable improvement.
8. The platelet count often decreases at 36 to 48 hours after onset in severe cases, and platelets should be given if bleeding occurs or if the platelet count falls below $30 \times 10^{2}9$/l.
9. Operative surgical management should be avoided in the first 72 hours of the illness if at all possible. Infants, particularly very small infants, tolerate laparotomy very poorly in the acute phase, and the extent of the disease is ill-defined early on, and there is a risk of bowel being removed which might have become viable again later with conservative treatment.

   If perforation develops, a peritoneal drain should be inserted to decompress the abdomen. This can be done by a paediatric surgeon under local anaesthesia in the incubator. Laparotomy may be required in infants who develop signs suggestive of an abdominal abscess. These signs include lack of improvement after 48 hours, persisting high temperature, a palpable mass in the abdomen and leucocytosis.
10. Feeds should be withheld and TPN continued for 7 days in mild cases, and as long as 3 weeks in severe cases, particularly if surgery has been required in the acute phase or there is delay in return of peristalsis.
11. Feeds should be started cautiously after this time as soon as bowel sounds have returned, the abdomen is soft and the baby has passed stools. The feeds should be increased slowly to achieve full feeds and discontinuation of TPN in about 2 weeks after restarting enteral feeds.
12. Abdominal distension, pallor and green gastric aspirates and sometimes macroscopic blood in the stools during the reintroduction of enteral feeds suggest that a stricture has developed, usually in the colon. This can be demonstrated by a barium enema. Intestinal obstruction due to a stricture which is still 'young' (less than 3 weeks from onset of NEC) may spontaneously improve on conservative management after a further 1 to 2 weeks of TPN, avoiding the necessity for resection and reanastomosis which would otherwise be required. The above symptoms may indicate recurrence of NEC but this is very rare.
13. Despite the severity of the acute illness, the outcome for survivors is

generally good, with very few cases having malabsorption problems sufficient to affect growth. Neurological abnormalities if they develop are usually related to periventricular leucomalacia, presumably developing during the actue phase of shock and cerebral hypoperfusion.

References

Bauer, C.R., Morrison, J.C., Poole, W.K., Korones, S.B., Boehm, J.J., Rigalto, H. *et al.* (1984) A decreased incidence of necrotizing enterocolitis after prenatal glucocorticoid treatment. *Pediatrics*, **73**, 682–688.

Santulli, T.V., Schullinger, J.N., Heird, W.C., Gougaware, R.D., Wisger, J., Barlow, B. *et al.* (1975) Acute necrotizing enterocolitis in infancy, a review of 64 cases. *Pediatrics*, **55**, 376–387

Touloukian, R.J., Kader, A. and Spencer, R.P. (1973) The gastrointestinal complication of neonatal umbilical venous exchange transfusion – a clinical and experimental study. *Pediatrics*, **51**, 36–43

Further reading

Brown, E.G. and Sweet, A.Y. (1980) *Neonatal enterocolitis*, Grune & Stratton, New York

Kosloske, A.M. and Musemeche, C.A. (1989) Necrotizing enterocolitis in the neonate. *Clinics in Perinatology*, **16**, 97–112

Lawrence, G., Bates, J. and Gaul, A. (1982) Pathogenesis of neonatal necrotizing enterocolitis. *Lancet*, **i**, 137–139

Moore, T.D. (ed.) (1975) Necrotizing enterocolitis in the newborn infant. *Report of 64th Ross Conference on Pediatric Research*, Ross Laboratories, Columbus, Ohio

Schullinger, J.N., Mollitt, D.L., Vincur, C.D., Santulli, T.V. and Driscoll, J.M. (1981) Neonatal necrotizing enterocolitis; survival management and complications – a 25 year study. *American Journal of Diseases of Children*, **135**, 612–614

Scheifele, D.W., Olsen, E.M. and Pendray, M.R. (1985) Endotoxinemia and thrombocytopenia during neonatal necrotizing enterocolitis. *American Journal of Clinical Pathology*, **83**, 227–229

Chapter 24

Genitourinary emergencies and ambiguous genitalia

Genitourinary emergencies

Failure to pass urine

Over 90% of infants pass urine within 24 hours of delivery; failure to do so requires investigation. Apparent failure to micturate may be due to inadequate observation since many infants pass urine at or shortly after birth and this may be unnoticed or unrecorded.

Genuine failure to micturate within 48 hours of delivery may be due to:

1. Dehydration, with normal renal function.
2. Non-functioning kidneys of congenital origin.
3. Severe obstruction to the urinary outflow.
4. Renovascular accidents due to perinatal hypoxia or shock.

Recognition

Dehydration, with normal renal function
This may be due to:

1. Inadequate fluid intake due to poor sucking from any cause or to insufficient milk.
2. Excessive fluid losses through the skin, due to phototherapy or radiant heat warmers.
3. Abnormal losses from persistent vomiting from any cause or diarrhoea.

Non-functioning kidneys, of congenital origin
Common causes are:

1. Bilateral renal agenesis. This may have been suspected before delivery, because of oligohydramnios. Ultrasound may confirm the absence of kidneys and of a bladder containing urine, but in renal agenesis the adrenals are often abnormal in site and shape and may be mistaken for kidneys. True oligohydramnios is usually accompanied by amnion nodosum, and by Potter's syndrome (flattened face, with large, low set ears, compression deformities of the limbs, particularly talipes equinovarus, and dislocation of the hip). There is usually difficulty in inflation

of the hypoplastic lungs, causing pneumothorax or pneumomediastinum. Renal agenesis can be confirmed postnatally by abdominal ultrasound examination.

2. Polycystic disease of the infantile (AR) variety. The diagnosis can usually be suspected prenatally, because of the huge size of the abdomen, and confirmed by ultrasound. Postnatally, an intravenous urogram (IVU) may show speckled opacities in the cysts.
3. Severe bilateral multicystic disease of the kidneys. Renal masses are usually palpable but the condition is often asymmetrical. The diagnosis can be confirmed by ultrasound and by IVU.

Severe obstruction to the urinary outflow

This may be due to:

1. In the male, bladder neck obstruction from urethral valves. If the obstruction is severe enough to prevent completely the passage of urine pre- and post-natally, the clinical picture, including oligohydramnios, may be similar to that in renal agenesis (see above). Occasionally there is abdominal distension from urinary ascites (see also p. 264), but in most cases the distension is due to bilateral hydronephrosis. The enlarged and hypertrophied bladder may be visible and palpable above the symphysis pubis and feels hard and muscular, like a small uterus. Confirmation of the diagnosis is provided by catheterization of the bladder and ultrasound.
2. The 'prune-belly' syndrome. In its complete form, this is confined to males; there is a variable degree of hypoplasia of the muscles of the abdominal wall, enormous dilatation of the bladder and ureters, and undescended testes. Urinary ascites may be present, particularly if there is a meatal atresia or stenosis, which may also be associated with a patent urachus and the discharge of urine through the umbilicus. The diagnosis is obvious clinically.
3. Atresia of the posterior urethra in the male. This is associated with severe renal dysgenesis. This condition may not be compatible with life.
4. Sacrococcygeal teratoma (p. 258).

Renovascular accidents

These are due to hypoxia or shock or a combination of both factors. The most common causes are severe perinatal hypoxia, or acute blood loss and less commonly an acute septicaemic illness present before delivery (p. 192). The conditions which may result are:

1. Renal tubular (medullary) necrosis. There is usually an anuric or severely oliguric phase lasting 2–3 days, followed by a polyuric phase with severe electrolyte (mainly sodium) losses. IVU during the early stages may show opacification of the medullary pyramids.
2. Renal cortical necrosis. The initial oliguric phase is similar to that in tubular necrosis but there is no polyuric phase. Slow recovery of renal output may occur but complete recovery of glomerular function may not occur. A retrospective diagnosis may be made by the demonstration of cortical calcification on a plain film 4–6 weeks after the event.

Management

Dehydration with normal renal function
Management consists in the treatment of the cause.

Non-functioning kidneys of congenital origin
There is no treatment for renal agenesis or polycystic kidneys and neither condition is compatible with life.

Severe obstruction of the urinary outflow
As soon as the diagnosis is clear the infant should be transferred to a paediatric surgical unit specializing in urological disorders. If there is no urinary outflow, the infant should be managed before transfer in the same way as the anuric infant (see below).

Renovascular accidents
The cause of the shock should be treated (pp. 71–79). If there is no urinary output, checked by catheter or suprapubic puncture, within 4 hours of re-establishment of adequate tissue perfusion as judged by the peripheral circulation, it is likely that cortical or tubular necrosis has occurred. However, a flow of urine can sometimes be started by i.v. frusemide (5 mg per kg). In resistant shock with persisting oliguria, dopamine in **low dosage** (5 μg/kg per minute) should be tried (p. 000). If there is no response to this or output is <0.5 ml/kg per hour, treatment by peritoneal dialysis will be required and transfer should be arranged to an appropriate unit. While this is being arranged, the fluid intake should be limited to 50 ml/kg per 24 hours, or to 25–30 ml/kg if oedema has already developed. Attempts to induce a diuresis by flooding the circulation with an excess of fluid can be dangerous. If there is hyperkalaemia (>8 mmol/l) the risk of cardiac arrhythmia or arrest can be reduced by a slow intravenous infusion of 10% calcium gluconate (0.5 ml/kg) using ECG control (Barratt, 1971). The serum potassium can be reduced temporarily by 8.4% sodium bicarbonate (containing 1 mmol of $NaHCO_3$/ml of solution) in a dose of 2 ml/kg; this should not be given unless there is a metabolic acidosis. A combination of glucose and insulin will also reduce hyperkalaemia temporarily; 0.5–1.0 units of a short-acting insulin should be given with 10–20 ml of glucose 50%. Blood glucose (or glucose strip estimations should be monitored at half-hourly intervals.

Dribbling of urine and retention

Though it is easier to detect an abnormal stream of urine in males, female infants can produce quite a forceful jet of urine which can be easily distinguished from any of the conditions described below.

Recognition

1. Bladder neck obstruction from urethral valves. The infant appears constantly wet from repeated dribbling of urine forced out of the

urethra by the hypertrophied bladder. The dribbling is not affected by a rise in intraabdominal pressure but can be increased by gentle pressure on the fundus of the bladder.
2. A neurogenic bladder occurs in meningomyelocele and sacral agenesis (p. 216) and in severe hypoxic-ischaemic encephalopathy. There is constant dribbling from a distended but not hypertrophied bladder. Urine is expressed from the bladder during crying or by light suprapubic pressure. Rarely, retention with overflow may develop in infants with cervical cord damage from a breech delivery (p. 50).
3. Transient retention, rarely with overflow, may occur in any ill infant.
4. Other causes of retention with overflow are obstruction of the urethra by hydrocolpos in girls (p. 265) or by an ectopic ureterocele in either sex.
5. Dribbling from an empty bladder indicates either a grossly incompetent vesical sphincter in a normal site, bilateral single ectopic ureters entering below the sphincter (Williams and Lightwood, 1972) or an incompetent sphincter opening into a persistent cloaca, as in some forms of masculinization in adrenal hyperplasia (pp. 267–272).

Management

1. Bladder neck obstruction, see p. 261.
2. Neurogenic bladder. The mother should be taught how to express the bladder at regular intervals (2-hourly in an infant) to avoid overdistension and to reduce the likelihood of infection, also intermittent catheterization.
3. Transient retention can be relieved by catheter or suprapubic aspiration if it requires any treatment at all.
4. Incontinence from hydrocolpos, ureterocele or ectopic ureter requires transfer to a specialist paediatric surgical unit.

Passage of urine from an abnormal site

Recognition

1. Absence of the penis is obvious; urine is passed from an opening into the anus.
2. In girls with a persistent cloaca, urine is passed from the common orifice, often with dribbling (see above).
3. A patent urachus causes urine to be passed from an opening in the inferior part of the umbilical ring, and may be associated with severe or complete obstruction to vesical outflow.

Urine with an abnormal smell

Urine infected with a coliform organism frequently has a fishy smell, while an infection with a urea-splitting organism such as a proteus causes the urine to smell of ammonia. For other abnormal smells, see p. 285.

Urinary ascites

Recognition

This is present at delivery as with ascites for other causes (p. 274) and must be distinguished from hydrops fetalis by the absence of generalized oedema, anaemia and hepatosplenomegaly (p. 117). The diagnosis of urinary ascites can usually be suspected by the presence of a major abnormality of the external genitalia and by the failure to pass urine after

Table 24.1 Causes of urinary ascites

Posterior urethral valves*
Spontaneous rupture of the bladder
Urethral atresia (sometimes with 'prune-belly' syndrome)
Neuropathic bladder
Bladder neck obstruction
Pelviureteric junction obstruction (bilateral)
Anterior urethral valves
Ureterocele
Obstructed megaureter (sometimes with 'prune-belly' syndrome)

delivery. The causes of urinary ascites (Kay *et al.*, 1980) are given in Table 24.1. The diagnosis can usually be confirmed by an IVU which shows extravasation of the contrast medium in the perirenal area, beneath the renal capsule or from a ruptured bladder.

Management

In many cases renal function is so poor that prolonged survival is impossible, but it is important to establish the exact cause of the condition since the ascites may be associated with completely normal function, as with spontaneous rupture of the bladder. Where an obstructive lesion is present, prompt decompression and urinary diversion should be carried out as soon as possible in a unit specializing in neonatal surgery. Until a flow of urine has been established, fluid intake should be limited and the urea and electrolytes should be estimated at frequent intervals, as water intoxication with hyponatraemia is a danger. After decompression there may be a transient phase of excessive loss of sodium and potassium.

Abdominal masses of renal origin

Recognition and management

Bilateral renal masses
Present at birth These may be due to polycystic disease (AR) (p. 261), bilateral hydronephrosis due to bladder neck obstruction (see above), bilateral obstruction at the pelviureteric junction or lower ends of the ureter, or multicystic disease of the kidneys (p. 261).
Masses developing after birth In acute pyelonephritis the kidneys may become sufficiently enlarged to be easily palpable, though perhaps not

strictly renal masses. Bilateral renal-vein thrombosis should also be considered; this must be differentiated from acute adrenal haemorrhage (p. 77).

Unilateral renal masses
Present before birth These may be due to hydronephrosis, multicystic disease, a congenital Wilms' tumour or the relatively benign mesoblastic nephroma which may be associated with polyhydramnios. Renal tumour must be distinguished from a congenital neuroblastoma.
Developing after birth These may be due to renal-vein thrombosis, renal or adrenal tumour, or acute adrenal haemorrhage (p. 77).

The investigation of renal masses may require merely an IVU and ultrasound, or more sophisticated investigations. Adrenal conditions can usually be distinguished from renal masses by the flattening of the upper calyces on IVU, and the depression of the kidney. Apart from a unilateral renal-vein thrombosis, which is usually treated conservatively, all the other conditions described above require transfer to a specialist unit.

Lower abdominal masses

Recognition

These are usually central and may be due to:

1. An enlarged and hypertrophied bladder from urethral obstruction or possibly urethral atresia (see above).
2. A distended neurogenic bladder (see above).
3. Urachal cyst; this does not usually communicate with the bladder or umbilicus. Infection may occur and cause peritonitis.
4. Hydrocolpos or hydrometrocolpos. This can usually be recognized by the presence of a greyish mass protruding through the vaginal opening; a distended bladder may result, with overflow incontinence (see above).
5. An ovarian cyst may present as a swelling arising from the pelvis, if torsion occurs there may be bleeding into the peritoneal cavity.

Management

For bladder neck obstruction and neurogenic bladder, see p. 262. Infants with urachal cyst, hydrocolpos, hydrometrocolpos or ovarian cyst should be transferred to a neonatal surgical unit. A twisted ovarian cyst is a surgical emergency.

Swellings in the genital region

Recognition and management

Hymenal tag

This is common; it is an oedematous tag of hymen protruding from the vagina. It has a yellowish appearance and can be seen to arise from the membrane of the hymen. No treatment is required as the tag retracts as the oedema associated with delivery subsides. A careful examination will exclude the possibility of sarcoma botryoides.

Swollen testis
This may be due to:

1. Pressure from a breech delivery. There is usually an accompanying hydro- or haematocele. The diagnosis is obvious because of the obstetric history and the accompanying swelling and bruising of the whole of the genital area. A variable degree of testicular atrophy may result.
2. Torsion: this may occur pre- or post-natally and may be unilateral or bilateral. The testis is swollen and the scrotum red, but appears painless when torsion has occurred before birth. Exploration of any swollen testis except when due to breech delivery must be undertaken as soon as possible to minimize the amount of atrophy.
3. Torsion of a testicular appendix: this usually occurs postnatally. The appearance is similar to torsion of the testis, but the amount of swelling is less, and the congested appendix may be felt as a pea-like swelling at the upper pole of the testis.

Inguinal hernia
Simple hernia This is more common in males than females and in pre-term as compared with term infants. The history of an intermittent swelling in the inguinal region or going down into the scrotum or labium should be accepted as being adequate proof that a hernia exists, provided that it was seen by a reliable observer. Since incarceration or obstruction is common, even an uncomplicated inguinal hernia should be operated on before the infant returns home from a maternity unit.

Incarcerated hernia Incarceration is common in inguinal hernia in the newborn infant, especially in the pre-term infant. Strangulation is rare but in unrecognized incarceration, the blood supply of the intestine may be sufficiently impaired to cause a Gram-negative septicaemia; a rare complication is vascular obstruction to the testis. The hernia is tense and tender and cannot be reduced by firm pressure. Symptoms of incarceration are:

1. Crying, due to intestinal colic.
2. Vomiting, which is bile-stained in about one-third of cases.
3. Diarrhoea, if the obstruction is incomplete.

The importance of these symptoms is that they may easily be mistaken for gastroenteritis: therefore all infants with vomiting and diarrhoea should be carefully examined to exclude incarcerated hernia. Forcible attempts at reduction should **not** be made; however, in some cases elevation of the infant's buttocks with a gallows splint may cause spontaneous reduction. Even if this has been achieved, operation is a matter of urgency.

Ambiguous genitalia

The birth of a child with ambiguous external genitalia gives rise to two emergencies:

1. Parental anxiety about the sex of the child. This should be resolved as clearly and quickly as possible, but not at the expense of accuracy of diagnosis. A wrong decision may have very serious consequences for the child.
2. A proportion of these infants will be found to be sodium-losers who may develop a sodium-losing crisis in the neonatal period or later. If untreated these crises can be fatal, but adequate diagnosis and treatment should prevent them from occurring.

It is important that five objectives should be clearly defined.

1. The range of abnormalities which should be included within the definition of ambiguous genitalia.
2. A plan for the initial clinical examination of the infant which will yield the maximum amount of information.
3. A plan for diagnostic investigations which involves:
   (a) Short-term investigations within the capability of most paediatric units;
   (b) The identification of infants requiring referral to a specialist diagnostic unit;
4. Genetic advice to the parents on the risk of recurrence of the condition in subsequent children.
5. Long-term arrangements for the support of parents and child through puberty, including decisions on hormonal treatment, removal of abdominal testes at puberty to avoid the risk of malignant change or to prevent virilization at puberty, and advice on reproductive potential.
6. If possible, a conclusion as to the sex for rearing should be reached before the age of 6 weeks as the birth details must (in the UK) be registered within that period. If this is not possible, the Registrar will agree to delay the registration if he is informed of the difficulty.

Recognition of the anatomical defect

The following abnormalities should be included under the definition of ambiguous external genitalia.

1. All infants whose external genitalia are abnormal to the extent that it is impossible to be certain, on inspection, whether the child is a boy or a girl.
2. Infants with the following abnormalities.
   (a) Hypospadias and impalpable testes;
   (b) An enlarged clitoris with otherwise normal external genitalia, or with partial fusion of the labia;
   (c) A micropenis with or without palpable testes;
   (d) A common urogenital sinus (an opening in the position of a vagina, but which also contains the urethral orifice).

Isolated hypospadias with normal testes should not be included in this category of ambiguous genitalia.

Causes of ambiguous genitalia

In most instances the condition can be seen to be in one of two categories.

1. A genetic female (46XX) infant in whom masculinization of the external genitalia has occurred; the degree of masculinization ranges from enlargement of the clitoris alone, through perineal hypospadias and a variable degree of fusion of the labia, to a completely formed penile structure with a urethral opening at the tip, with complete fusion of the labia majora to form a scrotum-like structure. However, gonads are never palpable in the labia or inguinal regions and further investigation shows that there are normal ovaries and uterus.
2. A genetic male (46XY) infant with incomplete masculinization of the external genitalia. In its extreme form, the external genitalia are female in type with a normal or slightly enlarged clitoris and a blind vaginal orifice; the urethra may be in the normal female position or there may be a urogenital sinus. Usually the testes are palpable in the labia majora or in the inguinal regions. There is of course no uterus.

Less commonly there are:

1. 46XX phenotypic males in whom the external genitalia are recognizably male but there is hypospadias and incompletely descended gonads which are found to be testes with rudimentary seminiferous tubules.
2. A genuine hermaphrodite, usually of 46XX genotype or with XX/XY mosaic. The appearance is that of a male with hypospadias and cryptorchidism. Exploration may show bilateral ovotestes or a testis on one side and an ovary on the other. Turner mosaic, XY/XO.

The common causes of ambiguous genitalia are given in Table 24.2.

The family and maternal history in ambiguous genitalia

As soon as an infant has been recognized as having abnormal external genitalia a full history should be taken, with special reference to the following points.

1. Whether any other sibs have abnormal genitalia or are known to have congenital adrenal hyperplasia (CAH) or other endocrine disorder. In particular whether deaths in the neonatal period have occurred, especially if abnormal genitalia were noted.
2. Whether there is anyone in the family, especially older sibs, with precocious puberty with short stature, absent testes in the 'males' or virilization or hirsutism in female relations or sibs.
3. Whether there are maternal aunts (mother's sisters) who are infertile, or who have been investigated for amenorrhoea or incomplete sexual development, or who have been found to have an unusual type of inguinal hernia (testicular feminization syndrome, XR).

Defect	*Male genotype*	*Female genotype*	*Sodium loss*	*Hypertension*	*17-OHP*	*17-Ox*
Congenital adrenal hyperplasia						
21-Hydroxylase (AR) (severe)	N	Variable masculinization	+	0	↑	↑
21-Hydroxylase (AR) (mild)	N	As above	0	0	↑	↑
11-β-Hydroxylase (AR)	N	As above	0	±	↑ (moderate)	↑
17-α-Hydroxylase (AR)	Incomplete masculinization	N	0	+	0	N or ↓
3-β-Hydroxysteroid dehydrogenase (AR)	As above	N or slight masculinization	+	0	0	As above
20,22-Desmolase (AR) (lipoid hyperplasia)	As above	N	+	0	0	0
Errors in testosterone action or metabolism						
Androgen-binding defect (XR)	Complete testicular feminization (external female genitalia)	Does not occur; normal female sibs	0	0	N	N
Incomplete androgen-binding defect (XR)	Incomplete masculinization	As above	0	0	N	N
Target tissue failure of testosterone conversion (AR) (5α-reductase deficiency)	As above: virilization at puberty	Confined to males; normal female sibs	0	0	N	N
Miscellaneous causes						
Endogenous (maternal) androgens	N	Variable masculinization	0	0	N	N
Exogenous drugs (androgens, progestagens) in pregnancy	N	As above	0	0	N	N
Danazol treatment in pregnancy*	N	As above	Transient	0	?	?
Turner's syndrome, some cases	Genotype XO or mosaic		0	+ if coarctation	N	N
True hermaphrodites (intersexes): mixed gonads	Variable combinations of ambiguous genitalia		0	0	N	N
Some patients with autosomal chromosomal disorders	Incompletely masculinized genotypic males		0	0	N	N

Abbreviations: 17-OHP, 17-hydroxyprogesterone (plasma); 17-Ox, 17-oxo(keto)steroids (urine); N, normal; ↑, raised; 0, absent; ↓, low.
*Castro-Magana *et al.* (1981).

4. Whether there are any sibs who have been brought up as girls but who have virilized and changed to a male gender identity at puberty (5α-reductase deficiency, AR).
5. Whether the mother shows any evidence of masculinization or virilization or has received any androgenic drugs or other drugs such as danazol (which are known to have side effects on the adrenal gland (Castro-Magana *et al.*, 1981).

Management and investigation

Both parents should be seen by a consultant, as soon after the birth as possible, to explain the plan of investigations. It is important not to be pushed into making a premature decision about the sex in which the child should be reared.

Clinical investigation

This should be done with great care and the findings should be recorded in the notes and signed. Particular points to be noted are:

1. Phallus: size, maximum length on stretching; presence of chordee, position of urethral opening.
2. Labia or scrotum: the degree of fusion of the labia, whether the scrotum is bifid, the size and rugosity of the scrotal sac.
3. Gonads: the presence or absence of gonads in the scrotal sac. If absent, whether they can be felt higher up or in the inguinal canal; the presence of gonads in the labia majora.
4. Vaginal orifice: whether this appears normal or whether there is a common urogenital sinus containing the urethral orifice.
5. On rectal examination, whether the cervix or uterus can be felt.
6. The presence of other malformations (autosomal chromosomal disorders).

Biochemical investigation

It should be made clear to the parents that the average neonatal unit has limited facilities for the investigation of infants with ambiguous genitalia and that any infant in which the diagnosis cannot be made with any degree of certainty will require investigation elsewhere or examination of a 24-hour urine by a specialist endocrine laboratory. About 80% of infants with CAH have the 21-hydroxylase defect which can be confirmed by the presence of a high plasma 17-hydroxyprogesterone (17-OHP)* and an increased amount of pregnanetriol in the urine and in such cases transfer may not be necessary. However, it is unwise to rely for the final diagnosis only on raised levels of 17-OHP or 17-oxosteroids, and abnormal metabolites specific to the various defects should always be looked for in

*The plasma 17-OHP is somewhat raised immediately after delivery in the normal newborn; investigation should therefore be delayed until the second day of life. Very ill infants may also have a raised 17-OHP level.

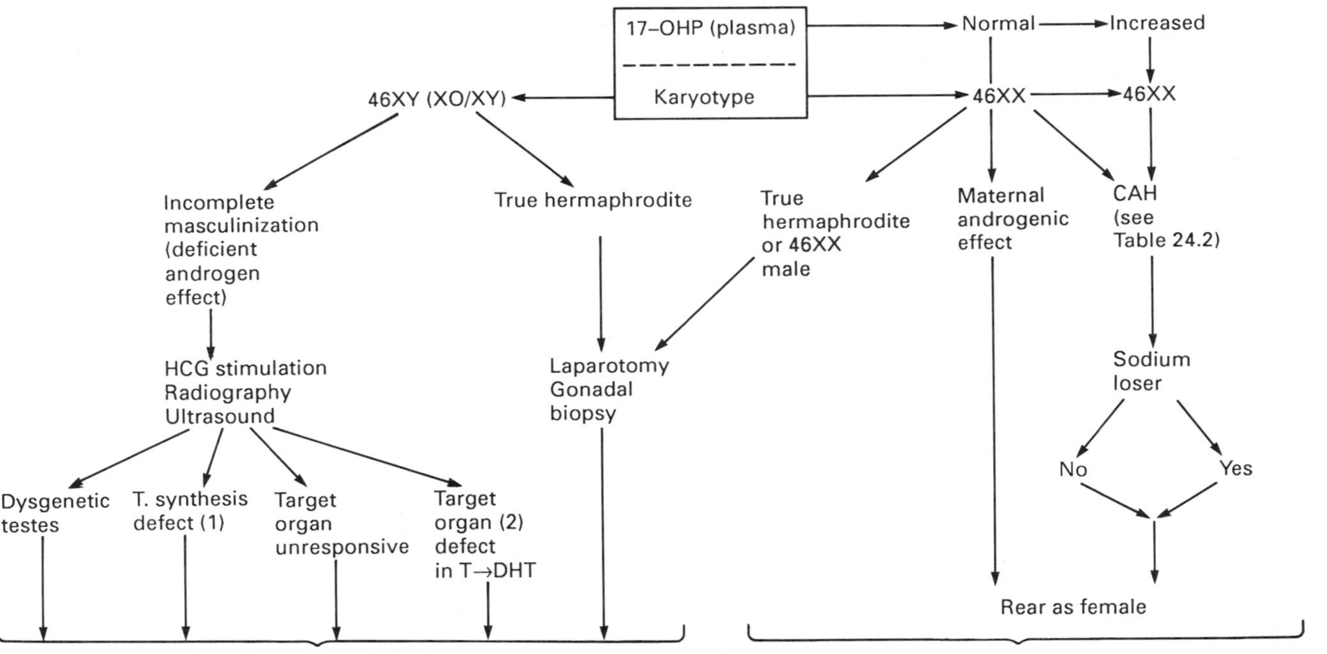

Figure 24.1 Investigation of infants with ambiguous genitalia. Abbreviations: DHT, dihydroxytestosterone; HCG, human chorionic gonadotrophin; 17-OHP, 17-hydroxyprogesterone; T, testosterone. (1) includes some forms of CAH which are sodium-losers. (2) 5α-reductase deficiency

a 24-hour urine collection. The investigation of incompletely masculinized genotypic males or possible true hermaphrodites is particularly difficult and requires transfer to a specialized unit. Figure 24.1 (modified from Hughes and Davies, 1980) gives a simplified plan of investigation.

Recognition of sodium-losers

This is dealt with in pp. 232–233 as this constitutes a metabolic emergency and occurs in a variety of conditions other than adrenal hyperplasia. It is important to bear in mind that infants with certain rare forms of CAH, in which the males are incompletely masculinized and the females have normal genitalia, are salt-losers, (3β-hydroxysteroid, and 20,22-desmolase deficiencies, see Table 24.2). The clinical picture in 20,22-desmolase deficiency (lipoid hyperplasia) is peculiar in that the affected infants develop a curious honey-coloured pigmentation shortly after birth (Hamilton, 1972); however, they rarely survive beyond infancy even with apparently adequate treatment.

General clues to the likely diagnosis

1. Micropenis alone or with undescended testes is likely to be due to hypopituitarism: lack of growth hormone may cause hypoglycaemia in the neonatal period.
2. Gonads in the scrotum, lower inguinal regions, or in the labia are generally testes.
3. An infant with ambiguous genitalia and no palpable gonads is generally a masculinized female.

Decision on sex of rearing

1. In difficult cases this decision should not be made until all the facts are available. The genotypic sex is not of crucial importance; for example, a 46XX infant with a scrotum, partially descended testes and a well-formed phallus should be brought up as a male, with repair of hypospadias and orchidopexy where necessary; and an XY infant with female external genitalia (as in the testicular feminizing syndromes) should be brought up as a girl. In 5α-reductase deficiency, the genotypic males have predominantly female external genitalia and should be brought up as girls but will require orchidectomy before virilization starts at puberty (Peterson *et al.*, 1977).
2. Where masculinization of the female is very complete, there will, however, be normal ovaries and uterus; a plastic surgeon should attempt to construct a vagina, with partial clitoridectomy. It is a serious mistake to make a decision without knowledge of the internal genitalia.

References

Barratt, T.M. (1971) Renal failure in the first year of life. *British Medical Bulletin*, **27**, 115–121

Castro-Magana, M., Cheruvansky, T., Collipp, P.J., Ghavami-Maibodi, Z., Angulo, M. *et al.* (1981) Transient adrenogenital syndrome due to exposure to danazol *in utero. American Journal of Diseases of Children*, **135**, 1032–1034

Hamilton, W. (1972) *Clinical Paediatric Endocrinology*, Butterworths, London, p. 120

Hughes, I.A. and Davies, D.P. (1980) *Clinics in Endocrinology and Metabolism*, **9**, 597–599

Kay, R., Brereton, R.J. and Johnson, J.H. (1980) Urinary ascites in the newborn. *British Journal of Urology*, **52**, 451–454

Peterson, R.E., Imperato-McGinley, J., Gautier, J. and Starla, E. (1977) Male pseudohermaphroditism due to steroid 5 alpha-reductase deficiency. *American Journal of Medicine*, **62**, 170–191

Williams, D.I. and Lightwood, R.G. (1972) Bilateral single ectopic ureters. *British Journal of Urology*, **44**, 267–273

Further reading

Brook, C.G.D. (1978) *Practical Paediatric Endocrinology*, Academic Press, London

Brook, C.G.D. (ed.) (1981) *Clinical Paediatric Endocrinology*, Blackwell Scientific, Oxford

Hamilton, W., Hutchison, J.H., Fraser, D., Koch, S.W. and Farquhar, T.W. (1984) Disorders of the endocrine glands. In *Textbook of Paediatrics*, 3rd edn, (eds J.O. Forfar and G.C. Arneil), Churchill Livingstone, Edinburgh, pp. 1106–1196

Lister, J. and Irving, I.M. (eds) (1990) *Neonatal Surgery*, 3rd edn, Butterworths, London

Chapter 25

Hydrops fetalis

In this condition there is generalized pitting oedema, often with ascites and occasionally with pleural effusions. The abdomen is usually grossly distended from the ascites and sometimes from hepatomegaly or hepatosplenomegaly, depending on the cause.

Recognition

The hydropic fetus can be recognized prenatally by its large size, the distension of the abdomen and splayed limbs and the large placenta which can be seen on ultrasound. Where the possibility of hydrops is suspected because a previous infant has been affected or in known blood group isoimmunization (predominantly due to rhesus incompatibility) or where both parents are known to be heterozygous for α°-thalassaemia, prenatal investigation is essential. Polyhydramnios commonly accompanies hydrops fetalis. Occasionally hydrops may recur, even in circumstances where the obvious causes have been excluded (Etches and Lemons, 1979); therefore the mother should be fully investigated (Table 25.1) if she has produced a previous infant with hydrops. Hydrops should be distinguished from ascites without oedema (p. 264). Hydrops from rhesus isoimmunization is probably best treated by transfusion into the fetal circulation by cordocentesis if the necessary expertise is available (p. 26). Fetal arrhythmias can sometimes be treated transplacentally by giving the mother appropriate treatment (p. 26).

Prenatal investigation of the mother

Table 25.1 Prenatal investigation of mother for hydrops fetalis (Etches, 1986)

Ultrasound
- Hydrops (fetus, placenta, amniotic fluid)
- Malformation
- Fetal heart (rate and structure)
- Multiple pregnancy

X-ray if needed
Blood group (ABO, Rh, minor antigens)
Antibodies (AB, Rh, minor antigens)

Kleihauer (before amniocentesis)
Syphilis serology
TORCH antibodies
α-Fetoprotein
Haemoglobin concentration
Haemoglobin electrophoresis
Glucose-6-phosphate dehydrogenase
Glucose tolerance test
Amniocentesis (optical density; lecithin/sphingomyelin ratio, chromosomal analysis)

The placenta

This should be examined by the naked eye for evidence of fetomaternal haemorrhage or other major abnormality, and should be kept for subsequent histological examination.

The hydropic infant

Some indication as to the possible cause of the condition may be obtained from clinical examination.

1. Severe anaemia with hepatosplenomegaly suggests blood group isoimmunization, fetomaternal haemorrhage, α°-thalassaemia, G-6PD deficiency, or in twins, twin-to-twin haemorrhage.
2. Hepatosplenomegaly without severe anaemia suggests an intrauterine infection (p. 179).
3. Hepatomegaly alone is not of great significance since the hepatic enlargement may be due to the generalized oedema, or raised venous pressure from a number of possible causes (Table 25.4).

Investigation of the hydropic infant (depending on other evidence and clinical signs)

Table 25.2 Investigation of the hydropic infant

Percentage haemoglobin and blood film (all cases), platelet and reticulocyte count
Blood group
Direct Coombs' test (suspected isoimmunization)
Haemoglobin electrophoresis and supravital staining for red cell inclusions (suspected α°-thalassaemia)
Test for G-6PD deficiency
Electrolytes, creatinine
Liver function test (for hepatitis)
X-ray of skull, abdomen, long bones
ECG with or without echocardiogram
Blood for bacterial and viral cultures and serology (pp. 181–193)
Serology for syphilis, cytomegalovirus, rubella, toxoplasmosis
Chromosome analysis (particularly in the presence of multiple malformations)

Dependence of the incidence of various causes on the ethnic origin of the parents

This may help in the investigation.

Table 25.3 Occurrence of hydrops fetalis in relation to ethnic group

Group	*Possible cause of hydrops*
Western European (Caucasian)	Rhesus isoimmunization
Mediterranean area	G-6PD deficiency with maternal ingestion of haemolytic agent (Mentzer and Collier, 1975)
Chinese and related races	i) As above, G-6PD deficiency ii) α°-Thalassaemia
Finnish	Congenital nephrotic syndrome

Table 25.4 Causes of hydrops fetalis

Infections
Toxoplasmosis
Cytomegalovirus disease
Leptospirosis
Chagas' disease
Syphilis
Chronic hepatitis
Parvovirus infection (p. 183)

Chronic anaemia
Blood group incompatibility
α°-Thalassaemia ([1])
G-6PD deficiency ([2])
Gaucher's disease
Leukaemia
Twin-to-twin transfusion
Chronic fetomaternal transfusion

Cardiac diseases
Bradyarrhythmias: heart block
Calcifying myocarditis (Coxsackie virus)
Acute myocarditis
Tachyarrhythmias: paroxysmal supraventricular tachycardia, atrial flutter
Truncus arteriosus
Subaortic stenosis
Right or left ventricular endocardial fibroelastosis and mitral insufficiency
Congenital insufficiency of pulmonary valve
Premature closure of foramen ovale
Premature closure of ductus arteriosus
Arteriovenous fistula
Uhl's anomaly ([4])
Cardiac neoplasm
Acardia

Renal diseases
Congenital nephrotic syndrome
Renal vein thrombosis

Malformations and congenital tumours
Pulmonary hypoplasia
Haemangioendothelioma
Chorangioma of placenta
Aneurysm of umbilical artery
Angiomyxoma of umbilical cord
Congenital hepatoblastoma ([3])
Congenital neuroblastoma
Leukaemia
Cystic hygroma
Cervical teratoma
Pulmonary lymphangiectasia
Cystic adenomatoid malformation of the lung
Down's syndrome
Achondroplasia
Trisomy 18
Turner's syndrome
Multiple malformations

Miscellaneous
Diaphragmatic hernia
Chylothorax
Idiopathic arterial calcification
Multiple placental infarcts
Multiple pregnancy with parasitic fetus
Fetal retroperitoneal fibrosis
Umbilical vein thrombosis
Intrauterine intracranial haemorrhage
Storage diseases
Small bowel volvulus
Meconium peritonitis
Tuberose sclerosis

Maternal disorders
Diabetes mellitus
Pre-eclampsia

Unknown cause

Table modified, with additions, from Giacoia (1980) reproduced by kind permission of author and publisher. Other references are given below. Etches (1986) gives a more comprehensive list of causes.
1. Bryan *et al.* (1981).
2. Mentzer and Collier (1975).
3. Benjamin *et al.* (1981).
4. Parchment heart with atrophic right ventricle (Corazza *et al.*, 1981).

Rarer causes of hydrops

The list of possible causes or associated conditions is enormous (Giacoia, 1980), but it is important to make a correct diagnosis because this may influence treatment (e.g. congenital syphilis) and also because of the genetic implications of some of the causes. Table 25.4 gives a classified list of causes and Table 25.5 a suggested plan for the pathophysiology of hydrops.

Table 25.5 Pathophysiology of hydrops fetalis

Possible mechanisms	*Specific disturbance*	*Aetiological examples*
Haemodynamic disturbance	Primary myocardial failure	Myocarditis (e.g. Coxsackie) Arrhythmias (e.g. supraventricular tachycardia) Premature closure of foramen ovale Severe anaemia Twin-to-twin transfusion
	High output failure	Arteriovenous fistula Severe anaemia Haemangioendothelioma Twin-to-twin transfusion
	Obstruction of venous return	Cystic malformation of the lungs Fetal retroperitoneal fibrosis Vena caval thrombosis
Decreased plasma oncotic pressure	Decreased albumin formation	Rhesis isoimmunization
	Increased albumin excretion	Congenital nephrotic syndrome
Increased capillary permeability	Hypoxia	Placental oedema Capillary damage (congenital infection)
Altered water homeostasis (fetus–placenta–amniotic fluid compartment)		

Table reproduced and modified from Giacoia (1980) with permission of author and publishers.

Management

1. Full-scale resuscitation should be started as soon as the infant is delivered, including intubation and IPPV with 100% oxygen and heart rate monitoring. A high inspiratory pressure is frequently required because of poor lung compliance (30–50 cm H_2O).
2. If the heart rate does not improve after 1 minute, emergency paracentesis of the abdomen in the right lower quadrant should be undertaken using a 20 ml syringe, three-way stopcock, and 18 guage Teflon catheter (e.g. Abbocath or Jelco).
3. Bilateral chest paracentesis may also be required. Precautions should

be taken not to cause pneumothorax. Ultrasound examination immediately before delivery may provide useful information about the presence and volume of fluid in both sides of the chest and the abdomen.

4. If the infant has Rhesus isoimmunization or anaemia from some other cause a cautious partial exchange with packed cells should be carried out with attention to the CVP (p. 131).
5. If there is a persisting tachyarrhythmia, emergency cardioversion may be required.
6. Failure to respond to the above management in the first half hour suggests that the infant may have hypoplastic lungs as a result of chronic pleural effusion *in utero*, or other intrinsic pulmonary disease.
7. The infant should be stabilized in an intensive care unit, with insertion of an umbilical arterial catheter, a chest X-ray, and the appropriate investigations initiated.
8. Respiratory management is usually difficult because of lung fluid and possible pulmonary hypoplasia.
9. Fluid intake should be conservative (40 ml/kg daily) usually 10% glucose, provided the blood glucose is maintained. No additional sodium should be given in the first few days, apart from sodium bicarbonate as required.
10. Frequent albumin infusions are of value in mobilizing tissue fluids.
11. Disseminated intravascular coagulation is common (for management see p. 91).

References

Benjamin, E., Lendon, M. and Marsden, H.B. (1981) Hepatoblastoma as a cause of intrauterine fetal death. *British Journal of Obstetrics and Gynaecology*, **88**, 329–332

Bryan, E.M., Chaimongol, B. and Harris, D.A. (1981) Alpha-thalassaemic hydrops fetalis. *Archives of Disease in Childhood*, **56**, 476–478

Corazza, G., Soliani, M. and Bava, G.L. (1981) Uhl's anomaly in the newborn. *European Journal of Pediatrics*, **137**, 347–352

Etches, P.C. (1986) Hydrops fetalis. In *Textbook of Neonatology* (ed. N.R.C. Roberton), Churchill Livingstone, Edinburgh, pp. 484–494

Etches, P.C. and Lemons, J.A. (1979) Non-immune hydrops fetalis. *Pediatrics*, **64**, 326–332

Giacoia, G.P. (1980) Hydrops fetalis (fetal edema). *Clinical Pediatrics*, **19**, 334–339

Mentzer, W.C. and Collier, E. (1975) Hydrops fetalis associated with erythrocyte G-6PD deficiency and maternal ingestion of fava beans and ascorbic acid. *Journal of Pediatrics*, **86**, 565–567

Further reading

Carlton, D.F., MacGillivray, B.C. and Schreiber, M.D. (1981) Non-immune hydrops fetalis: a multidisciplinary approach. *Clinics in Perinatology*, **16**, 839–851

Perlin, B.M., Pomerance, J.J. and Schifrin, B.S. (1981) Non-immunologic hydrops fetalis. *Obstetrics and Gynecology*, **57**, 584–588

Chapter 26

The floppy infant

The floppy or hypotonic infant is a common problem in the neonatal period. An important distinction which should be made is whether the hypotonia is paralytic or non-paralytic; if the arms and legs can be moved against gravity, either spontaneously or after stimulation of the palms and soles, or the infant is able to maintain the position of a passively elevated limb, then there is hypotonia but no significant weakness (Dubowitz, 1980i). The possible cause of the hypotonia can often be inferred from evidence available prenatally or during delivery.

Prenatal evidence

Lack of or reduced fetal movements

Paralytic conditions

1. Infantile spinal muscular atrophy (Werdnig–Hoffman disease) (AR).
2. Congenital poliomyelitis (usually with a clinically affected mother).
3. Dystrophia myotonica (AD but see also p. 23).
4. Congenital myasthenia (usually associated with affected mother).
5. Congenital myopathies.

Non-paralytic conditions

1. Prader–Willi syndrome (occasional familial cases, some due to unbalanced translocation between chromosomes 15 and 22).
2. Type II glycogenosis (Pompe's disease) (AR).
3. Non-ketotic hyperglycinaemia (AR) (usually with extreme ('rag doll') hypotonia).
4. Zellweger's syndrome (with hepatomegaly) (AR).

Associated with polyhydramnios

1. Myotonic dystrophy (AD) (p. 23).
2. Maternal treatment with anticoagulants (Warfarin syndrome) (Table 1.5).

Drugs given during pregnancy

1. Anticoagulants (p. 6).
2. Diazepam.
3. Lithium carbonate (Table 1.5).
4. Nitrazepam.

Intrapartum events

1. Severe intrapartum hypoxia.
2. Damage to cervical cord during difficult breech delivery.
3. Drugs given during delivery:
   (a) Sedatives or tranquillizers: diazepam, lorazepam, nitrazepam;
   (b) Magnesium sulphate for toxaemia (p. 225);
   (c) Alcohol for premature labour;
   (d) Local anaesthetics (p. 48);
   (e) Prolonged general anaesthetic (p. 230).
4. Hyponatraemia resulting from maternal hyponatraemia (p.000).

Conditions associated with recognizable clinical features

1. Prematurity below 34 weeks gestation.
2. Down's syndrome.
3. Maternal treatment with anticoagulants (p. 6).
4. Zellweger's syndrome, with hepatomegaly. Refer to standard paediatric texts for further details.

Hypotonia developing postnatally

1. Septicaemia or any severe infection.
2. Hypoxic-ischaemi brain injury.
3. Hyponatraemia from any cause (p. 226).
4. Various organic acidaemias associated with vomiting and metabolic acidosis developing within 24–48 hours of delivery (p. 284).
5. Botulism (see below).

Botulism

Botulism may occur during the neonatal period but more commonly somewhat later. The sequence of development of symptoms is an important clue to the diagnosis; these are usually as follows (L'Hommedieu and Polin, 1981):

1. Constipation, tachycardia.
2. Loss of head control, decreased spontaneous movements.
3. Depressed gag reflex.
4. Peripheral motor weakness.

5. Diaphragmatic weakness.

In addition, there may be ptosis, sluggish pupils, extraocular palsies and feeding difficulties. Tendon reflexes are reduced or absent. Few cases progress to respiratory failure.

Botulism must be distinguished from congenital myasthenia gravis with an affected mother, though symptoms in myasthenia are usually present at or shortly after delivery. In the familial form (AR) with an unaffected mother the onset may be in the neonatal period but is usually later. In myasthenia there is a clear response to edrophonium and neostigmine while in botulism there is none. Edrophonium (1.0mg) is given intravenously, with an almost immediate response in myasthenia, but lasts only a few minutes and is easily missed; neostigmine (prostigmin) (0.125mg) is given intramuscularly and the response occurs within 10–30 minutes and may last for 3–4 hours (Dubowitz, 1980ii).

In botulism the electromyogram (EMG) may be helpful, though the pattern is not specific to botulism (Johnson *et al.*, 1979). *Clostridium botulinum* can usually be cultured from the faeces but circulating toxin has only rarely been identified.

Management

Apart from infants needing respiratory support, tube feeding and frequent pharyngeal suction are usually required. There is a gradual improvement over the course of 2–3 weeks. There is no place for antibiotics or antitoxin. L'Hommedieu and Polin (1981) emphasize that aminoglycosides (gentamicin etc.) should not be given as they may potentiate the neuromuscular blockade; manoeuvres such as neck flexion for lumbar puncture or computerized tomography (CT) scan may precipitate respiratory arrest.

Muscle biopsy in congenital myopathies

Muscle biopsy between 4 and 8 months will establish the diagnosis and prognosis.

References

Dubowitz, V. (1980) *The Floppy Infant*, 2nd edn, Spastics International Medical Publications, William Heinemann Medical Books, London and J.B. Lippincott, Philadelphia, (i) p. 13; (ii) pp. 87–89

Johnson, R.O., Clay, S.A. and Arnon, S.S. (1979) Diagnosis and management of infant botulism. *American Journal of Diseases of Children*, **133**, 586–593

L'Hommedieu, C. and Polin, R.A. (1981) Progression of clinical signs in severe infant botulism; therapeutic implications. *Clinical Pediatrics*, **20**, 90–95

Further reading

Dubowitz, V. (1980) *The Floppy Infant*, 2nd edn, (ed. Spastics International Medical Publications, William Heinemann Medical Books, London and J.B. Lippincott, Philadelphia

Chapter 27

Metabolic emergencies and inborn errors of metabolism

These can be differentiated into two groups:

1. Disorders arising in a potentially normal infant as a result of influences which may operate before, during or after delivery; these are considered elsewhere as indicated.

Hypocalcaemia, pp. 219–221	Hypermagnesaemia, pp. 224–225
Hypercalcaemia, pp. 221–222	Hypoglycaemia, pp. 207–212
Hyponatraemia, pp. 226–235	Hyperglycaemia, pp. 212–214
Hypernatraemia, pp. 235–238	Pyridoxine dependence, pp. 287
Hypomagnesaemia, pp. 223–224	Sodium (salt)-losing crisis, pp. 228

2. Those caused by genetically determined disorders which are considered below under the heading of 'Inborn errors of metabolism'. With a few exceptions these are inherited as autosomal recessives (AR).

Inborn errors of metabolism (IEM)

Some of these conditions can be lethal if untreated (e.g. some types of hyperammonaemia, some of the organic acidaemias, galactosaemia, fructose intolerance, maple-syrup urine disease, non-ketotic hyperglycinaemia) or result in severe mental retardation if treatment is delayed or inadequate. In Muslim families from the Indian subcontinent and some parts of the Middle East, first-cousin marriages are more common than in Caucasians and the incidence of IEMs is correspondingly higher. In predominantly Caucasian communities the most common IEMs are the various types of hyperammonaemia (see Table 27.3) followed by the organic acidaemias and the primary lactic acidoses; the incidence of galactosaemia is low (between 1 in 40000 and 1 in 60000 live births), and fructose intolerance is probably even less common, though a frequency of 1 in 20000 has been reported for Switzerland (Baerlocher *et al.*, 1980).

Facilities for investigation

As it is impossible for every neonatal unit to have its own facilities for the investigation of rare and complex disorders, each unit should know where advice on investigation and emergency treatment is available, and where to transfer the baby if necessary. However, the most important factor in early diagnosis is an awareness in every neonatal unit of the symptoms that suggest the possibility of an inborn error of metabolism.

Clues that suggest that an infant may have an IEM

Family history

1. A previous infant or infants dying from unknown cause in the neonatal period, particularly if the illness developed after a symptom-free period of 1 to 3 days. Specific symptoms such as jaundice or fits may be recalled which may narrow down the possibilities.
2. A surviving sib with mental retardation of unknown cause. This may be due to phenylketonuria (PKU) or maternal PKU untreated during pregnancy (p. 25), goitrous cretinism and a wide variety of other IEMs.

During pregnancy

1. Prenatal testing may already have confirmed (or excluded) the presence of an affected fetus: this can only be done where a specific condition, or group of conditions, is anticipated. Prenatal diagnosis should always be confirmed after delivery. Many IEMs can now be detected prenatally; this is important where prenatal treatment (p. 25) is possible or the condition is untreatable and lethal, and a termination may have to be considered. (For a list of IEMs that can be diagnosed prenatally, see Appendices in Whittle and Connor (1989).)
2. The occurrence of fits in the fetus suggests pyridoxine dependence (p. 287).
3. Absent or reduced fetal movement may raise the possibility of non-ketotic hyperglycinaemia or Zellweger's syndrome if a previous sib has had one of these conditions or had extreme hypotonia from birth (see also Chapter 26).

At delivery

1. Ambiguous genitalia suggest one of the forms of congenital adrenal hyperplasia (CAH) or defective androgen effect (Chapter 24).
2. A goitre raises the possibility of goitrous cretinism but other possibilities such as drug or particularly iodide-induced goitre must be considered.
3. Fits occurring immediately after a normal delivery in an infant of normal appearance that appears well between fits may be due to pyridoxine dependence (p. 287).
4. Hepatomegaly may be present at birth in glycogen storage disease (Type I), the severe form of tyrosinaemia and other rare conditions such as the infantile form of Gaucher's disease or Zellweger's syndrome (refer to any standard major text of paediatrics for further information).

After delivery

The development of symptoms of IEM can be as follows:

1. It is characteristic of those IEMs that cause metabolic emergencies that the infant appears normal at birth and that symptoms usually develop

on the second or third day of life, as a result of the accumulation of toxic metabolites which were previously dialysed into the maternal circulation by the placenta.
2. These symptoms disappear after stopping milk feeds and changing to a glucose saline mixture either orally or intravenously. Recovery may occur within a few hours or over the course of 1–2 days if the infant has been very ill. Where a septicaemia rather than an IEM has been suspected, the improvement may be wrongly attributed to antibiotics; however, the return of the same symptoms on reintroducing milk feeds should strongly suggest the possibility of an IEM.

Recognition

In general, there are two patterns of illness in the acute metabolic disorders that present in the neonatal period. In the first group, which is typical of the organic acidaemias, galactosaemia and fructose intolerance, a metabolic acidosis rapidly develops, with circulatory collapse, closely mimicking a septicaemia; neurological symptoms and fits are relatively late except in galactosaemia and fructose intolerance in which hypoglycaemia develops early. In the second group, predominantly the hyperammonaemias, there is progressively increasing drowsiness and hypoventilation, followed by fits which are not due to hypoglycaemia; metabolic acidosis develops late.

Symptoms that suggest an IEM
These are given in Table 27.1.

Fits due to hypoglycaemia may occur in the organic acidaemias (methylmalonic, propionic and isovaleric acidaemia), galactosaemia, fructose intolerance, maple-syrup urine disease, tyrosinaemia and glycogen storage disease (Type I). The tachypnoea of a metabolic acidosis is easily mistaken for a respiratory or cardiac condition.

Diarrhoea may be due to lactase deficiency (lactose intolerance), but occurs rarely in galactosaemia also.

Table 27.1 Symptoms suggestive of an IEM

Reluctance or refusal to feed	Drowsiness	Jaundice	Apnoeic attacks or respiratory failure
Vomiting	Coma	Oedema	Tachypnoea (metabolic acidosis)
Failure to thrive	Fits	Ascites	
Diarrhoea		Haemorrhagic state	Pulmonary haemorrhage in hyperammonaemia (Sheffield *et al.*, 1976)

Signs that suggest an IEM

1. Jaundice: hepatic type, and later obstructive in galactosaemia, and fructose intolerance (p. 288).
2. Hepatomegaly: in galactosaemia and fructose intolerance the liver is not enlarged at delivery but enlarges rapidly after the infant has received the toxic sugar. Conditions in which the liver may already be enlarged at delivery have already been considered on p. 283.
3. Cataracts may develop in galactosaemia by the age of 3–4 days (Danks, 1981i).

Initial investigations (Tables 27.2 and 27.3)

All investigations which depend upon the identification of an abnormal metabolite or a raised level of a normal metabolite as opposed to an enzyme (as in galactosaemia) must be done while symptoms are present and the infant is receiving milk feeds. Abnormal metabolites may disappear within a few hours of stopping milk feeds. When facilities do not exist for the rapid estimation by micromethods of blood ammonia and lactate (as important initial screening tests), suitable blood samples should be sent urgently to the nearest specialist unit (after consultation by telephone to ensure that the specimens are correctly collected and transported); or the infant should be transferred, if fit enough.

Urine

1. Smell: certain conditions are associated with a specific smell in the urine (e.g. maple syrup in maple-syrup disease, sweaty feet in glutaric acidaemia and isovaleric acidaemia, cat's urine in β-methylcrotonic aciduria and rancid butter in tyrosinaemia). It is most important not to disregard the evidence of the mother or nurse who reports that the baby or the napkin 'smells funny', but to investigate at once. Occasionally infants smell of foodstuffs or spice which has been eaten by the mother immediately before delivery (e.g. cumin, fenugreek, curry) (Hauser *et al.*, 1985).
2. Clinitest tablets give a positive reaction to glucose, galactose, lactose, fructose, xylulose (pentose) and to some glucuronated drugs. Clinistix and other test papers are specific for glucose.
3. Ferric chloride: any colour reaction however transient should be noted. The ferric chloride test and phenistix papers should not be used to exclude any specific condition as the metabolites giving the colour reactions are not necessarily present when acute symptoms develop.
4. Acetest tablets or Ketostix strips: these give a positive reaction to

Table 27.2 Possible significance of simple tests

Test	*Possible disease*
Urine: Positive Clinitest (see also Table 27.4)	Galactosaemia, galactokinase deficiency*, fructose intolerance. Liver damage from a variety of causes. Hyperglycaemia (glucose), various causes (p. 212); transient neonatal diabetes must not be overlooked
Positive Clinistix (see also Table 27.4)	Galactosaemia when glucose accompanies galactose, fructose intolerance if glucose accompanies fructose, hyperglycaemia (p. 212); see above for transient neonatal diabetes
Colour reaction to ferric chloride and Phenistix	see above
Positive Acetest or Ketostix (especially with metabolic acidosis)	Maple-syrup urine disease Isovaleric acidaemia Propionic acidaemia Methylmalonic acidaemia Glycogen storage disease Type I (with hepatomegaly)

*Asymptomatic in the neonatal period but cataracts develop in infancy.

Table 27.3 Some of the IEMs which may cause severe illness in the neonatal period (Danks, 1987)

Disease	*Methods of detection*	*Vitamin responsiveness in some cases*	*Inheritance*
Carbamyl phosphate synthetase deficiency	Blood ammonia	Nil	AR
Ornithine transcarbamylase deficiency	Blood ammonia	Nil	XL*
Citrullinaemia	Blood ammonia HVE of urine or serum	Nil	AR
Other forms of hyperammonaemia	Blood ammonia HVE of urine or serum	Nil	AR
Propionic acidaemia	Metabolic acidosis GLC of urine	Nil	AR
Methylmalonic acidaemia	Metabolic acidosis GLC of urine	B_{12}	AR
Maple-syrup urine disease	Metabolic acidosis HVE of urine or serum GLC of urine	Thiamin†	AR
Isovaleric acidaemia	Metabolic acidosis GLC of urine	Nil	AR
Non-ketotic hyperglycinaemia	Clinical features (p. 279) HVE of urine and serum	Nil	AR
Galactosaemia	Clinical features (p. 288) Positive Clinitest (galactose ± glucose)	Nil	AR
Hereditary fructose intolerance	Clinical features (p. 29) Positive Clinitest (fructose ± glucose)	Nil	AR
Tyrosinaemia, severe form	Clinical features HVE of urine or serum	Nil	AR
Pyridoxine-dependent fits	Clinical features Therapeutic response	Pyridoxine	AR
Congenital lactic acidosis	Metabolic acidosis GLC of urine	Thiamin†	AR

*The mother, as carrier, is usually asymptomatic, with a normal blood ammonia level except after a protein load; affected male infants usually die within a few hours of birth. Female infants are affected to a smaller degree but are often symptomatic in the neonatal period. This is probably the commonest form of hyperammonaemia.
†Noted only in mild cases presenting later in childhood.
GLC = gas–liquid chromatography.
HVE = high-voltage electrophoresis.

'ketone bodies'. A positive test for ketone bodies is most unusual in the newborn except as a result of an IEM.

Dextrostix (see footnote to p. 59) and blood glucose estimations Hypoglycaemia is an important symptom common to a number of conditions (p. 208).

Blood ammonia estimations These should be done as part of the initial investigation.

Acid–base state A metabolic acidosis which is not secondary to hypoxia, cardiac failure, infection, shock, or renal insufficiency is likely to be due to one of the primary lactic acidoses or an organic acidaemia. Where one of these conditions is a possibility an urgent estimation of blood lactate should be done. The distinction between a primary and a secondary lactic acidosis is difficult, as it may take 48–72 hours for the lactate level to return to normal after a severe hypoxic state; also in primary lactic acidosis severe arterial spasm and thrombosis sometimes occur which may be attributed to shock (D.M. Danks, personal communication).

Stools The presence of a reducing substance (lactose) is important evidence suggesting lactase deficiency (lactose intolerance). The fluid part of the stool should be tested with a Clinitest tablet (p. 248).

Blood count A leucopenia and/or thrombocytopenia may be found in methylmalonic, propionic and isovaleric acidaemias but are too inconstant to be of much diagnostic help.

Management (in sequence)

As soon as an IEM is suspected the following sequence should be started:

1. Obtain blood and urine before altering the diet. Obtain advice on quantities of blood required from the local or specialized laboratory, according to the investigation required (see Table 27.3).
2. In a desperately ill infant:
   (a) Do an exchange transfusion or peritoneal dialysis in suspected hyperammonaemia, or an exchange transfusion in suspected galactosaemia or fructose intolerance.
   (b) Start empirical treatment with a combination (Danks, 1981ii) of: thiamin, 50 mg; nicotinamide, 600 mg; folic acid, 15 mg; riboflavin, 50 mg; pyridoxine, 50 mg; ascorbic acid, 300 mg; biotin, 100 mg; vitamin B_{12}, 1 mg. These may have to be given parenterally in an ill infant. Vitamin B_{12} **must** be given intramuscularly.
3. In less severely ill babies, change to oral or intravenous glucose saline (0.18% sodium chloride in glucose 4.3%).
4. If the diagnosis is still uncertain, start feeds by bottle or tube using a mixture containing glucose 5% with glucose polymer 5% (Caloreen, Scientific Hospital Supplies) with the addition of fats as medium-chain triglycerides, so that the calorie intake is enough to prevent catabolism (additional vitamins and trace elements must be supplied if this is continued longer than 48 hours); alternatively a complete protein-free preparation containing no lactose, sucrose or fructose, with added vitamins (Nilprote, Mead-Johnson) can be used.
5. When all clinical and biochemical evidence of metabolic disorder has disappeared, protein should be reintroduced unless a specific disorder of amino acid metabolism requiring a special mixture (e.g. maple-syrup disease) has been discovered. In many of the urea cycle disorders (hyperammonaemias) and organic acidaemias, protein can often be tolerated up to 1.0–1.5 g per kg per day.
6. Referral to special centres: where there are centres with special expertise, both biochemical and clinical, the infant with a suspected

IEM should be transferred as soon as the acute symptoms have resolved and the infant is metabolically stable. However, most hospitals with a neonatal intensive care unit should be able to undertake the management of infants with galactosaemia and fructose intolerance. For this reason these two conditions are considered in some detail below.

Galactosaemia and fructose intolerance

Both disorders have much in common clinically and are inherited as autosomal recessives. In some families in which neonatal deaths have occurred from undiagnosed jaundice and liver failure both diagnoses may have to be considered in subsequent infants.

Symptoms suggesting galactosaemia or fructose intolerance

Recognition Symptoms develop a few hours after the infant has received the toxic sugar (lactose, converted into galactose in the intestinal mucosa; or sucrose, converted into fructose). Human and cow's milk and commercial cow's milk preparations contain only lactose but Wysoy (Wyeth) contains fructose in the form of sucrose and other infant milks produced outside the United Kingdom may also contain sucrose, and their composition should be carefully checked. Antibiotic syrups or vitamin preparations may contain sucrose, and tablets (given crushed to infants) may contain lactose. When taking a dietetic history it is essential to check everything that the infant has had in the 48 hours before the onset of symptoms. Additional bottle feeds are often given at night to apparently completely breast-fed infants and it is always possible that sucrose might have been added to such a feed.

The initial symptoms in both galactosaemia and fructose intolerance are vomiting followed by rapidly increasing jaundice, and enlargement of the liver. The infant may develop a shock-like state due to severe hypoglycaemia, which may be mistaken for septicaemia, though both conditions may co-exist. Oozing from puncture sites and spontaneous skin haemorrhages may occur when the diagnosis has been missed for a few days. Initially the hyperbilirubinaemia is unconjugated but within a few days the level of conjugated bilirubin also rises. As soon as the diagnosis of either condition is suspected a random sample of urine should be collected (for details of testing see below and Table 27.3), and blood taken for estimations of galactose and glucose and also fructose if this is considered possible on the feeding history. Most laboratories can identify these sugars in urine and blood fairly rapidly. An immediate Dextrostix (see footnote, p. 59) should also be done to detect hypoglycaemia, and an urgent assay of red cell galactose-1-phosphate uridyl transferase should be requested. All milk feeds should then be stopped and all oral preparations should be checked to see whether they contain lactose or sucrose. It is important to appreciate that if the infant has not received the toxic sugar during the previous half hour, or has become so ill as to require an intravenous drip of glucose saline, there will be no abnormal sugars in the urine or blood except possibly glucose in the urine; but the level of galactose-1-phosphate uridyl transferase in the red cells is of course unaffected by alterations in

Table 27.4 Investigations in galactosaemia and fructose intolerance

Clinitest	*Clinistix*	*Further investigations*	*Sugars that may be present*	*Interpretation*	*Confirmation of diagnosis*
+	–	Sugar chromatography to identify sugar in urine Attempt to identify galactose or fructose in blood Always estimate blood glucose	Galactose Fructose	Galactosaemia Fructose intolerance Traces of galactose or fructose occur in liver damage from other causes	Clinical improvement on withdrawal of toxic sugar and specific enzyme assay on red cells (galactosaemia) or liver or intestinal mucosa (fructose intolerance)
+	+	As above	Galactose or fructose with glucose	As above; glucose may result from liver damage, renal glucosuria or from hyperglycaemia on i.v. glucose drip	As above
+	+	Blood glucose; hyperglycaemia if on i.v. glucose drip; normal in renal glucosuria	Glucose alone	As above if on i.v. glucose drip and oral feeds have been stopped; does not exclude either diagnosis	Look for other causes of hyperglycaemia or glucose in the urine but meanwhile exclude lactose, sucrose and fructose, until a diagnosis has been made. Transient neonatal diabetes must not be overlooked

the diet. An abnormally low level of this enzyme is diagnostic of galactosaemia; a normal value suggests fructose intolerance or some other metabolic disorder. In fructose intolerance, symptoms can of course only develop if sucrose (or rarely fructose or sorbitol, see note on p. 291) has been given, and initial confirmation of the diagnosis is provided by finding fructose in urine and blood (Table 27.4).

Urine testing The urine should be tested first with Clinitest tablets and then with a Clinistix strip or other glucose-specific test. It is a serious and often fatal error to use a glucose-specific test only and to assume that a negative test has excluded either diagnosis; equally the finding of glucose alone in the urine does not exclude the diagnosis of galactosaemia or fructose intolerance (Table 27.4). A positive Clinitest reaction is given by a number of sugars but in the context of the ill infant only galactose, fructose and glucose are important. The possible results of urine tests are summarized in Table 27.4. In both galactosaemia and fructose intolerance renal tubular damage may cause glucose to be present in the urine as well as the abnormal sugar.

Management

As soon as the diagnosis of either condition is suspected and specimens of urine and blood have been obtained, all sources of lactose and sucrose (see note on p. 291) should be excluded from the diet. As an emergency measure, 0.18% sodium chloride in glucose 4.3% can be given intravenously or orally until a suitable milk can be obtained. Until a definite diagnosis has been made the following milks, which contain no lactose, fructose or sucrose, can be given: Pregestimil or Cow and Gate Formula S (Soya) Food; both are nutritionally complete.

1. Before giving blood or plasma or doing an exchange transfusion, blood should be taken and kept suitably preserved until further investigation can be done.
2. Hypoglycaemia if severe or symptomatic should be treated by a bolus injection of glucose 10%–25% (p. 211).
3. Oozing or bleeding should be treated by intravenous vitamin K_1 2 mg, or with fresh frozen plasma if multiple coagulation defects are suspected (p. 87). Whole blood may also be required, but stored blood will not correct coagulation defects.
4. A blood culture should be done in all severely ill infants and appropriate parenteral antibiotics should be given (Chapter 14).
5. Very severely ill infants may benefit from an exchange transfusion.
6. Failure to improve may be due to incomplete exclusion of the toxic sugar from the diet, which should be carefully reviewed.

Galactosaemia

As soon as the diagnosis has been confirmed a strict lactose-free diet should be started. Pregestimil or Cow and Gate Formula S (Soya) can be used.

The eyes should be examined by an ophthalmologist for early cataracts; these should resolve if treatment is prompt and adequate.

Fructose intolerance

Recognition

Jaundice may be less marked but vomiting, bleeding and hypoglycaemia are usually more severe in fructose intolerance than in galactosaemia. The onset of symptoms may, however, be delayed for weeks or months if the infant has been receiving only breast milk or an artificial milk containing only lactose. Obviously an infant which has thrived for weeks or months on a lactose-containing diet cannot have galactosaemia. A small amount of sucrose may be contained in antibiotic syrups or vitamin preparations. A provisional diagnosis can usually be made on urine and blood tests as in galactosaemia, but confirmation of the diagnosis should be done in a specialist unit as it requires a fructose tolerance test, and preferably a liver or intestinal biopsy (Streb *et al.*, 1981).

Management

Since the diagnosis can rarely be confirmed quickly, empirical treatment with a strict sucrose–fructose*-free diet is justifiable; the following milks are suitable: breast milk and any of the standard infant milks such as Gold Cap SMA, Premium or Osterfeed. Intravenous fructose should **never** be given to small infants as it may cause a fatal hypoglycaemia and metabolic acidosis in unrecognized fructose intolerance and a severe metabolic acidosis even in a newborn who is sick for some other reason.

References

Baerlocher, K., Gitzelmann, R. and Steinmann, B. (1980) Clinical and genetic studies of disorders of fructose intolerance. In *Inherited Disorders of Carbohydrate Metabolism* (Eds E.D. Burman, J.B. Holton and C.A. Pennock), M.T.P. Press, Lancaster

Danks, D.M. (1981) Diagnosis of metabolic diseases after birth; neonatal screening and the investigation of symptomatic patients or babies at genetic risk. In *Recent Advances in Paediatrics* (ed. D. Hull), Churchill Livingstone, Edinburgh, vol 6(i) p.62; (ii) p.63

Danks, D.M. (1987) Acute neonatal illness in inborn errors of metabolism. In *Paediatric Emergencies*, 2nd edn. (ed. J.A. Black), Butterworths, London pp. 708–715

Hauser, G.J., Chitayat, D., Berns, L., Braver, D. and Mulbauer, B. (1985) Peculiar odours in newborns and maternal prenatal ingestion of spicy food. *European Journal of Pediatrics*, **144**, 403

Sheffield, L.J., Danks, D.M., Hammond, J.W. and Hoogenraad, N.J. (1976) Massive pulmonary haemorrhage as a presenting feature of congenital hyperammonaemia. *Journal of Pediatrics*, **88**, 450–452

Streb, H., Posselt, H.G., Wolter, K. and Bender, S.W. (1981) Aldolase activities of the small intestine mucosa in malabsorbtion states and hereditary fructose intolerance. *European Journal of Pediatrics*, **137**, 5–10

Whittle, M.J. and Connor, J.M. (1989) *Prenatal Diagnosis in Obstetric Practice*, Appendices I–IV, Blackwell Scientific, Oxford

*Sucrose is converted into fructose by the small intestinal epithelium. Sucrose, also known as saccharose, is the ordinary domestic cane or beet sugar. Honey contains fructose, glucose and small amounts of sucrose, and fruit juices contain fructose. Fructose is also known as laevulose or invert sugar. Sorbitol is converted into fructose in the body.

Further reading

Danks, D.M. (1974) Management of newborn babies in whom serious metabolic disorder is anticipated. *Archives of Disease in Childhood*, **49**, 576–578

Danks, D.M. (1981) *Recent Advances in Paediatrics*, **6**, 51–69 (for full reference see under References)

Holton, J.B. (Ed.) (1987) *The Inherited Metabolic Diseases*, Churchill Livingstone, Edinburgh

Stanbury, J.B., Wyngaarden, S.B. and Frederickson, D.S. (eds) (1983) *The Metabolic Basis of Inherited Disease*, 6th edn, McGraw–Hill, New York

Stephenson, S.R. and Weaver, D.D. (1981) Prenatal diagnosis; a compilation of diagnosed conditions. *American Journal of Obstetrics and Gynecology*, **141**, 319–343 (with a comprehensive list of references)

Acknowledgements

I wish to thank Professor David Danks, Mrs Anne Green, and Dr Alex Mowat for their help and advice in the preparation of this chapter.

Chapter 28

Maternal drug dependence and neonatal withdrawal symptoms

Judith Dawkins BSc.(Hons), MB, BS
Registrar in Psychiatry, St George's Hospital, London

and

Elizabeth Tylden MA, MB, BCh.(Camb) MRCPsych.
Honorary Consultant Psychiatrist, Bromley Hospital,
Honorary Consultant Psychiatrist, University College and The Middlesex Hospital Medical School

Recreational drug use is extremely common, and has become more common in women and schoolgirls. The problem of drug misuse in Britain has not yet reached the incidence of 1 in 5 births for heroin addicts in New York and Chicago hospitals. It is, however, so frequent that it must be looked for in every pregnancy. Because of the fear that the baby will be taken into care if the problem is revealed, mothers often conceal their drug use from professionals, and the situation may only become apparent when the baby develops withdrawal symptoms after delivery. The ruling of the House of Lords in the Berkshire case (*The Times*, 1986) has unfortunately reinforced these anxieties despite the fact that the ruling referred only to a narrow point of law.* Abstinence syndromes arising out of intrauterine passive addiction to opiates are potentially lethal but easily treated and totally recoverable.

There are now hardly any 'single-drug' abusers. Most drug users will take anything they can obtain, although many have a 'preferred' drug. Drugs are frequently adulterated with anything from marmite to scouring powders or other drugs. Therefore a mother may not know what she has

*Under the child care legislation (*Children and Young Persons Act* 1969, as amended), for a child to be taken into care there must be both primary and secondary grounds; the primary ground is that 'the child's proper development is being considerably prevented and neglected', and the secondary ground is that the child is 'in need of care and control'. In the Berkshire case the mother continued to use drugs throughout pregnancy, knowing that by doing so she could endanger the fetus; the child developed withdrawal symptoms after birth and was kept in hospital for 6 weeks, and a Care Order was taken out.

This case was unusual in that the primary grounds referred to events (pregnancy and delivery) in the past which could not recur, and it was this point only which was considered by the Law Lords. It was also considered that the child was 'in need of care and control' because the mother continued to use drugs after the birth of her child and these grounds were not disputed. This case was the subject of much misinformed and misleading comment in the media, and does not provide a precedent for taking out a Care Order on every newborn infant whose mother has taken drugs during pregnancy. Each case needs to be considered on its merits, and the ability of the mother to look after her child in a responsible manner must be assessed, whether she continues to use drugs after delivery or not.

Table 28.1 Commonly abused drugs

Drug			*Routes*
Official name	*Trade name*	*Slang names*	
Opiates			
Buprenorphine	Temgesic	Temmies	Intravenously Subcutaneously or intramuscularly ('skin popping') Inhaled (chasing the dragon) Smoked Snorted Oral
Codeine		Linctus	
Codeine and aspirin	Codis		
Dextromoramide	Palfium		
Dihydrocodeine	DF118	DFs	
Dipipanone and cyclizine	Diconal	Dikes	
Fetanyl	Sublimaze		
Heroin		Smack, skag, dry amps	
Methadone	Physeptone	Meth	
Papaveretum	Omnopon		
Pentazocine	Fortral		
Pethidine			
Hypnotics		Downers	
Barbiturates		Barbs	
Amylobarbitone	Amytal	Ammies	Injected Oral
Butobarbitone	Soneryl		
Quinalbarbitone	Seconal		
Quinalbarbitone and amylobarbitone	Tuinal		
Benzodiazepines			
Diazepam	Valium		Intravenously Oral
Lorazepam	Ativan		
Temazepam	Normison	Temazie	
Other related drugs			
Stimulants*			
Amphetamines		Speed	Injected Snorted Smoked Oral
Amphetamine sulphate		Sulphate	
Dexamphetamine	Dexedrine	Dexes	
MOMA and MDA	Ecstasy	Coke	Injected Snorted Smoked
Cocaine		Crack (very potent)	
Free based cocaine			
Psychedelics			
Cannabis		Black, Congolese, Durban, Ganja, Hashish, Kif, Marijhuana, Paki, Pot, Shit	Smoked Oral (cake)
Lysergic acid diethylamine^{25} (LSD^{25})		LSD^{25}, Acid	Oral
Phencyclidine†		PCP, Angel Dust	Usually snorted Injected
Alcohol‡			Oral
Solvents	Tipp-Ex, lighter fuel, aerosols etc.		Inhaled Oral

*Dexamphetamine (dexedrine) is a controlled drug in Britain, only to be used under supervision for treatment of narcolepsy and hyperkinesis in children. A powder form of amphetamine sulphate is produced illicitly.

†Not available in Britain.

‡See p. 6 for fetal alcohol syndrome.

actually taken (Choudry and Doe, 1986). Heavy cigarette smoking and/or alcohol use are commonly associated with drug usage.

Table 28.1 lists drugs commonly abused today with their 'slang', trade names and usual routes of administration. Many abuse benzodiazepines, drugs that are not always enquired about when a drug history is taken (Perera *et al.*, 1987).

Maternal conditions related to drug abuse that may affect the infant

The lifestyle associated with chronic drug abuse predisposes a woman to a number of complications. Drugs are expensive, so she may spend all her money on drugs, cigarettes and alcohol, at the expense of food. Some addicts are severely malnourished. Money is frequently obtained by prostitution, stealing or dealing.

Table 28.2 lists the main problems that may affect the infant's well-being. Early recognition and treatment of these is beneficial to both mother and infant.

Irregular menstrual cycles mean that a woman may not realize she is pregnant until the pregnancy is well advanced. This, with the fear and mistrust of hospitals, doctors and social workers, means that the drug abuser frequently attends late, irregularly or not at all for antenatal care (Fraser, 1976). She may present unbooked in labour. Hence there is an increased incidence of prenatal and perinatal problems in addition to those described above (Neuberg *et al.*, 1972). The effects of cocaine, and particularly 'crack', on the fetus have also been described recently; these

Table 28.2 Maternal complications of drug abuse

Drug type	*Complications*
Any expensive drug of abuse	Poor diet leading to malnutrition, anaemia, vitamin deficiencies Sexually transmitted diseases including hepatitis B and HIV infection Injury from violence and accidents Arrest and imprisonment Prostitution
Injected drugs	Injections: abscesses, septicaemia, hepatitis B, HIV, infective endocarditis, phlebitis, injection ulcers. Acute poisoning episodes Rhesus reactions/immunization. Injection can cause ischaemic gangrene with loss of limbs
Smoked drugs	Bronchitis. Heroin and cocaine pneumonia. Fetal hypoxia and undernutrition
Sniffed drugs	Corrosion of nasal passages, naal inflammation and collapse of nasal septum
Solvent abuse	Inhalation bronchitis and pneumonia. Rashes around mouth and nose. Psychotic episodes. Suffocation and cardiac arrest. Central and peripheral neuropathies causing trauma, ataxia and brain damage
Cocaine and amphetamines	Cardiac arrest. Paranoia. Transient psychoses lasting 5–6 days (amphetamine). Spontaneous abortion, fetal growth retardation, placental abruption and premature labour (cocaine) Other effects of cocaine, see below
Cannabis, LSD[25] and mushrooms and MDMA	Transient psychoses

are intrauterine growth retardation, small head circumferance (Cherukuri *et al.*, 1988; Chasnoff *et al.*, 1989) and possibly malformations of the skull (Bingol *et al.*, 1987). Terminal limb deformities, intestinal atresias and cerebral infarction have also been described in association with maternal abuse of 'crack' during pregnancy.

The period during which withdrawal symptoms may occur

Pregnancy

Sudden withdrawal of the drug, especially narcotics, can result in fetal withdrawal symptoms. At least half an hour before the addict mother feels withdrawal the fetus becomes hyperactive and tracings show tachycardia or bradycardia. Unless the woman is given an opiate the baby may die (Liu *et al.*, 1976).

After delivery

The time of onset of withdrawal symptoms varies widely from a few hours to several weeks after birth depending on the nature of the drugs involved and the time of the last dose before delivery. The most common time for withdrawal symptoms to develop is within the first 48 hours. With heroin, the onset may be any time from birth to 10 days (Zelson *et al.*, 1971). However, with drugs with a long half-life and slow metabolism and excretion in the neonate, e.g. methadone, the onset may be as late as 2–4 weeks of age and may go unrecognized, leading in extreme cases to fits and death (Kandall and Gartner, 1974).

During breast feeding

The amount of drug found in breast milk varies and there is the theoretical possibility of withdrawal symptoms arising in this period. However, in practice, many heroin addicts have great difficulty in breast feeding and in maintaining lactation. Very few are discharged breast feeding. Many choose to bottle feed and though there may be problems in hygiene arising from this, it may be the best solution.

Late onset: several weeks after delivery

Generalized cerebral irritability may develop several weeks after delivery. Whether this is the explanation of the reported increase in sudden infant death syndrome (SIDS) remains unclear. SIDS has been described in the babies of mothers who have used cocaine (Chasnoff *et al.*, 1985), benzodiazepines (Rementería and Bhatt, 1977) and methadone (Pierson *et al.*, 1972).

Recognition of the drug-abusing mother

The known drug abuser

In some cases, the mother is already known by her general practitioner, social worker, drug dependency unit or obstetrician to be abusing drugs. She may be referred from prison.

Awareness of the possibility of drug abuse

This is the most important factor leading to the recognition of drug abuse. Because the prevalence of drug abuse is rising, routine enquiries about drug use should be made. This is particularly important since fewer drug users inject their drugs and therefore do not have the signs of intravenous drug use. In one recent survey of babies born in a district general hospital to mothers taking heroin, 20 out of 23 women were smoking heroin; only three were injecting (Klenka, 1986).

There should be a high degree of suspicion if a women books late or presents in labour, has no general practitioner, is obviously homeless, has had frequent changes of address, is malnourished, has chronic ill health or positive serology for hepatitis B (HBV), HIV or syphilis; these are common findings in mothers who abuse drugs.

Signs associated with drug use

The signs described in Table 28.2 should be looked for.

Urine testing

Because of the frequent use of multiple drugs and the inaccuracy of most drug histories, screening of urine to determine recent drug ingestion is useful in all suspected cases of drug abuse. This may be done using a thin layer chromatography or enzyme monitored immunoassay. It is only available in some centres and reports may take a long time.

Unexpected symptoms in the neonatal period

The possibility of withdrawal symptoms should be considered in any infant with unexplained general jitteriness, irritability, fits or other symptoms described below.

Recognition of symptoms of withdrawal in the newborn

Differential diagnosis

This includes hypoglycaemia, hypocalcaemia, hypomagnesaemia, intracerebral haemorrhage, meningitis, infection and infective diarrhoea.

Time of onset

This is usually within the first 24–48 hours, but is variable (see above).

Nature of the symptoms

This depends on the drug(s) used by the mother. The symptoms of withdrawal from drugs commonly abused are summarized in Table 28.3. It should be remembered that most mothers are polydrug abusers and their infants may be withdrawing from several substances.

Table 28.3 Withdrawal symptoms in the neonate

Drug	*Withdrawal symptoms*		*Reference*
Opiates Heroin, methadone, etc.	All lead to the same withdrawal symptoms Symptoms in order of frequency (%)		
	Irritability	66	Zelson *et al.* (1971, 1973) Rahbar (1975)
	Tremors	65	
	Vomiting	37	
	High pitched cry	23	
	Sneezing	26	
	Hypertonicity and hyperactivity	20	
	Respiratory distress	13	
	Fever	9	
	Diarrhoea	7	
	Mucus secretion	6	
	Sweating	5	
	Convulsions	3	
	Yawning	3	
	Scratching face	2	
	Poor feeding	1	
	Salivation	1	
	Stuffy nose	1	
	Hiccups	0.4	
	Dehydration	0.4	
	Hypothermia	0.4	
	Any of these may be the main presenting symptom; the main difference between heroin and methadone is in the time of onset; with methadone it is later, symptoms are more severe and fits are more common		
Barbiturates	(a) Early or acute symptoms: constant crying, tremors, sleeplessness, hiccups, mouthing (similar to opiate withdrawal but onset later and can be after baby has been discharged), fits (b) Subacute phase (months) hyperphagia, prolonged crying, irritability, sweating, hyperacusis		Desmond *et al.* (1972) Bleyer and Marshall (1972) Schweigert (1972)
Amphetamines	Temporary drowsiness in infants during first few months. Irritability		Billing *et al.* (1980)
Cocaine	Abnormal neurological behaviour (increased tremulousness and startle responses measured with the Brazelton neonatal behavioural scale)		Chasnoff *et al.* (1985)
Benzodiazepines	(a) Regular use in pregnancy (chronic intrauterine exposure) tremors, irritability, hyperactivity, hypertonicity, tachypnoea, vigorous sucking (resembles opiate withdrawal) (b) Use at term (in labour or to control hypertension). Both lorazepam and diazepam have depressant effects causing low Apgar score, apnoeic spells, hypotonicity, poor feeding		Rementería and Bhatt (1977) Whitelaw *et al.* (1981) Cree *et al.* (1973)
Phencyclidine	Irritability, poor feeding, tremors, nystagmus, hyperreflexia, diarrhoea, skin abrasions, increased appetite, abdominal distension, sweating		Bean *et al.* (1981)

Management

During pregnancy and in labour

Awareness of the possibility of drug use and its early recognition are important. Continuity of care is essential in enlisting the trust of these mothers, who are frequently wary of hospital services. Many are appropriately concerned for their baby's health, and the antenatal period can become a time of stabilization for the mother. Liaison between the different agencies involved, e.g. general practitioner, psychiatrist, drug dependency unit, antenatal clinic, paediatrician and neonatal unit, is vital.

Screening for the medical complications associated with maternal drug abuse is essential. The use of testing for HIV and HBV after counselling is an increasingly important aspect of this, as the viruses become more widespread among drug users.

Most opiate addicts are offered oral methadone therapy. This entails establishing the daily methadone requirement which may require a period as an in-patient followed by regular prescribing. The general aims are to give the lowest possible dose sufficient to prevent withdrawal symptoms and to withdraw the drug slowly and gradually. This is safest for both mother and baby.

The principles of the management of the drug abuser in pregnancy and labour are summarized in Table 28.4.

Table 28.4 The management of the drug abuser in pregnancy and labour (Stauber *et al.*, 1982)

Drug	*Management in pregnancy*	*Management in labour*
Opiates	Slow withdrawal of drug Check oestriols Acute withdrawal causes fetal irritability which can lead to intrauterine death	Mother needs opiate in labour to prevent fetal distress; also routine analgesia/anaesthesia
Barbiturates	Substitute a drug with a long half-life, e.g. phenobarbitone, during withdrawal to prevent fits	Phenobarbitone cover in labour with routine analgesia
Amphetamines and cocaine	Try to encourage her to stop taking them	Routine
Benzodiazepines	Use drugs with a long half-life during withdrawal	Watch fetus
Psychedelics	Try to stop Give phenothiazines symptomatically	Watch maternal pulse and blood pressure. May need phenothiazines
All intravenous drugs	Care in handling blood	HBV/HIV precautions

After delivery

Naloxone should not be used in resuscitation because it may cause sudden withdrawal symptoms in the infant if the mother has been on opiates or methadone.

A urine drug screen for both mother and infant can be helpful in ascertaining which drugs have been abused recently. The infant requires close observation for the onset of withdrawal symptoms in the first 48 hours and ideally longer. This should not necessarily mean keeping the infant apart from the mother. If mild symptoms occur, they can be managed by simple measures, e.g. swaddling and frequent feeds, which the mother can be involved in. However, if the infant develops more severe withdrawal symptoms, transfer to a special care baby unit or neonatal unit may be indicated.

A mother who wishes to breast feed may do so, although this is frequently unsuccessful.

All mothers should be warned about the possibility of neonatal withdrawal symptoms.

Indications for drug treatment

Drug treatment is usually started once the withdrawal symptoms can no longer be managed by simple nursing measures such as swaddling and demand feeding (Finnegan *et al.*, 1975*a*,*b*). This is usually because of the following symptoms: severe irritability, tremors interfering with feeding and sleep, diarrhoea and vomiting, convulsions, hypo- or hyper-thermia or tachypnoea interfering with feeding (Rosen, 1977). Scoring systems have been used to rate the severity of symptoms and their response to treatment (Finnegan *et al.*, 1975*a*,*b*)

Opiate withdrawal

This is viewed by some as an autonomic storm. It is probably due to hypersensitivity of endorphin receptors and the absence of the modulatory effects of endorphins on the autonomic nervous system. All drugs of abuse have effects on the endorphin and dopaminergic systems, and their withdrawal symptoms are probably produced by similar mechanisms. In classical withdrawal a reducing programme uses the drug of addiction; however, this is seldom practicable. Any hypnotic or sedative drug can control withdrawal symptoms, as can any major tranquillizer in appropriate doses. Antihistamine drugs are useful, as are anticholinergics, α-blockers and β-blockers.

A number of compounds have been used in the neonate to suppress or control withdrawal symptoms, including paregoric (tincture of opium), phenobarbitone, diazepam, chlorpromazine, phenytoin and various combinations of these. They are usually given in divided doses according to the infant's body weight. Usual starting doses are: chlorpromazine 0.5–1 mg/kg 6 hourly initially (occasionally up to 1.5 mg/kg may be required); phenobarbitone 20 mg/kg loading dose, then 5 mg/kg for 1 day in two divided doses (i.e. 12 hourly).

Chlorpromazine is usually the first-line drug used; it is a useful all-purpose drug which can control most of the symptoms resulting from polydrug abuse. However, if severe symptoms or fits occur a combination of chlorpromazine and phenobarbitone, or phenytoin, or diazepam may be required.

Duration of treatment

This is very variable and depends on the drugs abused by the mother and their half-lives in the infant. It can only be assessed by gradually reducing the dose of drug given and observing the effect, using a chart or some other means of recording symptoms.

Follow up

Close observation and follow up are essential. The possibility of late-onset withdrawal symptoms should be borne in mind by all caring for the mother and her baby. The mother should be encouraged to watch for these and bring her baby back if concerned.

The mothers often have severe psychosocial problems and appropriate attempts to deal with these should be made before the infant's discharge from hospital. A case conference should be called before discharge to coordinate the activities of the various agencies involved, including the general practitioner and health visitor (Riley, 1987).

Throughout infancy these children remain at risk. There is of course an additional risk of infection with HBV or HIV. Associations between maternal drug use and SIDS, failure to thrive, suspected non-accidental injury (Billing *et al.*, 1980) and impaired psychomotor development (Olofsson *et al.*, 1983) have been reported. This does not occur in children where mothers are off drugs or have a stable lifestyle; it is probably due to poverty and social deprivation.

References

Bean, X.D., Alexander, R.L. and Kahn-Variba, J. (1981) Abstracts of the American Pediatric Society. *Society for Pediatric Research*, **15**, 649

Billing, L., Eriksson, M., Larsson, G. and Zetterström, R. (1980) Amphetamine addiction and pregnancy III. One year follow-up of the children: psychosocial and pediatric aspects. *Acta Paediatrica Scandinavica*, **69**, 675–680

Bingol, N., Fuchs, M., Diaz, V., Stone, R.K. and Gromish, D.S. (1987) Teratogenicity of cocaine in humans. *Journal of Pediatrics*, **110**, 93–96

Bleyer, W.A. and Marshall, R.E. (1972) Barbiturate withdrawal syndrome in a passively addicted infant. *Journal of the American Medical Association*, **221**, 185–186

Chasnoff, I.J., Burns, W.J., Schnoll, S.H. and Burns, K.A. (1985) Cocaine use in pregnancy. *New England Journal of Medicine*, **313**, 666–669

Chasnoff, I.J., Griffith, D.R., Macgregor, S., Dirkes, S.K. and Burns, K.A. (1989) Temporal patterns of cocaine use in pregnancy: perinatal outcome. *Journal of American Medical Association*, **261**, 1741–1744

Cherukuri, R., Minkoff, H., Feldman, J., Parekh, A. and Glass, L. (1988) Cocaine ("crack"). A cohort study of alkaloidal use in pregnancy. *Obstetrics and Gynecology*, **72**, 147–151

Choudry, N. and Doe, J. (1986) Inadvertent abuse of amphetamines in street heroin. *Lancet*, **ii**, 817

Cree, J.E., Meyer, J. and Hailey, D.M. (1973) Diazepam in labour: its metabolism and effect on the clinical condition and thermogenesis of the newborn. *British Medical Journal*, **4**, 251–255

Desmond, M.M., Schwanecke, R.P., Wilson, G.S., Yasunaga, S. and Burgdorff, I. (1972) Maternal barbiturate utilization and neonatal withdrawal symptomatology. *Journal of Pediatrics*, **80**, 190–197

Finnegan, L., Kron, R., Connaughton, J. and Errich, J. (1975*a*) A scoring system for the evaluation and treatment of the neonatal abstinence syndrome: a new clinical and research tool. In *Basic and Therapeutic Aspects of Perinatal Pharmacology*, (eds P.L. Marnelli, S. Garatric and F. Seissic), Raven Press, New York

Finnegan, L., Kron, R., Connaughton, J. and Errich, J. (1975*b*) Neonatal abstinence syndrome: assessment and management *Addictive Diseases*, **2**, 141–158

Fraser, A.C. (1976) Drug addiction in pregnancy. *Lancet*, **ii**, 896–899

Kandall, S.R. and Gartner, L.H. (1974) Late presentation of drug withdrawal symptoms in newborns. *American Journal of Diseases of Children*, **127**, 58–61

Klenka, H.M. (1986) Babies born in a district general hospital to mothers taking heroin. *British Medical Journal*, **293**, 745–746

Liu, D.T., Tylden, E. and Tukel, S.H. (1976) Fetal response to drug withdrawal. *Lancet*, **ii**, 588

Neuberg, R., Fraser, A., Weir, J. and Priestly, B. (1972) Drug addiction in pregnancy. *Proceedings of the Royal Society of Medicine*, **65**, 867–870

Olofsson, M., Buckley, W., Anderson, G.E. and Friis-Hansen, B. (1983) Investigation of 89 children born by drug dependent mothers II: Follow-up 1–10 years after birth. *Acta Paediatrica Scandinavica*, **72**, 407–410

Perera, K., Tulley, M. and Jenner, F. (1987) The use of benzodiazepines among drug addicts. *British Journal of Addiction*, **82**, 511–515

Pierson, P.S., Howard, P. and Kleber, H.D. (1972) Sudden deaths in infants born to methadone-maintained addicts. *Journal of American Medical Association*, **220**, 1733–1734

Rahbar, F. (1975) Observations on methadone withdrawal in 16 neonates. *Clinical Pediatrics*, **14**, 369–371

Rementería, J.L. and Bhatt, K. (1977) Withdrawal symptoms in neonates from intrauterine exposure to diazepam. *Journal of Pediatrics*, **90**, 123–126

Riley, D. (1987) The management of the pregnant drug addict. *Bulletin of Royal College of Psychiatrists*, **11**, 362–365

Rosen, F. (1977) Infants of addicted mothers. In *Neonatal and Perinatal Medicine*, 2nd edn (ed. R.E. Benhan), C.V. Mosby, St. Louis

Stauber, M., Schwerdt, M. and Tylden, E. (1982) Pregnancy, birth and puerperium in women suffering from heroin addiction. *Journal of Psychosomatic Obstetrics and Gynaecology*, **1**, 128–138

Schweigert, B.F. (1972) Neonatal barbiturate withdrawal. *Journal of American Medical Association*, **221**, 1282

Times (1986) House of Lords judgement re D (a minor), December 5.

Whitelaw, A.G.L., Cummings, A.J. and McFadyen, I.R. (1981) Effect of maternal lorazepam on the neonate. *British Medical Journal*, **282**, 1106–1108

Zelson, C., Rubio, E. and Wasserman, E. (1971) Neonatal narcotic addiction: 10 year observation. *Pediatrics*, **48**, 178–189

Zelson, C., Lee, S.J. and Casalino, M. (1973) Neonatal narcotic addiction: comparative effects of maternal intake of heroin and methadone. *New England Journal of Medicine*, **289**, 1216–1220

Further reading

Brockington, I.F. and Kumar, R. (eds) (1983) *Motherhood and Mental Illness*, Academic Press, London, Chapter 9

Chasnoff, I.J. (ed.) (1986) *Drug Use in Pregnancy; Mother and Child*, M.T.P. Press, Lancaster

Department of Health and Social Security (1984) Medical Working Group on Drug Dependence. Guidelines of good clinical practice in the treatment of drug misuse. DHSS, London

Drug Dependence in Pregnancy: Clinical Management of Mother and Child (1978) Obtainable from US Department of Health and Welfare Services. Research Branch Division of Resource Development. National Institute for Drug Dependence, 5600 Fishers Lane, Rockville, Maryland, U.S.A.

Rementería, J. (1977) *Drug Abuse: Pregnancy and Neonatal Effects*, C.V. Mosby, St. Louis

Roenak, D., Diamant, Y.Z., Yaffe, H. and Hornstein, E. (1990) Cocaine: maternal use during pregnancy and its effects on the mother, the fetus and the infant. *Obstetrical and Gynecological Survey*, **45**, 348–359

Senay, E.C. (1983) *Substance Abuse Disorders in Clinical Practice*, John Wright, Bristol

Tylden, E. (1973) The effects of maternal drug abuse on the fetus and infant. *Adverse Drug Reaction Bulletin*, **38**, 120–123

Tyler, A. (1986) *Street Drugs*, New English Library, obtainable from Institute for the Study of Drug Dependence, 1–4 Hatton Place, Hatton Garden, London EC1N 8ND

Chapter 29

Practical procedures

Blood sampling techniques

Capillary blood sampling

Indication

For reliable results it is essential to obtain free-flowing blood from a warmed area. A capillary sample can be used for blood counts, biochemical estimations and, with suitable precautions, for pH, $P\text{O}_2$ and $P\text{CO}_2$ estimations.

Equipment

A sterile blood count lancet or a spring-loaded device can be used, with capillary collecting tubes appropriate to the estimation required.

Procedure

The area to be used should first be warmed by immersion for 2–5 minutes in a water bath at 38–40°C or by warm compresses; it is then dried and cleaned with an alcohol swab. To obtain droplets of blood which can be easily collected the area around the selected site should be wiped with a thin layer of sterile soft paraffin. In the newborn, the heel is the most satisfactory site. The foot is dorsiflexed, with the thumb and fingers round the calf and foot, and the heel protruding through the circle made by them (Lissauer, 1982). The area of the heel that should be used is shown in the hatched areas in Fig. 29.1; the central part of the heel should be avoided because of the risk of infecting the calcaneus. The incision or puncture should not be more than 2.4mm deep (Blumenfeld *et al.*, 1979).

Sources of error

1. Inadequate warming, producing sluggish non-arterialized blood.
2. Excessive squeezing, causing dilution with interstitial fluid.
3. Exposure to air or air bubbles during collection (blood gases).
4. Use of a site too near previous punctures.

Complications

1. Local sepsis.
2. Calcaneal necrotizing chondritis, with or without septicaemia (Blumenfeld *et al.*, 1979).

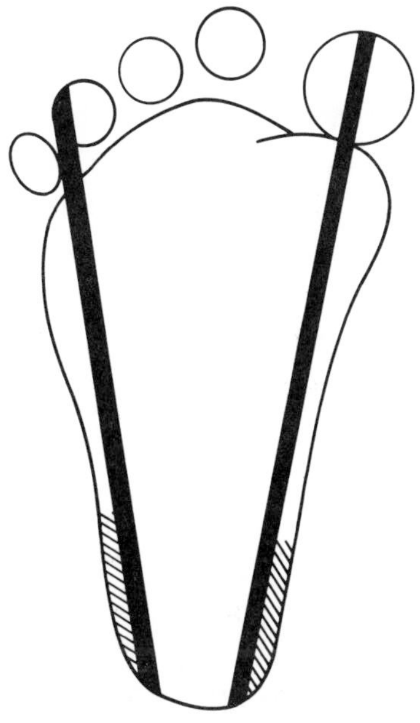

Figure 29.1 Side-to-side limits of calcaneus marked by line extending posteriorly from point between the 4th and 5th toes and running parallel to the lateral aspect of the heel and line extending posteriorly from the middle of the great toe and running parallel to the medial aspect of the heel. Heel punctures should be performed on the plantar surface of the heel, beyond lateral and medial limits of the calcaneus, marked by these lines (hatched areas). Reproduced from Blumenfeld *et al.* (1979) with permission of the authors and publishers

3. Calcified nodules in the heel.
4. Atrophy of calcaneal pad of fat if centre of heel is used.
5. Implantation dermoid.

Venepuncture

Indications

This is used to obtain blood samples of larger volume than are obtainable with capillary samples.

Equipment

A 23-gauge butterfly needle is most suitable for babies. Alternatively, a 2ml syringe may be used but it is difficult to avoid excessive suction.

Procedure

The antecubital fossa is the best site for venepuncture even in very small infants. One or more veins are usually palpable, particularly in small preterm infants with little subcutaneous fat. The infant should be held firmly on a flat surface, with the arm fully extended at the elbow. To achieve this a folded towel is placed under the point of the elbow; the elbow should rest on a firm flat surface. The assistant should maintain full extension of the arm, with one hand across the infant's palm, to prevent pronation and supination. The upper arm is firmly encircled by one hand; too tight compression obstructs the arterial flow and will reduce the venous return.

Complications

1. Local haematoma.
2. Local sepsis.
3. Thrombophlebitis.

4. Damage to the median nerve.
5. Damage to the brachial artery.

Arterial puncture

The radial artery is most commonly used; the right radial artery should be used for preference, because of its preductal origin. Brachial artery puncture should be avoided if at all possible, and should only be used for a single puncture; repeated attempts should not be made.

Indications
Arterial puncture is used mainly for pH and blood gas analysis.

Equipment
A 2ml syringe with a short 25-gauge needle should be used. Both syringe and needle should be flushed out with heparin in 0.9% NaCl. Alternatively a butterfly with a short 25-gauge needle can be used.

Procedure (Lissauer, 1982)
The radial artery can usually be found by palpation at the wrist, or by using a fibreoptic light source. An essential preliminary to insertion of the needle is the performance of Allen's test. In this test both radial and ulnar arteries are occluded by firm pressure until the hand is blanched. Maintaining pressure on the radial artery, the ulnar artery is released; if the whole hand flushes there is adequate collateral circulation and it is safe to proceed. Failure of the hand to flush on release of the ulnar artery indicates an absence or inadequacy of the ulnar artery.

After the skin has been cleaned, the needle is inserted, bevel up, along the line of the artery, at an angle of 30–45°, until slight resistance is encountered, indicating that both walls of the artery have been penetrated. Gentle suction is applied to the syringe and the needle is slowly withdrawn until blood flows into the syringe. At least 0.25ml of blood should be taken to avoid the effect of residual heparin on the acid–base balance. The puncture site should be compressed for 2–3 minutes after withdrawal of the needle. Repeated blood sampling by this method is likely to cause thrombosis of the artery or distal emboli (see below).

Complications of radial artery puncture

1. Haematoma.
2. Local sepsis.
3. Thrombosis of the artery.
4. Distal embolization in the digital arteries.
5. For other possible complications see under radial artery catheter insertion (p. 312).

Complications of brachial artery puncture
In addition to those listed under radial artery puncture, the use of the brachial artery may result in:

1. Damage to the median nerve in the antecubital fossa.
2. Repeated use of the same site or repeated attempts at puncture could

cause thrombosis of the artery, depriving the hand and forearm of their blood supply: in some instances loss of fingers or of part of the forearm have occurred.

Intravascular procedures

Exchange transfusion

See pp. 119–130.

Umbilical arterial catheterization

Indications

This provides central arterial access for blood gas and blood pressure monitoring using a pressure transducer, and a route for fluid infusion. If the infant is not of very low birth weight and is likely to have relatively mild respiratory problems, consideration should be given to the use of a peripheral intravenous infusion, saturation pulse oximetry, transcutaneous $P\text{O}_2$ and $P\text{CO}_2$ monitors, and capillary blood gases, to avoid the potential complications of umbilical arterial catheterization. This is frequently appropriate for infants over 30 weeks.

Equipment

1. Full sterile precautions, including gown, gloves and mask.
2. Umbilical arterial catheterization pack with umbilical arterial dilator and a pair of curved iris forceps.
3. 3.5 and 5FG umbilical catheters (or Searle intra-arterial oxygen monitor catheter).
4. Three-way tap.
5. 10ml syringe.
6. Suture material.
7. Flushing solution (0.9% Nacl with 0.5 unit of heparin/ml at an infusion rate of 1ml/hr (see also p. 309).

Procedure

1. Restrain the infant gently by all four limbs with the hips abducted at 45°. Connect to a cardiorespiratory monitor because much of the baby will be obscured by the drapes. If ventilation is going to be needed, intubate and ventilate the infant before the procedure to ensure a stable condition during the handling necessary to insert the catheter. Although this can be carried out in an incubator, it is much easier under a radiant overhead heater.
2. Scrup up, put on gown and gloves. Connect the syringe to the flushing solution, three-way stopcock and catheter, and flush through with heparinized saline to exclude air bubbles. Organize the instruments. Put the needle and stitch into the stitch holder, ready for use. Determine the length of the umbilical arterial catheter to be inserted (Fig. 29.2). In all except very small infants the 'low' insertion distance

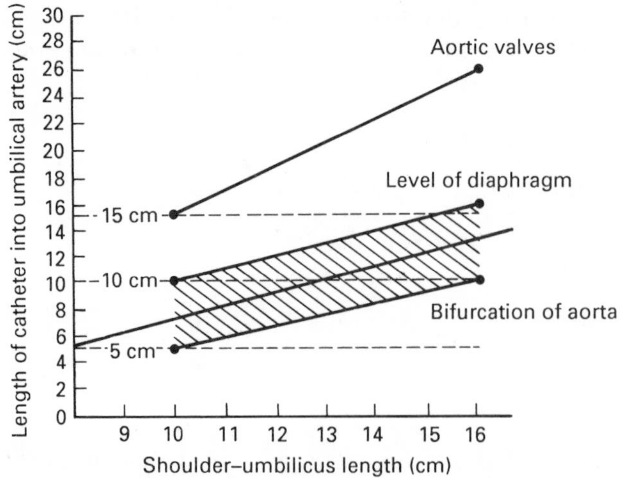

Figure 29.2 Umbilical artery catheterization guide. End-hole catheter marked at 5, 10 and 15 cm from the tip. Total length 38 cm. Reproduced from Swyer (1975) with permission of the author and publishers

is probably preferable; the 'high' insertion distance seems to be better tolerated by small infants.

3. Cleanse the area around the umbilicus with antiseptic and drape the abdomen, allowing the umbilicus to project through the drapes (for care with alcoholic antiseptic, see below).
4. Tie a piece of umbilical cord tape loosely around the umbilicus, just above the skin margin, to prevent bleeding from the umbilicus.
5. Fix two small artery forceps to the membranous edge of the cord, just above the cord tape on either side; these are to provide a good grip of the cord if bleeding starts, and to steady the cord stump when dilating the artery and inserting the catheter.
6. With a scalpel, slice cleanly through the cord 1–2 cm above the skin margin. The two arteries will be seen as firm string-like structures projecting slightly from the Wharton's jelly, usually at 4 o'clock and 8 o'clock at the level of the skin margin. They do not usually bleed, but there may be a tiny red dot of blood marking the place of the constricted lumen. The vein is a larger thin-walled flattened vessel, which oozes dark blood and is at 12 o'clock. Bleeding from the umbilical vein can easily be controlled by pressing on the skin of the abdominal wall just above the umbilicus, as the umbilical vein runs up towards the liver just under the skin.
7. Gently and patiently, using the weight of the umbilical dilator and no force, dilate up one of the arteries until it will accept the end of the umbilical catheter.
8. Insert the catheter gently, easing it in for the required distance (Figure 29.2). There is often some resistance at about 2 cm at the junction of the umbilical artery with the internal iliac artery. Gentle manipulation can usually negotiate this bend, but sometimes the anatomy makes this impossible. It may also be impossible on the other side. In this

situation it is likely that the umbilical artery meets the iliac artery at 90°. Correct insertion of the catheter is apparent from the pulsatile nature and free flow of blood. It is usually possible also to feel the catheter under the skin going inferolaterally in the umbilical artery, on its way to meet the iliac artery in the groin.

9. Fix the catheter with a stitch to the edge of the cord, then tie it firmly, but not tightly, several times around the catheter, just where the catheter enters the artery. Leave 1–1.5 cm tails on the suture to aid removal. Put a purse-string suture through the membranous part of the cord and tie firmly, leaving 2.5–4 cm tails.
10. Connect up the catheter to the intra-arterial infusion. It is desirable to run 1 ml of flushing solution/hour 'piggybacked' on to the main fluid line (usually glucose 10% plus additions; see p. 330), if the baby is not being fed. Alternatively, the heparin can be given with the glucose 10%. To clear the catheter when a sample has been taken, the 0.9% NaCl plus heparin solution should be used. In very small infants (<1.0 kg or <28 weeks) in order to avoid excessive addition of sodium from frequent flushing through of the catheter after taking blood samples, a flushing solution of lower sodium concentration (e.g. 0.18% NaCl in glucose 4.3%) should be used. This solution should also be used for the constant flushing solution, but at a rate of 0.5–1 ml/hour; rates of <0.5 ml/hour are inadequate to prevent clotting of the artery.
11. Observe frequently the circulation to the legs, as arterial spasm is common in the first few hours after insertion.
12. Take an X-ray to check the position of the catheter tip, which should be at either around L4 (just above the aortic bifurcation) or T10 (thoracic aorta) and well away from the origins of the coeliac, renal and superior mesenteric arteries (L1 to L3).

Prevention of complications of catheterization of the umbilical artery
Although the placing of a catheter in a major vessel can never be without risk, there are a number of precautions that should be taken; these are given below.

1. Experienced operator, or supervised if inexperienced.
2. Remove the catheter as soon as persisting blanching of the toes occurs.
3. The catheter must not be left *in situ* longer than is absolutely necessary.
4. Meticulous sterile precautions during insertion of the catheter.
5. Change the tubing and infusion solutions every 24 hours.
6. Avoid the use of hypertonic solutions; if a hypertonic solution has to be given, then give it very slowly.
7. Remove a damaged or contaminated catheter immediately.
8. Culture the tip of the catheter after removal.
9. Flushing of the catheter should be done cautiously, using 1–2 ml of the flushing solution over 5–10 minutes. Flushing more rapidly or using larger volumes causes retrograde flow in the arterial system and perfuses the brain with the flushing solution instead of with blood.
10. Different units permit different solutions to be infused up the umbilical arterial catheter. In some units the artery is used solely for sampling

and Po_2 monitoring: in others it is used as a route for fluid infusion and drug administration, including hypertonic glucose and amino acid solutions. Intralipid should not be infused because of fat embolization. Hyperosmolar solutions of $NaHCO_3$ or calcium gluconate should be diluted and given very slowly.

Complications

Insertion of the catheter
1. Traumatization of the artery and aorta; stripping of the intima of the umbilical artery.
2. Inadvertent entry into the peritoneum (see under 'The catheter *in situ*' below)
3. Blood loss.
4. Alcohol burns to fragile skin in extremely premature infants.
5. Infection of the umbilical stump.
6. Umbilical granuloma if the remnants of the stitches are not removed before discharge home.

The catheter in situ
1. Inadvertent misplacement of the catheter down the leg, into the carotid artery or one of the mesenteric arteries.
2. Clot on the end of the catheter, which may propagate into the coeliac, mesenteric or renal artery, or into the leg. Embolization of the renal artery may cause oliguria or abdominal distension, with hypertension as a late complication. Embolization of the mesenteric artery causes gastrointestinal haemorrhage and abdominal distension.
3. Arterial spasm in the legs, with blanching of the toes, and absent pulses in the foot.
4. Erythema, then necrosis, of the buttock, due to a misplaced catheter.
5. Perforation of the aorta, or of the umbilical or iliac arteries, with shock, haemoperitoneum and abdominal distension.
6. Oozing round the catheter.
7. Embolization by air bubbles.

Umbilical vein catheterization

Indications

1. Central venous access for exchange transfusion (p. 124).
2. Venous access when cannulation of a peripheral vein has failed.
3. Emergency injection of drugs during resuscitation (p. 41) and at other times.
4. Emergency transfusion of blood or infusion of other fluids.

For details of technique, see p. 124, and for complications, see pp. 127–130.

Infusion into the peripheral veins

Indications
This is the standard method for maintaining fluid balance in infants who are too ill to tolerate enteral feeding and who need a route for intravenous drugs (e.g. antibiotics).

Equipment

1. Antiseptic.
2. Swabs.
3. Adhesive tape.
4. 21-, 23- and 25-gauge short butterfly needles.
5. Peristaltic infusion pump.
6. Abbott T-connector.
7. Teflon intravascular catheters, sizes 22 and 25 gauge.
8. Gloves.

Procedure

1. Choose an appropriate intravenous fluid, make any necessary electrolyte additions and run the fluid through the tubing to exclude all air bubbles. A volumetric pump should be used for the infusion, capable of accurately delivering 1–50 ml/hour. A flexible piece of tubing with a 90° angle just before the Luer connector, such as an Abbott T-connector, is the best way of connecting the intravenous tubing to the cannula to permit effective fixation and the least chance of dislodgement.
2. Locate a suitable vein on the scalp or limbs. In the limbs the veins most distally situated should be used first, and on the scalp the veins on the top of the head should be used first. It may be important to avoid the area of the fontanelle if cranial ultrasound is likely to be requested in the next few days. Finding a suitable vein is facilitated by gentle venous occlusion by a hand or a tourniquet, or in the case of the scalp, by a rubber band around the head. The forehead below where the hairline will develop should not be used.
3. Clean the skin over the vein with antiseptic and choose the most appropriate cannula. Butterfly needles are best for scalp veins, and Teflon catheters, such as Jelco or Abbocath, are better for limb veins.
4. If a scalp vein needle is to be inserted, flush through with intravenous fluid solution from a 2 ml syringe. Disconnect the syringe, insert the tip of the needle through the skin next to the vein, then enter the vein. Blood usually runs back into the clear plastic tube after entering the vein. Once the tip is in the vein, it is sometimes possible to pass the needle gently up the vein for 3–4 mm. Flush through gently with the syringe and connect up to the Abbott T-connector and intravenous fluid line.
5. If a Teflon catheter is to be inserted, carefully inspect it, to make sure that there are no irregularities at the tip where it is near the central needle. Remove any plug which may be provided by the manufacturer in the Luer end of the needle. Insert the tip of the needle/catheter assembly through the skin beside the vein and advance it through the wall of the vein so that blood comes back up the needle. The volume of blood from a small vein may be very small, but the blood can sometimes be seen by looking up the open end of the Luer fitting. Without moving hand, and particularly without withdrawing the needle, even ½ mm, gently advance the catheter over the needle with the other hand and up the vein as far as it will go. Gentle rotation of the cannula between thumb and index finger helps to overcome any friction.

Remove the needle and connect up the Abbott T-connector and the intravenous line.
6. Fix the needle or cannula with tape (or plaster of Paris, if preferred, on the scalp), leave the vein proximal to the catheter/needle easily visible. Fix the intravenous tube so that accidental traction on the tubing will not dislodge the cannula or needle.
7. Immobilize the limb with a splint and keep the tubing well away from the other limbs. Restrain other limbs if necessary.

Complications

1. Bleeding from accidental disconnection.
2. Local infection or thrombophlebitis.
3. Fluid and electrolyte problems from incorrect infusion rate or constituents of intravenous fluid.
4. Skin necrosis from continued infusion by the pump when the intravenous tube has extravasated, particularly if hypertonic glucose, amino acids or a calcium solution or vasoconstrictor drugs are being infused. Despite the presence of apparently quite good veins on the dorsum of the foot in small infants, this is not a good site to use for butterfly needle insertion as the smallest amount of extravasated fluid very quickly produces a sizeable area of skin necrosis which may heal very slowly.
5. Fracture of radius and ulnar and of the lower part of the femur have occurred after the insertion of intravenous lines in the wrist and foot in very-low-birth-weight infants (Phillips and Lee, 1990).
6. Damage to neighbouring radial or ulnar arteries causing digital ischaemia.
7. For complications of total parenteral nutrition, see p. 334.

Radial artery (posterior tibial) catheter insertion

Indication

This provides access to arterial blood for sampling and blood pressure measurement using a transducer in infants with respiratory problems.

This route is used when umbilical arterial catheter insertion is not possible, after the umbilical arterial catheter has been removed, or to avoid placing an umbilical arterial catheter because of the potential risks involved.

Equipment

1. Heparinized 0.9% NaCl flushing solution (heparin 0.5 unit/ml).
2. Antiseptic.
3. Swabs.
4. Infusion pump.
5. 23- and 25-gauge Teflon cannulae (e.g. Jelco or Abbocath).
6. Blood pressure transducer and pressure monitoring equipment, if desired.
7. Cold-light fibreoptic transillumination equipment.

Procedure

1. Set up the flushing system with heparinized saline as for umbilical arterial catheterization.

2. In a semi-darkened room or incubator, transilluminate the wrist from the dorsum using the intense cold-light fibreoptic transillumination equipment. On the anterior aspect of the wrist the radial and ulnar arteries will be seen as two dark pulsating linear streaks on the radial and ulnar side of the wrist. The remainder of the forearm structures appear as homogeneous red semitranslucent tissues. Veins may be visible, but the bones and tendons are not. If there is only one artery on the radial side of the wrist, and no ulnar artery is visible, **do not attempt to cannulate the radial artery, as there is no collateral circulation to the hand** (see below). Do not attempt to cannulate the ulnar artery, as it is close to the ulnar nerve, which is very important for intact hand function later on. The right radial artery is preferred because of its preductal origin. The posterior tibial artery, visible by transillumination on the medial side of the ankle, is an alternative site.
3. In a manner similar to inserting a Teflon catheter into a vein, insert a 23- or 25-gauge Teflon catheter into the artery.
4. Connect up to the flushing solution and immobilize as for intravenous infusion.
5. Run the flushing solution.
6. Observe the circulation of the hand (see p. 306, Allen's test).
7. Do **not** infuse any solution other than flushing solution into the radial artery.

Complications (also p. 306)

1. Skin loss of the forearm and around the base of the thumb from excessive flushing of fluid; this is sometimes accompanied, though rarely, by muscle contractures.
2. Skin burns at site of insertion, due to prolonged transillumination.
3. Haematoma or infection at site of insertion: occasionally carpal tunnel syndrome.
4. Distal arterial spasm (transient blanching of the fingers)*.
5. Bleeding from accidental disconnection.
6. Air embolism.
7. Arterial thrombosis or embolism*, occasionally with loss of finger tips, or the whole or part of the fingers; occasionally amputation of the forearm is required.

This procedure is generally safer than umbilical arterial catheterization but cannot be used for fluid infusions other than the perfusing solution, and does not permit continuous arterial $P\text{O}_2$ monitoring with an intravascular electrode.

Respiratory system

Laryngoscopy and intubation

See pp. 39–40.

*see Allen's test, p. 306.

Methods of resuscitation of the newborn

See pp. 39–41.

Chest transillumination

Indications

This is used to establish a diagnosis in cases of suspected pneumothorax or pneumopericardium. This procedure is reliable in infants weighing less than 1.80 kg but cannot be relied upon in infants above this weight.

Equipment

1. Cold light fibreoptic transillumination equipment.
2. Dark green towels or specially made 'black out' incubator cover to obtain near darkness.

Procedure

1. In a darkened environment, the fibreoptic light is placed against the chest wall and the pattern of illumination noted.
2. For pneumothorax the end of the light is placed anteriorly, and then laterally. If a pneumothorax is present, the whole hemithorax lights up, and is obviously different from the other side.
3. For pneumopericardium, the end of the fibreoptic cable is placed directly over the heart; if a pneumopericardium is present, the heart is seen as a dark round pulsatile object surrounded by a halo of light.

Complications

There are normally none. Skin burning is extremely rare, unless the heat filter in the light box is defective. Most units put a small polythene bag over the patient end of the fibreoptic cable to prevent the transmission of bacteria from one patient to another, as speed is very important.

Insertion of a pleural drain

Indications

1. Pneumothorax.
2. Drainage of pleural fluid (e.g. chylothorax).

Equipment

1. Sterile towels.
2. Antiseptic.
3. Swabs.
4. Local anaesthetic, lignocaine 0.5%.
5. Small artery forceps.
6. Scalpel with small blade.
7. Stitch holder.
8. 4-0 silk on curved cutting needle.
9. Tape.
10. Chest drains (e.g. Argyle or Vygon).
11. Connecting tubing.

12. Underwater seal drainage bottle (must be at least 8 cm in diameter and the tip of the tube 2 cm below the surface of the water); or 'Pleurevac'.
13. Suction.

Procedure

1. Identify the presence of a significant pneumothorax by X-ray, transillumination and clinical examination, particularly confirming the **side** of the lesion.
2. Assemble and set up the equipment, connecting the underwater seal drainage bottle and connecting tube, and connect the air outlet from the drainage bottle to continuous suction at −5 cm of water pressure.
3. Scrub up, and clean and drape the baby.
4. Choose an intercostal space in the mid-axillary line (T 6–8) and inject 0.5–1 ml of 0.5% lignocaine. Wait for 5 minutes, if this is possible.
5. Make a 1 cm linear incision in the skin and muscle in the line of the ribs in the mid-axillary line over the chosen intercostal space, nearer the top edge of the rib, because the intercostal nerve, vein and artery run along the lower edge of the ribs.
6. Grasp the tip of the intercostal drain with a pair of fine artery forceps so that the tip of the forceps and the tube have the same long axis.
7. Insert the chest tube into the pleural space via the incision, using the forceps, and ensure that at least 3 cm of tube is pushed into the pleural space to ensure that the side hole is well within the thorax. Direct the chest tube tip anteriorly if possible. Release and withdraw the forceps.
8. An alternative method is to use the trochar provided, but this is not recommended because of the risk of lung trauma, particularly if the lungs are very stiff and do not collapse down to any extent in the presence of a pneumothorax. If the trochar is used, an adequate incision must be made before its insertion to prevent sudden entry of the tip; the tip of the trochar must not be allowed to go beyond the parietal pleura, the catheter then being pushed over the trochar into the pleural space.
9. Connect up to the underwater seal the drain system and check drainage. An alternative, if the infant needs to be moved, is a Heimlich chest drain valve.
10. Stitch the two edges of the incision together on each side of the catheter ensuring the correct position and use the 'tails' of the stitches to tie round the catheter to secure it; then tape it in place.
11. Put plastic waterproof adhesive tape around the tubing junctions in the underwater seal drainage system and X-ray to check position.

Complications

1. Trauma to the lung, usually when using a trochar.
2. Insertion of chest drain into the wrong side, an unforgivable mistake.
3. Incomplete evacuation due to loculation of air, or obstruction of the catheter tip by lung parenchyma; the tube may need to be repositioned by manipulating the external part, or by insertion of a second chest tube elsewhere. More suction may be required if there is a large broncho-pleural fistula and the infant is being ventilated at high pressure.
4. Damage to the intercostal artery or vessels.

5. An unsightly tethered scar; this is particularly important in chest tubes inserted anteriorly. The area where the b reast will develop in girls must be avoided **at all costs** because a tethered scar in this area produces unsightly deformation and asymmetry of the developing breast and considerable psychological trauma. The method of suturing described here usually produces an inconspicuous linear scar, while suturing with a purse-string suture produces a puckered scar adherent to deeper tissues.

Gastrointestinal system

Insertion of a peritoneal drain

Indications

This may be required to deal with tension pneumoperitoneum or gross ascites with inadequate diaphragmatic movement and ventilatory failure. The opinion of a paediatric surgeon is recommended in abdominal conditions of a less urgent nature where drainage or surgical treatment might be contemplated.

Equipment

1. Sterile towels and equipment for aseptic technique.
2. Antiseptic swabs.
3. Local anaesthetic, 0.5% lignocaine.
4. Small artery forceps.
5. Scalpel.
6. Stitch holder with 4-0 silk suture with a curved, cutting needle.
7. Chest drain.

Procedure

1. The usual site for a peritoneal drain is in the left iliac fossa. If the spleen is very large, however, the right iliac fossa may be preferable, to minimize the risk of perforating an abdominal organ.
2. Scrup up, clean and drape the abdomen.
3. Inject 0.5–1 ml local anaesthetic into the skin of the abdominal wall at the site for drain insertion and wait 5 minutes.
4. Make a stab incision with the scalpel and insert the chest drain tube 3 cm into the peritoneal cavity, using small artery forceps.
5. Stitch and tape in place.
6. Attach chest drain tube to sterile container, such as a sterile urine bag, and seal with plastic tape. In some cases of pneumoperitoneum, due to a large air leak from the lungs, the peritoneal drain may have to be connected to continuous suction because of rapid reaccumulation of the tension pneumoperitoneum. An underwater seal drain, however, should not be required.
7. X-ray to confirm the position.
8. Seek a surgical opinion to rule out other abdominal pathology.

Complications

1. Perforation of hollow or solid abdominal organs.
2. Introduction of infection.
3. Fluid, electrolyte, nutritional and immunological problems where there is continued drainage of large volumes of fluid from the peritoneal cavity.

Cardiac procedures

Insertion of a pericardial drain

Indications
This is used to relieve tension pneumopericardium.

Equipment

1. Sterile towels and equipment for aseptic technique.
2. Antiseptic swabs.
3. 18–21-gauge, 6–8cm Teflon intravenous cannulae (e.g. Jelco or Abbocath).
4. 10ml syringe.
5. Three-way stopcock.
6. Underwater seal drain.

Procedure

1. Scrub, clean and drape the chest and upper abdomen of the infant.
2. Fit syringe, three-way stopcock and cannula together.
3. Insert the tip of the cannula through the skin in the space between the xiphoid cartilage and the costal margin on the left side.
4. Direct the tip of the cannula towards the left scapula and cautiously advance it while pulling back on the plunger of the syringe.
5. Initially the firm consistency of the diaphragm and diaphragmatic movement will be felt; then air will be sucked back into the syringe, indicating entry into the pericardium, usually after about 3cm.
6. Advance the catheter over the stylet into the pericardium.
7. Remove the stylet and fix the cannula with tape.
8. It is usually advisable to connect to an underwater seal drain with 5cm of water suction and treat like a pleural drain, as there is usually a small but continuous leak for 1–2 days.
9. Check X-ray to confirm the correct position.

Complications

1. Damage to the upper surface of the liver, and abdominal bleeding.
2. Perforation of the heart (very unlikely).
3. Survival is unusual and is likely to be associated with major neurodevelopmental sequelae because of the adverse effects of the tension pneumopericardium on cerebral perfusion.

Genitourinary system

Suprapubic bladder aspiration

Indications

This is used to obtain a definitive diagnosis of a possible urinary tract infection or as part of a complete infection screen. This procedure is also advisable for obtaining a urine sample for the latex co-agglutination test for group B streptococcal antigen, as false positives may occur with skin colonization in a bag urine specimen.

Equipment

1. Swabs.
2. Antiseptic.
3. Mask.
4. Gloves.
5. 22-gauge 4cm needle.
6. 10ml syringe.

Procedure

1. This is an easy procedure, with little trauma, if the infant has a full bladder. The chances of getting a good specimen are increased if the infant is fed 20 minutes beforehand. Gentle pressure may be maintained on the labia or penis to prevent inadvertent micturition between the feed and the time when the sample is taken.
2. The infant is restrained, with the legs abducted at 45°.
3. The lower abdomen is cleaned with antiseptic.
4. The needle is inserted 1–2cm above the pubic symphysis and directed straight backwards; the bladder is mainly an abdominal rather than a pelvic organ in neonates.
5. Urine is aspirated and sent to the laboratory in the syringe. Any organisms growing in a suprapubic urine specimen are likely to indicate an infection.

Complications

1. Occasional transient haematuria.
2. Inadvertent bowel perforation may occur, but this does not appear to cause any serious problems.

Central nervous system

Lumbar puncture

Indications

1. Suspected meningitis.
2. Suspected subarachnoid haemorrhage.
3. Cerebrospinal fluid (CSF) removal in communicating hydrocephalus.

Equipment

1. Full aseptic technique, including gown, gloves and mask.
2. Swabs.
3. Antiseptic.
4. Sterile saline.
5. Sterile drape.
6. Lumbar puncture needle 22 (21–23)-gauge 4 cm needle or 22-gauge butterfly needle with the plastic tube removed.

Procedure

1. Consideration should be given to the ventilation of unstable infants before the procedure.
2. A cardiorespiratory monitor and/or transcutaneous $P\text{O}_2$ monitor or saturation pulse oximeter is required because observation of breathing, colour and heart rate may be difficult under the sterile towel, particularly with the infant's trunk flexed forwards. The procedure must be carried out with adequate warming.
3. Correct position and effective, but gentle, holding are critical factors in a quick, successful and atraumatic lumbar puncture. The spine should be flexed forward to open the space between the vertebrae posteriorly, but care must be taken not to affect breathing adversely, which in infants is largely diaphragmatic. The conventional position is for the patient to be placed on the left side. A pack is not usually required in the newborn to keep the spine in longitudinal alignment. The spine must not be rotated and the plane of the infant's back must be perpendicular to the table. An alternative position is to hold the infant in the sitting position, flexed forward. CSF pressure in infants in the lumbar space is very low. The advantage of the sitting position is that the pressure is higher due to hydrostatic forces, and fluid appears in the needle hub as soon as the spinal canal is entered, reducing the risk of a dry or bloody tap. Particular care must be taken, however, to prevent restriction of respiration.
4. Scrub up, put on gown and gloves, clean and drape the baby. Care must be taken with alcohol-based antiseptics in small infants, less than 28 weeks, because of the risk of skin 'burns'. In particular, antiseptics must be used sparingly and care must be taken to prevent alcoholic antiseptic soaking into the pad on which the baby is lying. If the baby is held on top of a pool of alcoholic antiseptic for a few minutes, there will be skin damage and permanent scarring over the lateral part of the iliac crest. In black babies this produces an obvious area of depigmentation, which takes many years to disappear.
5. Carefully identify the landmarks and ensure that the baby is held straight and that the spine is flexed and not twisted. A line joining the highest points of both iliac crests identifies the L3/4 interspace. The L3/4 or L4/5 interspace should be used, and only in rare cases L2/3 as the spinal cord projects lower down the canal in neonates and preterm infants than in older children and adults.
6. With the bevel of the needle facing laterally (i.e. parallel with the fibres of the interspinous ligament), the needle is inserted through the

skin. The stylet is then removed so that a clear view is obtained of the needle hub and therefore of any fluid passing down the needle.

7. The needle is then slowly advanced, 1 mm at a time, until fluid is seen in the needle hub; the specimen is collected in three bottles for cell count, microscopy, and culture and protein and glucose estimation. It is not usually as easy to define the tissue planes while advancing the needle as it is in older children and adults. In infants under 1.0 kg the canal may be entered just a few millimetres below the skin surface. Firm resistance to the needle usually means that the canal has been crossed and that the needle is up against the posterior aspect of a vertebral body.
8. If no fluid flows back into the needle hub, rotate the needle because a nerve root may be obstructing the needle end.
9. If blood comes back before the canal is entered, the needle has entered an epidural vein. These are large and fragile in newborns, so a bloody tap is not uncommon.
10. Remove the needle and apply a dressing. Collodion may be used to seal the skin puncture but it does not prevent the leakage of CSF into the tissues.

Complications

1. Coning is an important risk after lumbar puncture in older children and adults with raised intracranial pressure. This should also be borne in mind with neonates, but because of the expansile nature of the neonatal skull, major elevations in intracranial pressure are rare in newborns and coning is very unusual, even in the presence of hydrocephalus or a posterior fossa haemorrhage.
2. Introduction of infection.
3. Cardiorespiratory deterioration during the procedure (e.g. apnoea), and hypothermia if inadequate precautions are taken to ensure adequate warming.
4. Implantation dermoid. This complication is very rare if a styletted needle is used when penetrating the skin.

Subdural tap

Indications

This is used to release subdural haematoma.

Equipment

1. Aseptic technique, gown, gloves, mask.
2. Sterile drape.
3. Razor.
4. Antiseptic swab.
5. 20-gauge short lumbar puncture needle.
6. 10 ml syringe.

Procedure

1. Shave the head in a 5-cm radius around the fontanelle.
2. Scrub up, put on gown and gloves. Clean the head with antiseptic (e.g.

Betadine, providone-iodine 10% in aqueous or alcoholic solution) over the fontanelle and for 7 cm along the coronal suture on either side, and drape.
3. The needle should be inserted through the skin at the lateral angle of the fontanelle; the stylet is then removed and the needle is advanced cautiously, 1 mm at a time until a popping sensation is felt as it penetrates the dura. The distance inserted is usually less than 1 cm. The fluid will drain passively, or gentle suction may be required.
4. If a dry tap is obtained, the procedure may be repeated 1 cm further laterally in the coronal suture, if the width of the suture permits entry of the needle.
5. Because of the high incidence of bilateral subdural collections, the procedure should be carried out on both sides as a small subdural may not have been detected by cranial ultrasound.
6. Repeat the cranial ultrasound and obtain the opinion of a neurosurgeon urgently.

Complications

1. The introduction of infection.
2. Entry of the subarachnoid space; this heals up by itself.

This procedure does not exclude anterior and posterior subdurals and a follow up ultrasound examination and computerized tomography (CT) scan are recommended if either of these is suspected.

Ventricular tap

Indications

1. Removal of ventricular fluid in acute hydrocephalus.
2. Sampling of ventricular fluid in ventriculitis.
3. Ventriculography.

Equipment

1. Aseptic technique, gown, gloves, mask.
2. Sterile drape.
3. Razor.
4. Antiseptic swab.
5. 10 ml syringe.
6. 20–23-gauge lumbar puncture needle 5 cm long.

Procedure

1. Shave the head in a 5 cm radius around the anterior fontanelle.
2. Clean and drape the head.
3. The point for insertion of the needle is at the lateral angle of the fontanelle or in the line drawn from the inner canthus of the eye to the coronal suture.
4. The needle is inserted parallel to the falx cerebri and directly downwards towards the base of the skull. The normal ventricle will be entered at a depth of around 4 cm and this depth can be estimated by ultrasound examination before the procedure. In patients requiring

ventricular puncture, the ventricle is frequently very large and it may be entered at 0.5–1 cm or less.

5. The stylet is withdrawn every 0.5 cm and the needle advanced slowly until CSF is obtained. The needle should not be advanced more than 4 cm if fluid has not been obtained.
6. CSF is removed slowly with the syringe. About 15–20 ml or more can be removed to decompress acute hydrocephalus. The rapid removal of an excessive volume of CSF is accompanied by signs of shock, pallor, and sweating, and sometimes apnoea. This may be corrected by injecting a small amount of saline back through the needle, or by giving more fluid parenterally.
7. The needle is removed and an adhesive dressing is applied.

Infants likely to need repeated ventricular taps should have a ventriculostomy reservoir inserted under the skin to avoid the necessity of repeated ventricular punctures, unnecessary trauma to the brain and risk of infection and serious fluid and electrolyte disturbances.

References

Blumenfeld, T.A., Turi, G.K. and Blanc, W.A. (1979) Recommended site and depth of newborn heel skin punctures based on anatomical measurements and histopathology. *Lancet*, **i**, 230–233

Lissauer, T. (1982) Practical procedures in children (1). *Hospital Update*, **8**, 1423–1432

Phillips, R.R. and Lee, S.H. (1990) Fractures of long bones occurring in neonatal intensive therapy units. *British Medical Journal*, **301**, 225–226

Swyer, P.R. (1975) The intensive care of the newly born. *Monographs in Paediatrics*, **6**, 188, Karger Basel

Further reading

Fletcher, M.A., MacDonald, M.G. and Avery, G.B. (eds) (1983) *Atlas of Procedures in Neonatology*, Lippincott, Philadelphia

Wilkinson, A. and Calvert, S. (1986) Practical procedures. In *Textbook of Neonatology*, (ed. N.R.C. Roberton), Churchill Livingstone, Edinburgh, Chapter 31, pp. 817–835

Chapter 30

Iatrogenic complications and accidents

The complications arising from procedures carried out in the newborn are so numerous that it is impossible to describe them all. However, an attempt has been made to cover the most important ones. Where a procedure is described in detail in a previous chapter, the associated complications are included with the description of that procedure; these are listed in this chapter, with page references.

Although it is not possible to prevent complications arising, it is important to be aware of the more common ones, so that they can be recognized at an early stage and treated quickly and effectively.

The question of litigation inevitably arises after a serious complication or accident. It is essential that all complications and mishaps related to treatment are accurately and honestly recorded in the notes and signed, with the time and date, by the doctor concerned. At the same time the consultant in charge of the patient should be informed. Where appropriate, a sketch should be made in the notes and a photograph should be taken as soon as possible. In the event of a serious accident which may involve permanent disability or death, the consultant should see the parents at the earliest opportunity and explain what happened and why it happened; a prognosis should also be given. If the parents are not satisfied with the explanation given, they should be offered a second opinion, by someone of their own choice, or by another consultant who has not been previously concerned with the case in any way. In the U.K., it is a matter of common observation that the majority of cases of litigation appear to arise because of inadequate communication the parents feeling that they were not told the whole truth, and that important facts were kept from them.

Intravascular procedures

Reduction of complications (arterial catheterization)

General measures aimed at reducing the complications of intravascular procedures are:

1. The artery should be located by Doppler (temporal artery) or transillumination (radial and posterior tibial arteries).

2. The catheter should be inserted percutaneously rather than by cut-down.
3. A continuous flow should be used rather than intermittent infusions.
4. The catheter should be removed if the flow is inadequate or there is extravasation of fluid.
5. Bolus injections should be avoided, particularly of calcium gluconate, vasoconstrictors or hypertonic solutions.
6. No solution other than heparinized 0.9% NaCl (0.5 unit heparin/ml), without glucose, should be used in a peripheral arterial catheter.

Capillary blood sampling (p. 304)

Venepuncture (p. 305)

Arterial puncture

Exchange transfusion

Umbilical artery catheterization (pp. 309–310)

Umbilical vein catheterization (pp. 127–130)

Radial artery catheterization (p. 313)

Posterior tibial artery catheterization (p. 313)

Temporal artery catheterization

The following complications have been recorded:

1. Sloughing of the skin at or near the site of insertion, with consequent scarring.
2. Loss of the tip of the ear.
3. Septicaemia.
4. Cerebral embolism, with fits and hemiplegia.

Peripheral vein infusions (p. 312)

Cardiac procedures

Insertion of pericardial drain (p. 317)

Gastrointestinal system

Insertion of peritoneal drain (p. 317)

Tube feeding

Tube passed through the nose

1. Increased airway resistance.
2. Infection, nasopharyngeal discharge.

Nasogastric or orogastric route

1. Aspiration of gastric contents into lungs.
2. Perforation of oesophagus.
3. Perforation of the pharynx.
4. Pyloric obstruction by the tube.
5. Accidental insertion of a nasogastric tube into the lung, usually the right lower lobe bronchus.

Nasojejunal (transpyloric) route

1. Perforation of oesophagus or pharynx.
2. Perforation of the duodenum, usually associated with stiffening of polyvinyl chloride (PVC) tubes due to the action of the intestinal secretions; unlikely or much less common with silicone rubber tubes.
3. Intussusception.
4. Difficulty in withdrawal of the tube, especially PVC tubes.

Insertion of rectal thermometer

The following complications have been described: rectal bleeding and perforation causing peritonitis or pneumoperitoneum.

Genitourinary system

Suprapubic bladder aspiration (p. 318)

Central nervous system

Lumbar puncture (p. 320)

Subdural tap (p. 321)

Ventricular tap (p. 321)

Respiratory system

These can be divided into local complications produced by the procedure itself and those related to the effects of gases used in resuscitation or ventilation.

Transillumination of the chest (p. 314)

Insertion of pleural drain (p. 315)

Mechanical ventilation (Table 12.3 p. 141)

Intubation

Early complications

1. Acute transient swelling of the vocal cords caused by the trauma of inexpert intubation or attempts to force the tube through a closed glottis. Symptoms are inspiratory stridor and a hoarse or weak cry.
2. Perforation of the larynx or trachea: cause, as above.
3. Intubation of the oesophagus and overdistension of the stomach with the possibility of gastric perforation (rupture) (p. 253).
4. Collapse of the right upper lobe by the endotracheal tube inserted into the right main bronchus.
5. Overinflation of the right lung, also due to malposition of an endotracheal tube. There is a risk of pneumothorax.
6. Perforation of a segmental bronchus during suction of secretions through an endotracheal tube.

Late complications

1. Subglottic stenosis.
2. Infective tracheobronchitis, usually due to Gram-negative bacilli.
3. Pneumonia, particularly with *Pseudomonas aeruginosa.*
4. Necrosis, adhesions scarring of the vocal cords with permanent alteration of the voice.
5. Stricture of the nasal airway.

Continuous positive airway pressure (CPAP)

CPAP with face mask

1. Facial trauma and skin ulceration.
2. Corneal abrasion which may be complicated by *Pseudomonas* or *Proteus* conjunctivitis or panophthalmitis (Cole *et al.*, 1981). All infants on CPAP by mask who develop conjunctivitis should be investigated immediately and should be examined with fluorescein by an ophthalmologist if Gram-negative organisms are found on a film of the discharge. Treatment with appropriate antibiotics (depending upon the known sensitivities of *Pseudomonas* in the unit) should be given locally, parenterally and possibly by the subtenon route (Golden and Coppel, 1970).
3. Gastric distension if a tube is not kept in the stomach; there is a risk of gastric perforation.

CPAP with nasal prongs or shortened endotracheal tube

1. Increased airway resistance, contributing to respiratory distress.
2. Ulceration and partial destruction of the nasal system; stricture formation.
3. Accumulation of solidified secretions in the pharynx, with airway obstruction.
4. Gastric distension, as above.

CPAP with head box

1. Ulceration of the skin of the neck.

2. Hydrocephalus, thought to be due to partial obstruction to the venous return by compression of the neck.
3. Gastric distension as above.

CPAP with mask

Intracranial haemorrhage, especially of the cerebellum (p. 97).

Negative pressure ventilators

1. Pressure ulceration of the skin of the neck or pelvis.
2. Gastric distension, as above.
3. Cooling of the infant due to an inefficient seal.

Effects of ventilation

Effects of inspired oxygen

1. Bronchopulmonary dysplasia, which appears to be related to high inspired oxygen concentration and high peak inspiratory pressure.
2. Retinopathy of prematurity (retrolental fibroplasia) which is probably related to high arterial Po_2 and the duration of oxygen therapy, low birthweight and the degree of prematurity.

Effects of high pressure system, particularly intermittent positive pressure ventilation

1. Pneumothorax.
2. Mediastinal emphysema.
3. Pulmonary interstitial emphysema.
4. Overhydration (hyponatraemia, p. 227) due to humidified oxygen.
5. Damage to the lungs from overheating of the humidification system.

Miscellaneous

Local skin applications

1. Sensitivity reactions from adhesive tape with the risk of skin sepsis or septicaemia.
2. Skin trauma from removal of adhesive tape.
3. Skin burns from heated electrodes.
4. Skin trauma from ECG electrodes, monitoring probes etc.
5. Haemorrhagic necrosis from application of iodine or alcohol preparations used for skin sterilization in very low birthweight infants. Iodine should not be used, and alcohol should be wiped off immediately after application. Absorption of alcohol from the skin causes potentially dangerous levels of alcohol in the blood.
6. Hexachlorophane in high concentrations, if not washed off, causes fits and cystic encephalomalacia.

Phototherapy

1. Bronzing when phototherapy is used for the reduction of unconjugated hyperbilirubinaemia in the presence of high levels of conjugated bilirubin (as in severe cases of rhesus isoimmunization).
2. Increased insensible water loss.
3. Hyperthermia.
4. Conjunctivitis from eye pads.
5. Nasal obstruction or apnoeic attacks from displaced eye pads.

High-intensity light transillumination

Skin burns may be produced if a cold-light source of illumination is not used in the localization of the radial artery or the diagnosis of pneumothorax. Even with a cold-light source, skin burns may be produced by prolonged application.

Fractures of the long bones and ribs

In very low birthweight infants (<28 weeks gestation), fractures may be produced by quite minor procedures, such as the insertion of an intravenous catheter at the wrist or foot (Phillips and Lee, 1990). Ribs may be fractured during chest physiotherapy.

References

Cole, G.F., Davies, D.P. and Austin, D.J. (1980) Pseudomonas ophthalmia neonatorum: a cause of blindness. *British Medical Journal*, **281**, 440–441

Cole, G.F., Chaudhuri, P.R. and Carroll, L.P. (1981) Mask for continuous positive airway pressure: does it cause corneal abrasions? *British Medical Journal*, **284**, 19

Golden, B. and Coppel, S.P. (1970) Ocular tissue absorption of gentamicin. *Archives of Ophthalmology*, **84**, 792–796

Kanto, W.P. and Parrish, R.A. (1977) Perforation of the peritoneum and intra-abdominal haemorrhage: a complication of umbilical vein catheterization. *American Journal of Diseases of Children*, **131**, 1102–1103

Miller, D., Kirkpatrick, B.V., Kodroff, M., Ehrlich, F.E. and Salzberg, A.M. (1979) Pelvic exsanguination following umbilical artery catheterization in neonates. *Journal of Pediatric Surgery*, **14**, 264–269

Phillips, R.R. and Lee, S.H. (1990) Fractures of long bones occurring in neonatal intensive therapy units. *British Medical Journal*, **301**, 225–226

Further reading

Fletcher, M.A., MacDonald, M.G. and Avery, G.B. (eds) (1983) *Atlas of Procedures in Neonatology*. Lippincott, Philadelphia.

Rao, H.K.M. and Elhassani, S.B. (1980) Iatrogenic complications of procedures performed on the newborn: part 1, intravascular procedures. *Perinatology–Neonatology* (Sept.–Oct.) **4**, 25–32

Rao, H.K.M. and Elhassani, S.B. (1980) Iatrogenic complications of procedures performed on the newborn; part 2, respiratory procedures. *Perinatology–Neonatology* (Nov.–Dec.) **4**. 43–52

Rao, H.K.M. and Elhassani, S.B. (1981) Iatrogenic complications of procedures performed on the newborn; part 3, phototherapy, tube feeding and others. *Perinatology–Neonatology* (Mar.–Apr.) **5**, 23–31

Chapter 31

Meeting nutritional requirements in newborn infants; practical aspects

Requirements for term infants

During the first week of life the term newborn is physiologically adapted to receiving smaller amounts of energy and water than are required later, has ample supplies of glycogen and fat, and is well hydrated at birth. During this period of low intake, fat is metabolized to form water, and there may be, after an abnormal or hypoxic delivery, a short period of antidiuresis (Finberg *et al.*, 1982).

Energy (average intake)

Day 1	30 kcal/kg per 24 hours (126 kJ/kg per 24 hours)
Day 2	40–90 kcal/kg per 24 hours (168–378 kJ/kg per 24 hours)
Day 3	65–100 kcal/kg per 24 hours (273–420 kJ/kg per 24 hours)
Day 4	80–100 kcal/kg per 24 hours (336–420 kJ/kg per 24 hours)
Day 5	100–110 kcal/kg per 24 hours (420–462 kJ/kg per 24 hours)

Water

The water requirements during the first week are normally supplied from breast milk, or modified cows' milk formulae, with or without supplements of glucose water. The average requirements during the first week are shown in Figure 31.1.

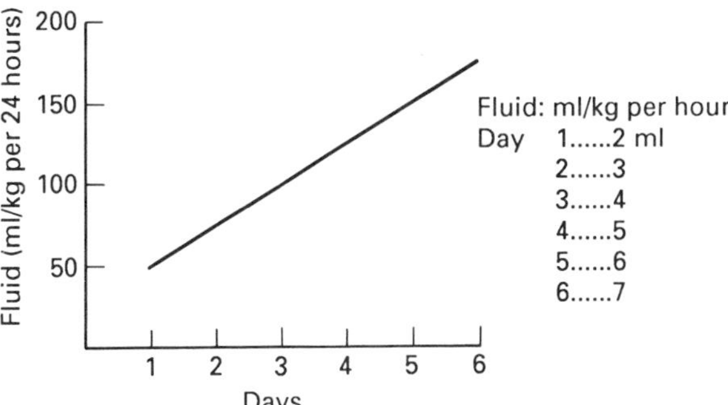

Figure 31.1 Water requirements in the first week of life. Reproduced from Jones and Owen-Thomas (1971) with permission of authors and publishers

Electrolytes

Sodium	2.5 mmol/kg per 24 hours
Potassium	2.0 mmol/kg per 24 hours
Calcium	2.0 mmol/kg per 24 hours

Daily intakes of fluid and electrolytes must take account of previous accumulated deficits in water and electrolyte intake and renal function.

Protein

2.5 g/kg per 24 hours

Requirements for low birth weight infants

Pre-term and small for gestational age infants, particularly those below 1.25 kg birth weight, have very little nutritional reserve and the timely provision of adequate nutritional support is second only in order of priority to ventilatory support.

Energy requirements

The approximate energy requirements for well enterally fed appropriately grown infants of birth weight 1.25 kg are (Swyer *et al.*, 1978):

	kcal (kJ)/kg body wt per 24 hours	
Basal metabolism	55	(230)
Activity	15	(63)
Specific dynamic action of food	10	(42)
Faecal losses	11	(46)
Growth	30	(126)
	121	(504)

These parameters are subject to considerable variation, however, and are not well established in term infants (Rubecz *et al.*, 1981). An infant would need to tolerate 180 ml of milk/kg per 24 hours containing 68 kcal (285 kJ)/100 ml to retain 30 kcal (126 kJ)/kg per 24 hours for growth. The energy cost of growth is around 4.9 kcal (21 kJ)/g weight gain for such an infant, so 30 retained kcal (126 kJ)/kg per 24 hours would provide a modest incremental growth rate of 6 g/kg body weight per 24 hours.

A parenterally fed infant has a smaller obligatory calorie requirement because there are no faecal losses as all intravenously infused calories are retained. These calories may be produced by catabolism of protein (4.3 kcal (18 kJ)/g), fat (9.3 kcal (39 kJ)/g) or carbohydrate (4.1 kcal (17 kJ)/g), and energy in the form of carbohydrate or fat must be provided simultaneously with protein to encourage tissue anabolism instead of deamination of protein components and their use as an energy source ('protein-sparing effect').

Fat and carbohydrate requirement

Fat and carbohydrate are interchangeable as protein-sparing energy sources (Rubecz *et al.*, 1981). An adequate supply of essential fatty acids must be provided, contained in human milk or formula in enterally fed infants; or intralipid must meet at least 4% of total calorie requirement in parenterally fed infants (Tashiro *et al.*, 1976).

Protein requirement

The amount required is 2.5–4.0 g/kg per 24 hours (Seashore and Seashore, 1976). Term infants require around 2.5 g/kg per 24 hours for adequate nitrogen retention and growth, while premature infants have a variable requirement, but should not receive more than 4 g/kg per 24 hours enterally or parenterally because of the risks of neurodevelopmental consequences of hyperammonaemia and hyperaminoacidaemia.

A detailed consideration of the nutritional requirements including minerals and vitamins is beyond the scope of this book. For further consideration of fluid and electrolyte management of very low birthweight infants see Chapter 4.

Nutritional formulations available

Enteral

Human milk (71 Kcal (298 kJ); 1.5 g of protein, 0.8 mmol of calcium, 0.9 mmol of sodium per 100 ml)
Human milk is the best nutrient for term infants, for nutritional, immunological, bacteriological and social reasons. Although the milk of mothers of pre-term infants contains more calories, electrolytes and protein than the milk of mothers delivering at term, the composition becomes more dilute after the first few weeks after delivery and may be less than adequate in protein, calories, sodium and calcium for a rapidly growing small pre-term infant. This has led to attempts to enrich human milk by fractionation or by the addition of a fortifier (e.g. Enfamil, human milk fortifier).

Pooled donated human milk (from mothers delivering at term) is considered inadequate for very low birthweight pre-term infants, and those fed only on the mother's own breast milk require 180–200 ml/kg per 24 hours and supplementation with sodium (1 mmol/100 ml) and calcium (2 mmol/kg per 24 hours) to sustain adequate growth.

Infant formula (68 kcal (285 kJ); 2.3 g of protein, 1 mmol of calcium, 0.9 mmol of sodium per 100 ml)
Most standard infant formulae have a 60:40 whey/casein protein composition and a low sodium content, like human milk. As with human milk, a large intake of 180 ml/kg per 24 hours or more and similar sodium and calcium supplementation required to meet the needs of a very low birthweight infant.

Pre-term infant formula (81 kcal (340 kJ), 2.8 g of protein, 2 or more mmol of calcium and 2 mmol of sodium per 100 ml)
A number of such formulae have recently become available, designed for very low birthweight pre-term infants and, despite some initial problems, appear to meet the nutritional needs of these infants, particularly in those that cannot tolerate a high fluid load (e.g. infants with bronchopulmonary dysplasia).

Parenteral

Glucose 10% and electrolytes (e.g. 2.0 mmol of NaCl, 1.5 mmol of Kcl, 0.5 mmol of calcium gluconate per 100 ml)
This is the basic intravenous fluid for sick infants to maintain fluid and electrolyte balance, with frequent appropriate adjustments being made to the electrolyte content. Glucose 5% may have to be used if the blood glucose rises consistently above 10 mmol/litre (180 mg/100 ml). Glucose 10% (150 ml/kg per 24 hours) provides 61 kcal (256 kJ)/kg per 24 hours which just covers basal energy requirements; but infants maintained on this alone develop progressive incremental protein catabolism, negative nitrogen balance and essential fatty acid deficiency. Such a solution is satisfactory only for a short time only (e.g. 5–7 days in infants previously in good nutritional state, and 2–3 days in infants in poor nutritional state or extremely small pre-term infants). Glucose 5% at the same infusion rate leaves a major energy deficit in addition, necessitating more rapid tissue catabolism and protein breakdown to meet energy demands.

Vamin-Glucose
This is a commercially available synthetic crystalline aminoacid mixture containing 7.0 g of amino acids (equivalent to 6.1 g of protein), 10 g of glucose, 5 mmol of sodium, 2 mmol of potassium and 65 kcal (275 kJ) per 100 ml and is the most commonly used amino acid preparation for total parenteral nutrition (TPN) in infants. A dosage of 35–40 ml/kg per 24 hours provides 2.1–2.4 g of protein/kg per 24 hours.

Intralipid 10% or 20%
This is an energy-rich soya bean oil fat emulsion stabilized with egg lecithin 1.2 g and glycerol 2.5 g/100 ml, buffered to pH7. Intralipid 10% contains 10 g of fat and 100 kcal (420 kJ)/100 ml while Intralipid 20% contains 20 g of fat and 200 kcal (840 kJ)/100 ml. The particle size is slightly larger in Intralipid 20%. Some 85% of the fat is made up of unsaturated and polyunsaturated triglycerides; 0.5 g of fat as Intralipid/kg per 24 hours provides basic essential fatty acid requirements during TPN (Tashiro *et al.*, 1976). A dosage of 15–20 ml/kg per 24 hours provides 1.5–2.0 g of fat and 15–20 kcal (62–84 kJ)/kg per 24 hours with Intralipid 10%, and 3.0–4.0 g of fat and 30–40 kcal (126–168 kJ)/kg per 24 hours with Intralipid 20%. The fat infusion rate must be increased no faster than the disappearance rate from plasma and the infusion should be continuous throughout 24 hours without 'catch-up' periods at a higher rate, which may induce lipaemia (Whitfield *et al.*, 1983; Kao *et al.*, 1984). Dosage should start at 0.5–1 g/kg per 24 hours and should be increased by 0.5 g/kg every 24 hours

depending on the triglyceride level. Serum triglyceride levels should not exceed 2.25 mmol/litre (200 mg/100 ml) if the effects of fat overdosage are to be avoided. Opalescence of the plasma is an unreliable guide to lipaemia. Major contraindications to the use of Intralipid are moderate to severe jaundice, thrombocytopenia, signs of septicaemia and respiratory problems of critical severity.

Ped-El
This is an electrolyte and trace element solution containing calcium, magnesium, iron, zinc, manganese, copper, fluoride, iodine, phosphate and chloride, and is used to cover uncompensated daily losses of these electrolytes and trace metals; it is added to Vamin-Glucose in a dose of 4 ml/kg per 24 hours.

Solivito
This is a water-soluble vitamin preparation which is added to the daily requirement of glucose 10% during parenteral nutrition in a dose of 0.5 ml/kg per 24 hours. The solution must be protected from light by using aluminium foil.

Vitlipid Infant
This is a fat emulsion similar to Intralipid 10% containing fat-soluble vitamins (A, D_2, K_1), which is added to Intralipid 10 or 20% in a dose of 4 ml/24 hours.

Vamin-Glucose, Intralipid, Solivito, Ped-El and Vitlipid Infant are marketed in the U.K. by KabiVitrum* and the reader is referred to the appropriate data sheets for detailed composition.

Risks and benefits of enteral and parenteral feeding in neonates and infants

Enteral feeding

In all situations, enteral feeding is preferable to parenteral feeding if enteral feeding is tolerated, absorbed and supports a satisfactory rate of growth.

Advantages of enteral feeding

1. Milk constitutes 'total enteral nutrition' meeting all the nutritional needs of the infant (except perhaps in some extremely premature infants).
2. Use of the gastrointestinal tract is physiological and stimulates enterohormonal and digestive maturation.
3. Infection risk is low.
4. Enteral feeding is cheap.

*KabiVitrum Ltd, KabiVitrum House, Riverside Way, Uxbridge, Middlesex UB8 2YF. Tel: Uxbridge (0895) 5144.

Disadvantages of enteral feeding

1. Risks of regurgitation and pulmonary milk aspiration, delay in gastric emptying, exacerbation of respiratory status and apnoeic attacks, hypoperistalsis and constipation.
2. Malabsorption of (a) fat, due to functional bile salt deficiency in premature newborns, (b) carbohydrate, due to lack of adequate intestinal lactose, and (c) glucose/galactose malabsorption.
3. Although the relationship of enteral feeding to necrotizing enterocolitis (NEC) is not fully understood and NEC can occur before any enteral feeding has been offered, enteral feeding none the less appears to be a promoter of the disease process, perhaps by supplying substrate for bacterial overgrowth in infants at risk.

Gastrointestinal feeding is only an available option if the gastrointestinal tract is intact and functions normally.

Alternative method of enteral feeding

Continuous nasogastric feeding has been used to increase the amount of milk tolerated in the first weeks of life (Valman *et al.*, 1972), and to reduce the effects of feeding on respiratory mechanics, but the risk of feed aspiration remains. Some small infants who will not tolerate intermittent feeding will tolerate slowly increasing continuous feeding. The potential advantages of continuous over conventional feeding have not, however, been systematically evaluated in small infants.

Transpyloric feeding (duodenal or jejunal), using continuous milk infusion via a silicone rubber preweighted tube (e.g. Vygon), has been used in small infants to establish early feeding, combining the advantages of continuous nasogastric feeding with, theoretically, less risk of feed aspiration. This technique has not been adequately evaluated in infants below 1.0 kg; tube dislodgement, malabsorption and resultant poor growth appear to be the major disadvantages (Whitfield, 1982).

Parenteral feeding

Advantages

1. Absorption is certain because the nutrient is delivered parenterally.
2. Integrity of the gastrointestinal tract and its absorptive function are not necessary.

Disadvantages and complications

1. Delivery of nutrients which are potentially toxic directly into the systemic circulation.
2. Risk of systemic infection at infusion sites.
3. Risk of infusion of nutrients at a faster rate than they can be assimilated, with resultant metabolic disorders (hyperammonaemia, hyperaminoacidaemia, lipaemia, hyperglycaemia).
4. Nutritional deficiencies due to relative lack of a particular nutrient in the solution. Requirements for many substances are not clearly established in the newborn, e.g. copper, zinc and other trace metals, carnitine, taurine (see below).

5. Cholestatic jaundice (p. 114).
6. Investigational anaemia from repeated blood tests for TPN monitoring and the risks of repeated transfusions (e.g. transfusion-acquired cytomegalovirus or HIV infection).
7. Lack of stimulus to maturation of the gastrointestinal tract if feeding is withheld (Lucas *et al.*, 1983).
8. Expensive.
9. Prescription errors.

Practical aspects of administration of parenteral nutrition

Parenteral feeding is required when nutritional requirements cannot be met by enteral feeding. TPN is required if no enteral feeding is tolerated and all the nutritional needs of the infant must be met parenterally. When some enteral feeding is tolerated, the remainder of the nutritional requirements must be provided by supplementary parenteral nutrition (SPN) to promote tissue anabolism and growth. The composition of the infusate is the same for TPN and SPN, a smaller volume being used for SPN depending on enteral intake and absorption.

Because of the risks of infection and dosage errors, it is most desirable to have parenteral nutrition prescriptions made up daily in the pharmacy in sterile conditions using a laminar flow hood. Such facilities are not generally available, so a 'do-it-yourself', 'cookery book' method is given below. The equipment required is given in Table 31.1 and shown in Figure 31.2. Details of the dosage schedule are given in Table 31.2, and the final infusate constitution at full dosage is given in Table 31.3. The reader is also referred to KabiVitrum data sheets on the components and references (Panter-Brick, Wagget and Dale; Shaw, 1973).

1. Before starting TPN, correct fluid and electrolyte balance, acid–base status, check adequacy of urine output (2ml/kg per hour). Consider relevant contraindications, particularly to the use of Intralipid (moderate to severe jaundice, septicaemia, thrombocytopenia, critical pulmonary disease), and review caloric requirement for TPN.
2. Using Table 31.2, calculate the requirements of Vamin-Glucose and add a volume of Ped-El to the Vamin-Glucose bottle sufficient to provide 4ml of Ped-El/kg with the daily allowance of Vamin-Glucose.
3. Calculate glucose 10% and NaCl requirement and add a volume of dipotassium hydrogen phosphate and Solivito to give 1mmol/kg and 0.5ml/kg respectively in the calculated daily dose of glucose 10% and NaCl.
4. Attach the bottle containing Vamin-Glucose plus Ped-El and bottle containing glucose 10% plus additives, each to a burette input limb of the Travenol paediatric TPN set.
5. Calculate the hourly infusion rate for the daily allocations of Vamin-Glucose plus Ped-El and glucose 10% plus additives together, given over 24 hours and calculate the volumes of these two solutions that must be mixed in the burette to deliver the appropriate volumes. Run through and exclude air bubbles from TPN set tubing ('aqueous line').

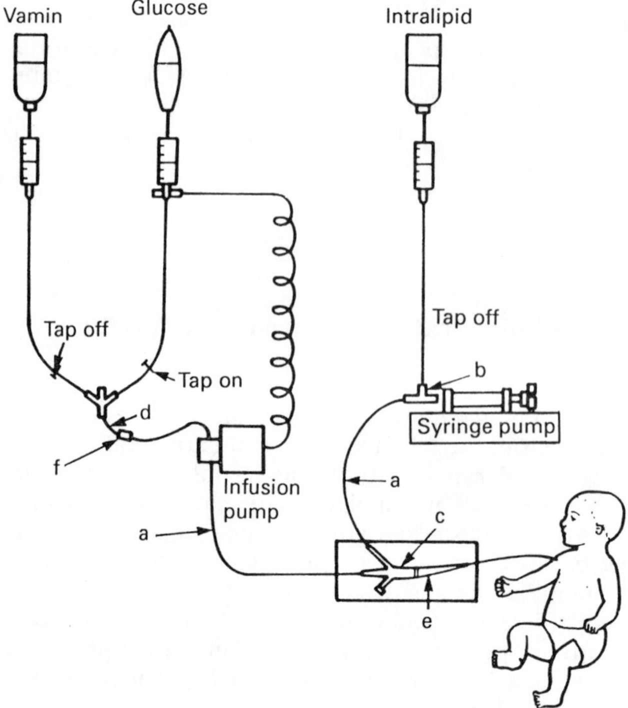

Figure 31.2 Equipment for delivery parenteral nutrition. a, Extension set; b, three-way stopcock; c, dual injection site; d, L-S connector; e, intravenous cannula; f, Millipore filter. Reproduced from Candy (1980) with permission of author and publishers

Table 31.1 Equipment for total parenteral nutrition in infants

Solutions	Vamin-Glucose, 100 ml bottle Glucose 10%, 500 ml bag Intralipid 20%, 100 ml bottle Ped-El, 20 ml vial Solivito ampoule (to be reconstituted with the addition of 5 ml glucose 10%) Vitlipid Infant, 10 ml vial 30% (hypertonic) NaCl (5 mmol/ml) Dipotassium hydrogen phosphate (1 mmol/ml)
Disposable infusion equipment	Travenol paediatric TPN set (Alternative is a standard paediatric giving set with a 100 or 200 ml burette, the additional bottle being connected to the burette using an adult giving set inserted through the rubber injection port in the burette, using a 21-gauge needle.) Millipore filter Luer Y-connector 30–50 ml syringe to fit syringe pump (see below) Narrow bore anaesthetic extension tubing (e.g. Travenol)
Infusion pumps	Volumetric infusion pump which can deliver accurately 2–20 ml/hour (e.g. IVAC cassette-type infusion pump) Syringe pump capable of delivering 0.1–4 ml/hour (many commercially available, e.g. Sage, Vickers)

Table 31.2 Schedule for introduction of total parenteral nutrition in neonates and infants, and resultant nutritional intake

Day of TPN	*Nutrient solution* (ml/kg daily)			*Infused intake/bodyweight per day*					
	*Vamin-9-Glucose**	*Intralipid 20%†*	*Glucose 10% + NaCl 2 mmol/100 ml**	*Total fluid* (ml)	*Total calories* (kcal)§	*Protein equivalent*	*Fat* (g)	*Na* (mmol)	*K* (mmol)
0 (Glucose and electrolytes only)	0	0	150	150	62	0	0	3.0	2.3
1	12	5	133	150	73	0.7	1	3.3	2.2
2–4	25	10	115	150	83	1.5	2	3.4	2.5
5 onwards (full dosage)	40	15–20	95–90	150	95–102	2.4	3–4	3.6–3.7	2.8

Total fluid intake may be increased by increasing glucose 10% intake in infants who will tolerate the glucose and fluid load. Gastrointestinal losses can be compensated for by increasing the volume of glucose 10% and adding extra KCl or providing a separate gastrointestinal replacement solution which can be connected to the burette.

*Add Ped-El 4 ml/kg daily.

†Add 4 ml of Vitlipid Infant (dose of intralipid increased as permitted by triglyceride monitoring (see the text)).

‡When using glucose 10% and electrolytes only, add KCl 1.5 mmol/100 ml and calcium gluconate 0.5 mmol/100 ml. When using TPN, add dipotassium hydrogen phosphate (1 mmol/kg) and Solivito 6.5 ml/kg.

§1 kcal = 4.2 kJ.

Table 31.3 Total parenteral nutrition infusate composition (full dosage from day 5 onwards)

Carbohydrate and fat		*Vitamins*	
Glucose	13.0g	Thiamin	0.12mg
Soya bean oil	4.0*	Riboflavin	0.18mg
Egg lecithin	0.24g	Nicotinamide	1mg
Glycerol	0.5mg	Biotin	0.03mg
		Pyridoxine	0.2mg
Amino acids		Pantothenic acid	1mg
L-Alanine	120mg	Ascorbic acid	3mg
L-Arginine	132mg	Folic acid	0.02mg
L-Aspartic acid	164mg	Vitamin B_{12}	0.2μg
L-Cysteine/cystine	56mg	Vitamin A	400μg
Glycine	84mg	Calciferol (D_2)	400 Units
L-Histidine	96mg	Vitamin K_1	200μg
L-Isoleucine	156mg		
L-Leucine	212mg	*Minerals*	
L-Lysine	156mg	Sodium	3.6mmol
L-Methionine	76mg	Potassium	2.8mmol
L-Phenylalanine	220mg	Calcium	0.7mmol
L-Proline	324mg	Magnesium	0.16mmol
L-Serine	300mg	Chloride	4.1mmol
L-Threonine	120mg	Phosphate	1.4mmol
L-Tryptophan	40mg	Iron	2.0μmol
L-Tyrosine	20mg	Zinc	0.6μmol
L-Valine	172mg	Magnanese	1.0μmol
Glutamic acid	360mg	Copper	0.3μmol
		Fluoride	3.0μmol
Water to	150ml	Iodine	0.04μmol

Amounts are per kg body weight per 24 hours.
*50% of esterified fatty acids derived from linoleic acid.

6. The flow rate is controlled on the aqueous line by an accurate volumetric pump. Attach a Millipore filter, then one of the upper limbs of a Luer Y-connector ((d) in Figure 31.2) to the end of the aqueous line. Run through to exclude air (to the other upper limb of the Y-connector will be attached the lipid line (see below), and to the lower limb the patient's infusion administration cannula).
7. Calculate the daily requirement of Intralipid 20% and draw this volume plus 5 ml (for dead space) of Intralipid 20% into a syringe. Add 4 ml of Vitlipid Infant, connect to a narrow-bore anaesthetic extension tube and run through to exclude air ('lipid line'). Connect the lipid line to the vacant upper limb of the Y-connector. Run through to exclude air. Calculate lipid line infusion rate and set up the syringe in a syringe pump to deliver the lipid emulsion at that rate over 24 hours.
8. Ensure that all bubbles are excluded and that the infusion site is functional, then connect the distal limb of the Y-connector to the patient's intravenous cannula and start the pumps at the appropriate rate.

   It is necessary that all the above manipulations be conducted with appropriate aseptic precautions to reduce the risk of infection.

9. TPN monitoring
   (a) Daily for the first week, then twice weekly: plasma urea and electrolytes, plasma triglycerides;
   (b) Twice weekly: haemoglobin, white blood cells, platelets, calcium, magnesium and phosphate;
   (c) Weekly: bilirubin (direct and indirect), plasma proteins, alkaline phosphatase, transaminases;
   (d) Every 2 weeks: zinc and copper.
10. The dosage may be increased progressively as given in Table 31.2, paying due regard to the results of monitoring blood tests. Intralipid dosage can be increased by daily increments of 0.5g of fat/kg per 24 hours up to a total of 3–4g/kg per 24 hours (Barness *et al.*, 1981). Many infants will not tolerate this much, however, without significant lipaemia (Shennan *et al.*, 1977); triglyceride levels should not be permitted to exceed 2.25mmol/litre (200mg/100ml) because of the dangers of lipid deposition in the tissues (Pereira *et al.*, 1980; Halpin and Dahms, 1983). Sudden glucose and fat intolerance is usually a sign of septicaemia, the most likely source being the infusion site. Under these circumstances, the fat infusion must be stopped and the carbohydrate infusion rate halved until blood glucose results are available. Appropriate investigation for infection and appropriate antibiotic treatment should be initiated.

Nutritional management strategy in pre-term infants

Appropriately grown infants of more than 1.5kg (or 32 weeks gestation or more) without respiratory problems

The majority manage with enteral feeding only, and do not usually need intravenous fluids. Active sucking with coordinated swallowing begins at around 33 or 34 weeks gestation.

Plan: Initiate nasogastric feeding at 60ml/kg per 24 hours on the first day, increasing slowly to 150ml/kg per 24 hours by 5 days and then to 180–200ml/kg per 24 hours by 14 days.

Appropriately grown infants of 1.25–1.5kg (or 29–32 weeks gestation), small for gestational age, or larger infants with respiratory problems

These infants require intravenous fluids to maintain hydration, and blood glucose until feeds can be established.

Plan: Initiate glucose 10% and electrolytes plus calcium infusion at 60ml/kg per 24 hours (4mg of glucose/kg per minute) within the first hour of life. When there are bowel sounds and the baby has passed stools (perhaps with the assistance of a glycerine suppository), start enteral feeding around the third or fourth day of life by intermittent or continuous nasal, orogastric or transpyloric feeding. Aim to reach 150ml/kg per 24 hours by day 6 or 7 as tolerated, then increase slowly to 180–200ml/kg per 24 hours or transfer to premature formula or breast milk with fortifier. Failure to start enteral feeding by the third or fourth day of life or to reach 150 ml/kg per 24 hours by day 6 or 7 because of feed intolerance are indications for parenteral nutrition until full feeding can be established.

Appropriately grown or small for gestational age infants of 0.5–1.25 kg (24–28 weeks gestation)

Such infants have very small nutritional reserves and usually take several weeks to become fully established on enteral feeding, particularly the smallest infants who are at greater risk of feed intolerance, malabsorption and necrotizing enterocolitis, and frequently have severe respiratory and other complications. A period of TPN followed by SPN is required before feeding and growth are fully established.

Plan: Initiate intravenous fluids with glucose 10% and electrolytes (see also Chapter 4). Do not add potassium for the first 24 hours as some very immature infants develop symptomatic hyperkalaemia due to cell leakage and oliguria in the first 48 hours, presenting a difficult management problem. Sodium requirements in the first 24–48 hours are low, particularly if urine output is low. Great care must be taken to limit the volume of sodium-containing catheter flushings in the first few days of life; sodium bicarbonate should be used cautiously as low urine output and high transcutaneous water losses together may cause an abrupt rise in the serum sodium level to >150 mmol/litre within the first 24 hours after birth. Serum electrolyte levels should be measured twice in the first 24 hours of life in infants of <1.0 kg birth weight in order to take early corrective action if there are signs of a rapidly rising sodium level (increase fluid intake) or potassium level (calcium supplementation, ion-exchange resin enemata, glucose and insulin, exchange transfusion).

Most infants of <1.0 kg birth weight require around 90, 150 and 180 ml of fluid/kg per 24 hours on the first, second and third day of life respectively to keep the sodium level normal. This is because of large transcutaneous water losses through porous gelatinous skin. Usually this has to be given as glucose 5% because the infant cannot tolerate the glucose load of such a volume of glucose 10% because of lack of effective insulin receptors.

By the end of the first week of life the skin has become parchment-like and more waterproof and the urine output has improved, but a large sodium diuresis develops because the immature tubules cannot reabsorb filtered sodium. This results in a considerable sodium and water depletion which is shown by a large weight drop and poor skin turgor. Urine sodium and water losses should be measured at the end of the first week and appropriate supplementation given. This usually requires an **additional** sodium intake of 3–7 mmol/kg per 24 hours. Care must be taken to avoid overloading with sodium and water, however, or this will aggravate the developing signs of a patent ductus arteriosus which usually appear in the second week of life.

In well infants with bowel sounds who have passed stools, enteral feeding may be started in the first 3 days but must be increased very cautiously as tolerated (e.g. 0.5–1.0 ml/kg per feed increase every 24 hours). By 3 days of life, TPN should be introduced and increased as tolerated to full dosage (see Table 31.2), then subsequently tailed off as milk intake becomes sufficient to meet the baby's needs.

Prolonged TPN (beyond 3 weeks) in such infants presents major technical problems. A central venous line may have to be used and should be inserted before suitable peripheral sites are exhausted, and nutritional deficiencies may occur. Recent studies suggest that the trace element composition of the schedule given is inadequate for long-term use and will lead to zinc and copper deficiencies. The zinc requirement for small growing premature infants is around 6 μmol (400 μg/kg per 24 hours) (Lockitch *et al.*, 1983; Zlotkin and Buchanan, 1983), and copper requirement is 0.6 μmol (40 μg) (Lockitch *et al.*, 1983), compared with 0.6 μmol zinc and 0.3 μmol copper/kg per 24 hours provided by the schedule. Blood amino acid and ammonia levels should be measured in small infants on prolonged TPN who are inexplicably unwell. Requirements of taurine (Gaull and Rassin, 1980) and carnitine (Schiff *et al.*, 1979; Schmidt-Sommerfeld *et al.*, 1982; Orzali *et al.*, 1984), which are not present in current TPN solutions, are unknown but may be significant.

Nutritional strategy in infants requiring surgery

Term neonates and infants requiring major surgical treatment for gastrointestinal abnormalities may require TPN if enteral feeding has to be stopped for more than 5–7 days. Although nutritional requirements for term infants are not as well established as for pre-term infants, and the effects of surgery on tolerance of TPN components is largely uninvestigated, the schedule in Table 31.2 is satisfactory for such infants (Zlotkin, 1984).

Preoperative

Preoperative nutritional status appears to be an important determinant of postoperative morbidity in infants; those in poor nutritional condition in whom non-immediate surgery is planned benefit from several days of preoperative nutritional rehabilitation with TPN. TPN should be stopped on the day of the operation and replaced by glucose 10% and electrolytes to permit effective prompt perioperative adjustments of fluid and electrolyte status.

Postoperative

First 48 hours

Fluid intake should be reduced by about 30% (to 90–100 ml/kg per 24 hours) of glucose 10% and electrolytes. Electrolyte additions should be adjusted in accordance with postoperative electrolytes and urine output, and potassium should not be added in the first 24 hours postoperatively because of potassium release from tissue catabolism and low urinary output due to postoperative antidiuresis. Glucose 5% may be required if there is glucose intolerance.

After 48 hours

Fluids should be increased once the urine output has picked up (2 ml/kg per minute or more) and TPN started in infants in poor nutritional status in whom successful enteral feeding is not anticipated in the next few days (by 5–7 days postoperatively).

References

Barness, L.A., Dallman, P.R., Anderson, H., Collipp, P.J., Nicholson, B.L., Walker, W.A. *et al.* (1981). American Academy of Pediatrics Committee on Nutrition. Use of intravenous fat emulsions in pediatric patients. *Pediatrics*, **68**, 738–743

Candy, D.C.A. (1980). Perinatal nutrition in pediatric practice: a review. *Journal of Human Nutrition*, **34**, 287–296

Finberg, L., Kravath, R.E. and Fleischman, A.R. (1982) *Water and Electrolytes in Pediatrics*, W.B. Saunders, Philadelphia, p. 222

Gaull, G. and Rassin, D. (1980) Taurine in development and nutrition. *Ciba Symposium 72, Sulphur in Nutrition and Biology*, Excerpta Medica, Elsevier, Amsterdam and London, pp. 271–288

Halpin, T.C. and Dahms, B.B. (1983) Complications associated with intravenous lipids in infants and children. *Acta Chirurgica Scandinavica, Supplement*, **517**, 169–177

Jones, R.S. and Owen-Thomas, J.B. (1971) *Care of the Critically Ill Child*, Edward Arnold, London, p. 288

Kao, L., Cheng, M. and Warburton, D. (1984) Triglycerides, free fatty acids, free fatty acid/albumin molar ratio and cholesterol levels in serum of neonates receiving long term lipid infusions. Controlled trial of continuous and intermittent regimens. *Journal of Pediatrics*, **104**, 429–435

Lockitch, G., Godolphin, W., Pendray, M.R., Riddell, D. and Quigley, G. (1983) Serum zinc copper retinol binding protein, prealbumin and caeruloplasmin concentrations in infants receiving intravenous zinc and copper supplementations. *Journal of Pediatrics*, **102**, 304–308

Lucas, A., Bloom, S. and Aynsley-Green, A. (1983) Metabolic and endocrine consequences of depriving preterm infants of enteral nutrition. *Acta Paediatrica Scandinavica*, **72**, 245–249

Orzali, A., Maetzke, G., Donzelli, F. and Rubaltelli, F.F. (1984) Effect of carnitine on lipid metabolism in the neonate II. Carnitine addition to lipid infusions during prolonged total parenteral nutrition. *Journal of Pediatrics*, **104**, 436–440

Panter-Brick, M., Wagget, J. and Dale, G. (undated) *Intravenous Nutrition in Paediatrics* (KabiVitrum booklet available from KabiVitrum Ltd., KabiVitrum House, Riverside Way, Uxbridge, Middlesex UB8 2YF, U.K.

Pereira, G.R., Fox, W.W., Stanley, C.A., Baker, L. and Schwartz, J.C. (1980) Decreased oxygenation and hyperlipemia during intravenous fat infusions in premature infants. *Pediatrics*, **66**, 26–30

Rubecz, I., Mestyán, J., Varga, P. *et al.* (1981) Energy metabolism, substrate utilisation and nitrogen balance in parenterally fed post-operative neonates and infants. *Journal of Pediatrics*, **98**, 42–46

Schiff, D., Chan, G., Seccombe, D. and Hahn, P. (1979) Plasma carnitine levels during intravenous feeding in the neonate. *Journal of Pediatrics*, **95**, 1043–1046

Schmidt-Sommerfeld, E., Penn, D. and Wolf, H. (1982) Carnitine blood concentration and fat utilisation in parenterally alimented premature newborn infants. *Journal of Pediatrics*, **100**, 260–267

Seashore, J. and Seashore, M. (1976) Protein requirements of infants receiving total parenteral nutrition. *Journal of Pediatric Surgery*, **11**, 645–652

Shaw, J.C.L. (1973) Parenteral nutrition in the management of sick low birth weight infants. *Pediatric Clinics of North America*, **20**, 333–358

Shennan, A., Bryan, M. and Angel, A. (1977) The effects of gestational age on intralipid tolerance in newborn infants. *Journal of Pediatrics*, **91**, 134–137

Swyer, P.R., Putet, G., Smith, J.M. and Heim, T. (1978) Energy metabolism and substrate utilisation during total parenteral nutrition in the newborn. In *Intensive Care of the Newborn II*. (ed L. Stern, W. Oh and B. Friis-Hansen) Masson, New York, pp. 307–316

Tashiro, T., Ogata, H., Yokoyama, H., Mashima, Y. and Ittoh, K. (1976) The effect of fat emulsion (Intralipid) on essential fatty acid deficiency in infants receiving intravenous alimentation. *Journal of Pediatric Surgery*, **11**, 505–515

Valman, H., Heath, C. and Brown, R. (1972) Continuous intragastric milk feeds in infants of low birth weight. *British Medical Journal*, **3**, 547–550

Whitfield, M.F. (1982) Poor weight gain in the low birth weight infant fed nasojejunally. *Archives of Disease in Childhood*, **57**, 597–601.

Whitfield, M., Spitz, L. and Milner, R. (1983) Clinical and metabolic consequences of two alternative regimens of total parenteral nutrition in the newborn. *Archives of Disease in Childhood*, **58**, 168–175

Zlotkin, S.H. (1984) Intravenous nitrogen intake requirements in full term newborns undergoing surgery. *Pediatrics*, **73**, 493–496

Zlotkin, S. and Buchanan, B. (1983) Meeting zinc and copper intake requirements in the parenterally fed preterm and full term infant. *Journal of Pediatrics*, **103**, 441–446

Further reading

Winters, R. and Hasselmeyer, E. (eds) (1974) *Intravenous Nutrition of the High Risk Infant*, Wiley, New York

Heird, W., McMillan, R. and Winters, R. (1976) Total parenteral nutrition of the pediatric patient. In *Total Parenteral Nutrition* (ed. J.E. Fisher), Little Brown, Boston, pp. 253–283 (50 references)

Kanarek, D., Williams, P. and Curran, J. (1982) Total parenteral nutrition in infants and children. In *Advances in Pediatrics*, **29**, 151–181 (151 references)

Chapter 32

Talking to parents

Talking to parents about minor conditions in their baby

Explanations to the mother immediately after delivery must be given with great care. If the mother has been heavily sedated or has just had a general anaesthetic, she may appear to take in what has been said, but in fact may be too confused to understand or retain it. One must be prepared to repeat the explanation next day.

Apart from the more serious conditions which require a full explanation, there are many minor abnormalities or variations in an infant's behaviour that may appear trivial to the medical and nursing staff but which may cause the mother great anxiety unless a proper explanation is given (Table

Table 32.1 Conditions of no clinical importance that may cause parental anxiety

Skin lesions
- Strawberry naevi
- 'Stork bite' (nuchal or occipital capillary naevus)
- Milia
- Erythema toxicum
- Innocent pigmented naevi
- Epithelial pearls in the mouth

Cephalhaematoma
Subconjunuctival haemorrhage
Peripheral and traumatic cyanosis
Tongue tie
Diastasis recti
Protuberant xiphisternum
Hydrocele
Sacral dimple
Umbilical anomalies, e.g. hernia
Physiological jaundice
Snuffles
Periorbital oedema
Talipes calcaneo-valgus
Vaginal skin tag
Breast enlargement
Hooded prepuce

Reproduced from Roberton (1984) with the permission of author and publishers.

32.1). Discussions between the medical and nursing staff in front of the mother about feeding, weight gain and other routine matters should not take place as if she did not exist; the mother should be brought into the conversation and given a proper explanation of what is going on. Chance remarks by the staff, which are overheard by the mother, are often misunderstood or misinterpreted.

Pre-term infants

Parents should be reassured that the side-to-side flattening of the head, which is common in many pre-term infants, is not permanent and that the head will become normal in shape within a few months.

Before the infant goes home, the parents should receive accurate instructions about heating in the home, with particular attention to the infant's bedroom at night.

Follow-up arrangements should be explained to the parents, and the local health visitor or 'premature follow-up nurse' should be given the necessary details about the infant's delivery and subsequent progress. Any social difficulties should be discussed with the hospital social worker.

All infants

Night feeds

Most young infants require a night feed at or around 2a.m. If the night staff have been giving a night feed in hospital, the mother should be told about this before she takes the baby home.

Sleepy infants

Some infants sleep a great deal during the first week of life and it is difficult to get them to feed for longer than a few minutes at a time. They should be fed whenever they wake or appear hungry; it is useless to try to force them to feed.

Noisy breathing

Many newborn infants with a completely normal nasopharynx snort and snuffle during sleep. Although disturbing to anxious parents, the noise is quite harmless and does not indicate an impending cot death.

Loose stools

Many breast-fed infants pass unformed stools of the colour and consistency of scrambled egg. Small greenish brown loose or watery stools are usually evidence of underfeeding.

Frequency of stools

Most infants tend to pass a stool after a feed, and therefore pass up to six stools in the 24 hours. In breast-fed infants particularly, there is a great variation in the number of stools passed; some babies pass six or more and others one stool every 2–3 days. Provided that the infant is thriving and the stools are not hard there is no need to do anything.

Straining during defaecation

Most infants go red in the face when defaecating; no treatment is required unless the stools are hard and the infant screams during defaecation, which usually indicates a small anal fissure.

Blood in the stools

See p. 100.

Pink urine

See p. 100.

Vaginal bleeding

A small amount of vaginal bleeding occurs in some infants on the third or fourth day of life, and may continue for another 2–3 days. The bleeding is quite unrelated to any disorder of the blood, and is analogous to a miniature menstrual period.

Breast enlargement

Some enlargement of the breasts occurs in most term infants of either sex, usually towards the end of the first week. One breast may be more enlarged than the other. No treatment is required, and the swelling gradually resolves, though this occasionally takes 3 or 4 weeks.

Male circumcision

There are no medical indications for circumcision in the newborn; therefore the operation cannot be performed under the British National Health Service, and must be done privately, preferably by a paediatric surgeon. However, exceptions to this rule may be necessary under certain circumstances (see below).

There are certain groups who may wish to have their baby circumcised.

Jews

Normally, if not done at the hospital, a ritual circumcision is done by a rabbi. In Britain this is generally done skillfully and under satisfactory conditions.

Muslims
Although it is not essential from a religious point of view that circumcision should be done in the neonatal period, it is usually done at this time. In areas where there is not a large Muslim community, the facilities for circumcision are not always well organized, and infection and other complications may result from unskilled operators. In such circumstances, some paediatric surgeons have taken the view that more hospital time is taken up in dealing with the complications of an unsatisfactory circumcision than is occupied by doing the operation themselves under the National Health Service; they regard this as a form of preventive medicine.

North American
There are no religious reasons for circumcision in these two groups. Rather, these diverse societies seem to be imposing conformity and uniformity on their members by surgery. It is doubtful whether most North American parents are even dimly aware of the reduced incidence of carcinoma of the penis in circumcised individuals. Normally the operation is done privately, preferably by a paediatric surgeon.

Female circumcision

Although this may be requested by some African parents, they are usually well aware that opinion in Europe is strongly against the operation, even in its least mutilating form. The operation is illegal in the U.K.

Sticky eyes

A mild conjunctivitis is quite common in the first week of life and in most cases requires nothing more than cleaning with sterile cotton wool and saline or boiled water. A mild 'sticky eye' may be the first indication of a blocked or partly blocked lacrimal duct; in such cases the eye tends to 'water' excessively. In the majority of cases the blockage clears spontaneously but probing may be required if symptoms persist after the age of 6 months. For gonococcal and chlamydial conjunctivitis see pp. 184–185.

Mongolian blue spot

This inappropriately named condition is common in newborn infants of all brown-eyed black-haired races, and occurs in some infants of dark European parents, particularly those from the Mediterranean region. Usually this area of bluish–black pigmentation is confined to the lumbosacral region, but patches of pigmentation also occur in the scapular areas, and on the dorsal aspects of the upper arms and on the legs, including the posterior part of the ankles. By the age of 18 months to 2 years the pigmentation has either faded or has blended into the colour of the surrounding skin.

To the uninitiated, the Mongolian blue spot is occasionally mistaken for a bruise, and child abuse may be suspected.

Milia

Milia are minute white papules on the face. No treatment is required, and they disappear within a few weeks of delivery.

Toxic or eosinophilic erythema

These small lesions appear quite suddenly in the first few days of life. The appearance is that of a minute urticarial weal with a raised white centre surrounded by a red area. No treatment is required and the lesions disappear at or before the end of the first week.

Septic spots

Minute septic spots which are superficial will usually clear after washing with an antiseptic soap such as 'Sterzac' baby soap, which contains a low concentration of hexachlorophane.

Capillary naevi

The pale naevi, which can be blanched on pressure and occur on the forehead, upper eyelids and the occipital region, usually fade completely. Dark red, raised or pigmented naevi require separate consideration.

Reference

Roberton, N.R.C. (1984) The routine clinical examination. In *Antenatal and Neonatal Screening* (ed. N.J. Wald), Oxford University Press, Oxford, p. 259

Chapter 33

Stillbirths and neonatal deaths

It is now widely accepted that the needs of the parents after a stillbirth, a miscarriage or a termination are similar to those after a neonatal death. The facilities and advice that are offered to the parents of a stillborn child should be similar to those offered to the parents of a child that has died during the neonatal period, but with a few differences discussed below.

Stillbirths

Until recently, it was assumed that the parents of a stillborn child would prefer that the child's body be disposed of anonymously by the hospital, without a funeral service and in a communal unmarked grave. This procedure, although intended to spare the parents worry and distress, has been found to cause an abnormally prolonged and severe grief reaction in the mother, and less commonly in the father, due to the inability to come to terms with the child's death by way of the formalities and ritual of a burial service.

Now, most hospitals are ready to make arrangements with a local undertaker for a simple funeral service and burial in a marked grave, or for disposal by cremation.

In general, the later the stillbirth the greater the parental distress; death during labour or delivery is particularly distressing.

A photograph of the child should be taken, unless there is a totally unacceptable degree of maceration or deformity; many mothers will accept gratefully a photograph of even a severely abnormal baby; inkpad footprints, incubator card, name bracelet and a piece of hair may also be offered to the parents.

It is important that both parents should be given the opportunity to see the child before it is removed for burial or cremation, and that they should be allowed to hold the baby, if they wish. The parents should be reminded that siblings may wish to share in their grief, and that they can come to the hospital to see and hold the baby; however, this is an intimate family decision.

Registration and funeral arrangements

After a stillbirth the hospital or family doctor gives the parents a certificate to be taken to the Registrar of Births, Marriages and Deaths within 42 days (21 days in Scotland). The Registrar gives the parents a certificate for burial and a copy of the Stillbirth Certificate. If the baby was stillborn before 28 weeks, there is no requirement to register it as a stillbirth. There has recently been an increased demand for funeral arrangements, followed by cremation or burial, for the baby born dead before the 28th week of pregnancy. Since there is no Registrar's certificate for disposal or Coroner's certificate, there is no documentation to allow a legal burial or cremation. However, some local authorities will permit burial or cremation on production of a certificate or letter, signed by a medical attendant; for burial a written request signed by the parents is also necessary. It should be noted that there are no identifiable remains after the cremation of a pre-viable fetus. Further information can be obtained from the Stillbirth and Neonatal Death Society (SANDS; see Appendix 4 for the address), or from the Education Committee of the British Institute of Funeral Directors (see Appendix 4 for address), who publish a leaflet *Funerals for Foetal Remains*.

Post-mortem

Normally the parents should be asked to give their permission for a post-mortem examination, and the object of doing the examination should be carefully explained. In certain cases, when the cause of death is obvious and uncomplicated, as in hypoxia from a prolapsed cord, there is no need for a post-mortem; however, if the parents wish to have one done in such cases, their wishes should be respected. Unfortunately, the information from an autopsy in a stillbirth is usually much less helpful in establishing the cause of death than it is in a neonatal death.

Obviously, it is the responsibility of the obstetrician to see the parents as soon as a stillbirth has been delivered, but it is generally more appropriate for the paediatrician to see the parents afterwards to give them information about bereavement counselling and to arrange a follow-up appointment to discuss the post-mortem findings. The information which should be given to the parents after the post-mortem is discussed below.

Neonatal deaths

When it is apparent that an infant may die, the paediatrician should have a photograph of the baby taken; this can be given, or offered, to the parents if the need arises (see also under Stillbirths, p. 349). When a newborn infant is seriously ill, the parents and siblings should be encouraged to visit as often as possible.

A neonatal death must be registered by one of the parents; this requires a death certificate which is completed by one of the paediatric staff, and gives the presumed, or provisional cause of death. When a post-mortem is to be performed, the appropriate section on the back of the death certificate should be completed, indicating that further information will be available; if this is done the death certificate can be given to the parents without delay, since unnecessary delay is distressing.

The Coroner

Only in exceptional circumstances is a neonatal death reported to the Coroner. The reasons for doing so are:

1. The circumstances of death were such that a death certificate could not be completed, even with a provisional cause of death, without an autopsy ('sudden unexpected death'). This would be very unusual in a neonatal death.
2. When there is a possibility that mismanagement or negligence contributed to or caused the death of the infant.

The decision to notify the Coroner should be make on the facts of the case, and should never be used to obtain a post-mortem which has been refused, or is likely to be refused, by the parents. Normally, in a neonatal death the Coroner asks the hospital pathologist to do the post-mortem, unless there is a possibility of mismanagement or negligence by the hospital or its staff.

It should be understood that the Coroner does not need to have a post-mortem done in every case that is reported to him; he can authorize the clinician to issue a normal death certificate, endorsed on the back to say that the case has been reported to the Coroner. After an autopsy has been performed at his request, the Coroner issues a special form of death certificate.

The reporting of a case to the Coroner gives some protection to the relatives against a 'cover-up' by the hospital, and also to the medical staff against unreasonable complaints by relatives about management and treatment. The Coroner is in a position to discuss the circumstances of death with the relatives in an unbiased manner, since he had nothing to do with the clinical conduct of the case.

Follow up and counselling

Depending upon local arrangements, the obstetrician may hand over to the paediatrician the responsibility for seeing the parents of a stillbirth when the results of the post-mortem are available, and in neonatal deaths the paediatrician should see the parents as soon after the baby has died as possible, and arrange a subsequent appointment. In all maternity hospitals and units the parents should be given the address of the local branch of the Stillbirth and Neonatal Death Society who can advise on counselling and befriending services; the booklet *The Loss of your Baby at Birth or Shortly After* should be available to the parents. Information leaflets are also published by SANDS on *Diabetes in Pregnancy*, *Neural Tube Defects*, *Abruptio Placentae*, and *Respiratory Distress Syndrome*.

When the paediatrician has received the post-mortem report, he should see both parents together, and give them a full explanation of the events which led to the infant's death. The important points are:

1. The immediate cause of death.
2. Contributory factors.
3. Whether death occurred from a cause that would be unlikely to recur;

for example placenta praevia, abruptio placentae, or a rare congenital malformation without any known cause.

4. If there is a possibility that subsequent infants would be at risk from the same condition, it should be explained what the risk is and how it could be minimized. For example:
   (a) In genetically determined conditions the actual or statistical risk should be given, with an explanation of any pre-natal or post-natal investigations that can be done to detect the affected infant, and any early treatment that may be available. If a termination might be advised for an affected fetus, the risks of investigation of the fetus should be fully discussed;
   (b) For a maternal condition that has caused or contributed to a stillbirth or neonatal death (e.g. diabetes), the parents should be advised about changes of management in a subsequent pregnancy that would improve the outlook.

In all cases the paediatrician should write to the obstetrician and the family doctor, giving his findings and full details of what he has told the parents. A copy of this letter should be filed in the obstetric **and** paediatric notes. If it is likely that the parents may move to another area or another country, they should be given a copy of the paediatrician's report for their new doctor or hospital.

Requirements of various ethnic and religious groups

The number of different minority groups in Britain is so large that it would be impossible to cover all their requirements individually. However, hospital staff should be aware that ignorant or insensitive handling of the parents of a child who has just died is very distressing, particularly if the parents themselves are feeling insecure or uncertain.

Every hospital with a sizeable minority group in its area should have a list of the appropriate priests who can be contacted, and the names of community leaders, who can be called upon to help with difficult ethical or other problems. A list of reliable interpreters in the appropriate language should also be available.

Chapter 34

Social problems

In all social problems arising before or after delivery the medical and nursing staff must work closely with the parents, the social services and the primary health care team.

The unmarried mother

A child born to an unmarried woman is legally illegitimate. Even though the prejudice against illegitimacy is decreasing, the unsupported mother and her child may suffer financial and social discrimination. In the U.K. in 1990, approximately one in four births were illegitimate, and the number of such births has more than doubled over the past 15 years. However, three-quarters of illegitimate children were born to parents who were cohabiting at the time of delivery.

The circumstances in which a child may be born illegitimately are extremely diverse, and it is important that those concerned with the mother and baby should be fully informed about all aspects of the case. The main difficulties for the unmarried mother arise when she does not wish to marry or has no prospect of marrying the father of the child.

The birth certificate

The responsibilities for registering the birth of an illegitimate child fall on the mother if the father has not acknowledged paternity. In some hospitals the Registrar of Births pays a weekly visit to the maternity unit. The mother may prefer to use the shortened form of the birth certificate which does not require details of parentage or subsequent adoption.

The father

The father of an illegitimate child has no legal rights over the child unless he has been required to contribute to the child's maintenance through an Affiliation Order. If the relationship between the parents permits it, there is no reason why he should be prevented from visiting the mother and baby.

Special cases

Adolescent pregnancy (see also p. 9)
This is usually taken to mean that the mother is under the age of 18 years at the time of delivery; in the U.K., marriage under the age of 18 years requires parental permission and under 16 years it is illegal. Some of these pregnancies are concealed until a late stage or even until delivery, which may be unattended. Inadequate or absent antenatal care is common; if the delivery is unattended, the infant may suffer from hypoxia or hypothermia, or may be abandoned. Although adolescent pregnancies have a high incidence of risk factors such as smoking, pre-eclampsia and pre-term delivery, the actual outcome depends more upon socioeconomic conditions and lifestyle than any physiological immaturity. Many of the non-obstetric adverse factors can be reduced by adequate antenatal care and good support from the family. In the 10–15-year age group, however, the incidence of pre-eclampsia, pre-term delivery and small for gestational age infants remains high, even though these very young girls are more likely than the older adolescents to remain within the parental home. In all cases much support is required from the social worker, who may also be involved in helping the girl's parents. After delivery she may need advice on contraception.

A proportion of victims of rape are unmarried girls, often below the age of 16 years (see below).

The problems of the adolescent father have been neglected until recently. He may need support and counselling about his own role, and he may benefit from being involved in the girl's antenatal education and care.

Rape
The amount of physical and emotional distress and damage resulting from rape varies greatly, and is frequently underestimated in the courts. The emotional disturbance is likely to be greatest in the unmarried girl, particularly if she is a virgin. Appropriate support may be needed for a long time. In all cases the victim should be tested for gonococcal infection, syphilis, hepatitis B and HIV infection. If a pregnancy results, a termination is usually advised. If it is allowed to continue, the infant should be tested for syphilis and HIV, and should be given prophylaxis against hepatitis B (p. 188) if the mother has been shown to have been infected.

Various ethnic and religious groups
It is essential that everyone involved in the management of the unmarried mother should be aware of the different attitudes towards illegitimacy in the various minority groups in the U.K. Although British society in general has become progressively more tolerant towards the unmarried mother, in some Asian communities such an event is regarded as a disgrace to the family, and there is a risk that the girl may be disowned and ostracized by the community, particularly if the father belongs to a different faith or race. In such cases it may be helpful to enlist the help of a religious or community leader.

Infants of mixed race
Sometimes, as in adoption cases, it is helpful to be able to predict the amount of skin pigmentation in an infant. Most pre-term African and Asian infants are pink at birth, and some Asian term infants also have relatively little skin pigmentation. The amount of pigmentation of the nail beds at birth is of little use in predicting the future amount of skin pigmentation, and the presence of a Mongolian blue spot is not a good indication of how dark-skinned the infant may become, since it is sometimes found in infants of European parentage. Placement for adoption of infants of mixed parentage should be done with great care, particularly with regard to skin pigmentation, as this has great significance to many couples. It is usually possible to assess the amount of skin pigmentation by the age of 6 weeks. An infant with greater or less pigmentation than the adopting couple may be rejected or be at risk for abuse (Fuller and Geis, 1985). In recent years there has been much discussion about the view of some local authority social services departments that children should be placed with and adopted by parents of the same ethnic origin as the child; the view of the Department of Health in the U.K. is that this should only be one factor in deciding appropriate placement.

Alcoholism

Maternal alcoholism may or may not be known to the hospital staff before delivery, and the mother may attempt, successfully or not, to conceal it. The main problems arising from maternal alcoholism are as follows.

Social

Particularly if both parents are taking excessive amounts of alcohol, there may be financial difficulties, poor housing and unemployment. Alcoholism is a contributory factor in child abuse and it is an offence to be drunk in charge of a child. In some cases, it may be necessary to take out a Care Order or institute Wardship proceedings for the baby.

Fetal alcohol syndrome

The clinical characteristics of fetal alcohol syndrome are described on p. 7. Since there is no test for the condition, the diagnosis depends upon the clinical awareness of the paediatrician. If there is a reasonable certainty about the diagnosis, its implications must be carefully explained to the parents, with particular reference to intellectual impairment. The parents, or the mother, may respond to advice on treatment and agree to be referred to an appropriate helping agency and/or to Alcoholics Anonymous.

Drug abuse

The clinical symptoms and management of the neonatal abstinence or withdrawal syndrome arising from exposure of the fetus to drugs are described in Chapter 28. Drug dependence may produce the following problems.

Social

As in alcoholism, family life and the parents' competence may be impaired, particularly if both parents are using drugs, and care proceedings may be necessary; however a careful assessment is required of the competence of the couple to bring up a baby, rather than the rigid application of a set of rules; many couples, although using drugs, whether 'hard' or not, are socially and economically quite stable. There is no reason for taking a newborn infant into care solely because it suffered symptoms of drug withdrawal after delivery, and any care proceedings must be based upon an assessment of the risk to the infant of neglect or abuse on returning home.

Removal or temporary separation of the child from the mother

No baby should be removed from its mother unless there is no practicable alternative, and the mother has given her permission. In the following circumstances, however, there are good reasons for the removal of the infant.

Medical conditions affecting the mother

A serious maternal infection which may be transmitted to the baby
The usual indications are:

1. Active tuberculosis.
2. Chickenpox (varicella) or measles at delivery or in the puerperium.
3. Gastrointestinal infections.

In these situations removal is temporary and only necessary until the mother is no longer infective or the infant has been immunized and given time to develop immunity or has been protected against the mother's infection by appropriate antibiotic cover.

Any acute medical condition that makes the mother too ill to look after the baby
Normally, removal is only necessary for a few days; pneumonia or meningitis are such indications.

An acute condition related to pregnancy, labour, delivery or the post-partum period that causes the mother to be severely ill
Examples are pulmonary embolism, post-operative infection and severe post-partum haemorrhage.

Psychiatric conditions
These may be:

1. Long-standing, such as schizophrenia, acute hypomania or depression in a sufferer from manic-depressive psychosis.

2. Of recent onset, generally starting in the puerperium, such as an acute schizophrenic episode, depression, or less commonly a manic episode.

It should be emphasized that to take this action the disturbance must be extremely severe and such as to endanger the life or well-being of the baby or to make it impossible for the mother to look after it properly. In general, removal of the baby is likely to exacerbate the mother's condition, and the best solution is to admit them both to an adequately supervised mother and baby unit in a psychiatric unit.

If the mother has been on psychotropic drugs before delivery, the infant should be watched carefully for signs of the direct action of the drug, and for withdrawal symptoms (see p. 297).

Social reasons

The risk of child abuse

When a baby has just been delivered, the only grounds for its immediate removal are that there is clear evidence that another child in the same household has suffered abuse or injury necessitating its removal into care or wardship and that the circumstances necessitating the previous child's removal have not changed. This is a serious step which should only be taken if it is envisaged that separation will be permanent; the decision should have been fully discussed with the parents before delivery and no attempt should be made to remove the infant by subterfuge.

Detention of the mother in prison

The correct and humane procedure, with which the mother needs to agree, would be to arrange admission to a mother and baby unit in a women's prison; there are three such units in the U.K., in which the mother is allowed to keep her baby for up to 9 months and in certain circumstances up to 18 months. The sentencing judge has the power to forbid the mother from keeping the child with her in prison but can only recommend that the baby should accompany her. Normally a recommendation is made by the probation service, and is of course subject to the mother's agreement. If the mother is under 18 years she would be detained in a Young Person's Prison, where there are no facilities for her to keep the baby with her.

References

Fuller, R.L. and Geis, S. (1985) The significance of the skin color of a newborn infant. *American Journal of Diseases of Children*, **139**, 672–673

Further reading

McAnarney, E.R. and Greydanus, D.E. (eds) (1981) Adolescent pregnancy: a risk condition (includes an article on the adolescent father). *Seminars in Perinatology*, **5**, 1–103

Wright, T.J. and Topliss, T.J. (1986) Alcohol in pregnancy. *British Journal of Obstetrics and Gynaecology*, **93**, 201–202

Appendix 1

Abbreviations

AD: autosomal dominant
ADH: antidiuretic hormone
AFP: α-fetoprotein
AR: autosomal recessive
ARC: AIDS-related complex
AZT: azidothymidine
BP: blood pressure
BPD: biparietal diameter
BPD: bronchopulmonary dysplasia
CAH: congenital adrenal hyperplasia
CDH: congenital dislocation of the hip
CHD: congenital heart disease
CF: cystic fibrosis (of the pancreas)
CMV: cytomegalovirus
CPAP: continuous positive airway pressure
CT(CAT): computerized (axial) tomography
CVP: central venous pressure
CVS: chorionic villus sampling
DIC: disseminated intravascular coagulation
DMSA: dimercaptosuccinic acid
DNA: deoxyribonucleic acid
DOCA: deoxycortone (or desoxycorticosterone) acetate
DZ: dizygotic
ECF: extracellular fluid
ECM: external cardiac massage
ECMO: extracorporeal membrane oxygenation
EMG: electromyogram
ENL: erythema nodosum leprosum
ENT: ear, nose and throat
ETT: endotracheal tube
FFP: fresh frozen plasma
FiO_2: Fractional concentration of inspired oxygen
G-6PD: glucose-6-phosphate dehydrogenase
GFR: glomerular filtration rate
GLC: gas-liquid chromatography
HBV: hepatitis B virus
HIV: human immunodeficiency virus

HVE: high-voltage electrophoresis
IDM: infant of a diabetic mother
IEM: inborn error of metabolism
i.m.: intramuscular
IMV: intermittent mandatory ventilation
IPPV: intermittent positive pressure ventilation
IT: intrathecal
ITP: idiopathic thrombocytopenic purpura
i.v.: intravenous
IVH: intraventricular haemorrhage
IVU(P): intravenous urogram (pyelogram)
kPa: kilopascal (= mmHg/7.5 or Torr/7.5)
LP: lumbar puncture
MsAFP: maternal serum alpha-fetoprotein
MZ: monozygotic
NDI: nephrogenic diabetes insipidus
NEC: necrotizing enterocolitis
NICU: neonatal intensive care unit
NTD: neural tube defect
PAT: paroxysmal atrial tachycardia
PCV: packed cell volume (syn. haematocrit)
PEEP: positive end-expiratory pressure
PFC: persistent fetal circulation
PIE: pulmonary interstitial emphysema
PIP: peak inspiratory pressure
PKU: phenylketonuria
$P\text{O}_2$ (CO_2): partial pressure of oxygen (carbon dioxide)
PPF: plasma protein fraction
PROM: premature rupture of membrane
PVC: polyvinyl chloride
RDS: respiratory distress syndrome (also known as hyaline membrane disease)
$S\text{O}_2$: haemoglobin oxygenation %
SC(B)U: Special care (baby) unit
SFD: small for dates (same as SGA)
SGA: small for gestational age (same as small for dates)
SIADH: syndrome of inappropriate ADH secretion
SIDS: sudden infant death syndrome
SLE: systemic lupus erythematosus
SPN: supplementary parenteral nutrition
SVT: supraventricular tachycardia
THAM: tris-hydroxyaminomethane
TOF: tracheo-oesophageal fistula
TPN: total parenteral nutrition
VMA: vanillylmandelic acid
XD: X-linked dominant
XL: X-linked
XR: X-linked recessive
ZIG: zoster immunoglobulin

Appendix 2

Apt's test

A small amount of stool is mixed with water to lyse the red cells and to produce a haemoglobin solution. One part of the stool mixture is added to 5–10 parts of water; there must be a distinctly coloured fluid. The stool should be red and not tarry because in a tarry stool the oxyhaemoglobin has already been converted to haematin. The mixture is centrifuged at 2000 rpm for 1–2 minutes, and the pink haemoglobin solution is filtered ore decanted off. Then 1 ml of 0.25 normal (1%) sodium hydroxide solution is mixed with 5 ml of the haemoglobin solution, and the colour change is read at 2 minutes. With adult haemoglobin the solution will turn yellow–brown while with fetal haemoglobin the solution remains pink.

Reference

Apt, L. and Downey, W.S. (1955) Melaena neonatorum – the swallowed blood syndrome. *Journal of Paediatrics*, **47**, 6–12.

Appendix 3

Incidence and recurrence risks for come common conditions

Table A3.1 General population risks

Infant mortality rate* (1988:U.K.): 9.0 per 1000 live births
Neonatal mortality rate* (1988:U.K.): 4.9 per 1000 live births
Perinatal mortality rate* (1988:U.K.): 8.8 per 1000 live and stillbirths
Spontaneous miscarriage: 1 in 6 of recognized pregnancies
Sudden infant death syndrome: 2–4 per 1000 live births
Major malformation or genetic disorder: 2–5% of liveborn infants
Trisomy 21: 1 in 700 births†
Trisomy 18: 1 in 3000 births†
Trisomy 13: 1 in 5000 births†
Turner's syndrome: 1 in 2500 female births†

*Office of Population Censuses and Surveys (1990).
†From Connor and Ferguson-Smith (1984).

The empirical risks for some common disorders are listed in Table A3.2; these risks only apply to the population studied, in this case the U.K.

Table A3.2 Empirical risks for some common disorders (%)

Disorder	*Incidence*	*Sex ratio* M:F	*Normal parents having a second affected child*	*Affected parent having an affected child*	*Affected parent having a second affected child*
Anencephaly[a]	0.20	1:2	5[b]	—	—
Asthma	3–4	1:1	10	26	—
Cerebral palsy	0.20	3:2	1[c]	—	—
Cleft palate only	0.04	2:3	2	7	15
Cleft lip ± palate[a]	0.10	3:2	4	4	10
Club foot	0.10	2:1	3	3	10
Congenital heart disease (all types)[a,d]	0.50	1:1	1–4	1–4	10
Diabetes mellitus (juvenile insulin-dependent)	0.20	1:1	6	1–2	-
Dislocation of hip[a]	0.07	1:6	6	12	36
Exomphalos	0.02	1:1	<1	—	—
Epilepsy (idiopathic)	0.50	1:1	5	5	10

Table A3.2

Disorder	*Incidence*	*Sex ratio* M:F	*Normal parents having a second affected child*	*Affected parent having an affected child*	*Affected parent having a second affected child*
Hirschsprung's disease[a]	0.02	4:1			
short segment	—	—	3	2	—
long segment	—	—	12	—	—
Hydrocephalus[f] (isolated; not XR)	0.05	1:1	3[e]	—	—
Hypospadias (in males)	0.02	—	10	10	—
Manic depressive psychosis	0.40	2:3	10–15	10–15	—
Mental retardation (idiopathic)	0.30–0.50	1:1	3–5	10	20
Profound childhood deafness	0.10	1:1	10	8	—
Pyloric stenosis[a]	0.30	5:1	—	—	13
Male index			2	4	13
Female index			10	17	38
Renal agenesis (bilateral)	0.01	3:1			
Male index			3	—	—
Female index			7	—	—
Schizophrenia	1–2	1:1	10	16	—
Scoliosis (idiopathic adolescent)	0.22	1:6	7	5	—
Spina bifida[a,b]	0.30	2:3	5[a]	4[a]	—
Tracheo-oesophageal fistula	0.03	1:1	1	1	—

[a]Multifactorial: risks only apply to population studied.
[b]Risk for anencephaly or spina bifida.
[c]If associated with ataxia, symmetrical spastic diplegia or ethetosis, risk approx. 10%.
[d]See Table 1.15 for specific forms of cardiac malformation.
[e]Additional 1–2% risk of other neural tube defects.
[f]X-linked recessive hydrocephalus is associated with hypoplastic flexed thumbs.
Reproduced from Emery (1983) with permission of author and publishers.

Conditions that give rise to difficulties

Osteogenesis imperfecta (fragilitas ossium)

The classification is confusing, but a generally accepted one is as follows (Taitz, 1987):

Type I (AD): responsible for about 80% of all cases; blue sclerotics, intrauterine or birth fractures rare.
Type II (AR): severe, with intrauterine or birth fractures and early death.
Type III (AR): similar to Type II but less severe.
Type IV (AD): rare; similar in severity to Type III.

Ocular conditions

Before giving genetic advice to two blind individuals who wish to have children, it is essential to make an exact diagnosis in each case, since there are numerous genetically distinct causes of blindness which are inherited independently. An ophthalmologist can usually make a precise diagnosis. Ocular albinism is inherited as an X-linked recessive, but generalized albinism is a recessive condition; however, there are two types of generalized albinism which are inherited independently.

Only 10% of cases of congenital cataract are of genetic origin; most congenital genetically determined cataracts are due to an autosomal dominant gene, but recessive and X-linked forms also occur.

Retinitis pigmentosa is commonly recessive, but may be X-linked or AD. The Laurence–Moon–Biedl syndrome is AR.

Deafness (Reardon and Pembrey, 1990)
Non-genetic causes must be excluded. About 40% of the cases of genetically determined deafness are recessively determined, 10% are due to AD conditions and a few are XR. Particularly with the recessive forms, there are a number of different genes that are inherited independently. It is difficult to distinguish clinically between these various forms of recessively determined deafness but empirically deaf children only result from about 2% of marriages between deaf parents.

Congenital heart disease
See pp. 20–21.

Anorectal malformations (Boocock and Donnai, 1987)
An anorectal malformation associated with other minor abnormalities, such as abnormal ears or thumbs, may indicate a dominantly inherited condition with variable penetrance. But an anorectal malformation as part of a complex or multiple malformation may be due to a rare recessively determined condition or to a chromosomal abnormality. In doubtful cases a clinical geneticist should be consulted.

Prader–Willi syndrome
Although the majority of cases appear to be sporadic, familial cases do occur. Some of these have an unbalanced translocation between chromosomes 15 and 22; one parent may have a balanced translocation (Fernandez *et al.*, 1987). Chromosome analysis should be undertaken on a first affected child; high resolution cytogenetic techniques are required.

Conditions with low or negligible recurrence risk
Table A3.3 gives conditions that, when occurring as isolated defects, carry a very small risk of recurrence after the birth of an affected child.

Table A3.3 Low-risk conditions

Intestinal atresia (excluding cystic fibrosis)
Hypoplastic or dysplastic kidneys
Syndactyly (as a single abnormality)
Polydactyly (in Caucasians)
Klippel–Feil syndrome
Pierre–Robin syndrome
Sturge–Weber syndrome
VATER complex

References

Boocock, G.R. and Donnai, D. (1987) Anorectal malformations; familial aspects and associated anomalies. *Archives of Disease in Childhood,* **62**, 576–579

Connor, J.M. and Ferguson-Smith, M.A. (1984) *Essential Medical Genetics*, Blackwell Scientific, Oxford, p. 162

Emery, A.E.H. (1983) *Elements of Medical Genetics* 6th edn, Churchill Livingstone, Edinburgh, pp. 244–245

Fernandez, F., Berry, C. and Mutton, D. (1987) Prader–Willi Syndrome in siblings. *Archives of Disease in Childhood,* **62**, 841–843

Office of Population Censuses and Surveys (1990) *Population Trends,* **60**, 48

Reardon, W. and Pembrey, M. (1990) The genetics of deafness. *Archives of Disease in Childhood,* **65**, 1196–1197

Taitz, L.S. (1987) Child abuse and osteogenesis imperfecta. *British Medical Journal,* **295**, 1082–1083

Appendix 4

Useful addresses

Association for Spina Bifida and Hydrocephalus
22 Upper Woburn Place, London WC1
(071-388-1382)

Down's Children's Association/Down's Syndrome Association
12/13 Clapham Common, South Side, London SW4
(071-720-0008)

Education Committee, British Institute of Funeral Directors
11 Regent Street, Bristol

Foundation for the Study of Infant Deaths
35 Belgrave Square, London SW1
(071-235-1721)

Multiple Births Foundation
Queen Charlotte's and Chelsea Hospital, Goldhawk Road, London W6 0XG
(081-748-4666)

Sickle Cell Society*
Green Lodge, Barretts Green Road, London NW10
(081-961-7795)

Stillbirth and Neonatal Death Society (SANDS)
28 Portland Place, London W1
(071-436-5881)

Support after Termination for Abnormality (SAFTA)
20 Soho Square, London W1
(071-439-6124)

Thalassaemia Society, United Kingdom*
107 Nightingale Lane, London N8
(081-348-0437)

Twins and Multiple Births Association (TAMBA)
41 Fortuna Way, Ayelsbry Park, Grimsby, South Humberside DN37 9SJ

*Apply to these organizations for centres in other parts of the UK.

Index

Note: Where appropriate, a page reference highlighted in **bold** refers to the main entry for that heading (or sub-heading).